Pulmonary Hypertension

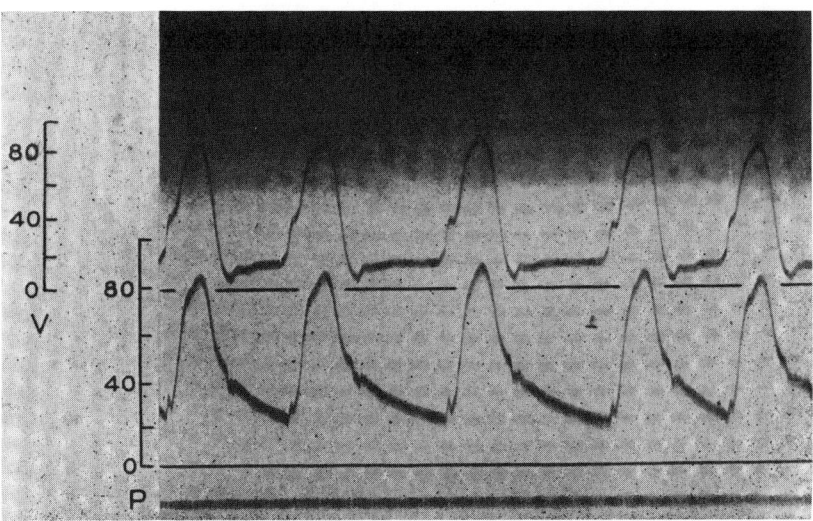

"... the first demonstration that the tip of a catheter was placed in the pulmonary artery of man in order to record pressure pulses." The pressure tracings on the cover are from the right ventricle (upper) and pulmonary artery (lower) in a case of "rheumatic valvulitis with hypertension in the lesser circulation." (Cournand A, Bloomfield RA, Lauson HD: Double lumen catheter for intravenous and intracardiac blood sampling and pressure recording. *Proc. Soc. Exp. Biol. Med.* 60:73–75, 1945, with permission.) The quotation is from: Cournand A. Description of the prize-winning work. In: Sourkes TL, *Nobel Prize Winners in Medicine and Physiology 1901–1965*. London, Abelard-Schuman, p. 366, 1966.

PULMONARY HYPERTENSION

edited by

E. KENNETH WEIR, M.D.
Associate Professor of Medicine, University of Minnesota
Director, Cardiac Catheterization Laboratory
Minneapolis V.A. Medical Center
Minneapolis, Minnesota

and

JOHN T. REEVES, M.D.
Professor of Medicine
Associate Director, Cardiovascular Pulmonary
Research Laboratory
University of Colorado Health Sciences Center
Denver, Colorado

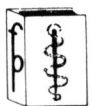 FUTURA PUBLISHING COMPANY, INC.
MOUNT KISCO, NEW YORK
1984

Copyright © 1984
Futura Publishing Company, Inc.

Published by
Futura Publishing Company, Inc.
295 Main Street
Mount Kisco, New York

L.C. No.: 83-082628
ISBN No.: 0-87993-206-6

All rights reserved.

No part of this book may be translated or reproduced in any form without the written permission of the Publisher.

Contributors

Alfred P. Fishman, M.D.
William Maul Measey Professor of Medicine
Director, Cardiovascular-Pulmonary Division
Department of Medicine
University of Pennsylvania
Philadelphia, Pennsylvania

Bertron M. Groves, M.D., F.A.C.C.
Associate Professor of Medicine
Director, Cardiac Catheterization Laboratory
University of Colorado Health Sciences Center
Denver, Colorado

Jan Herget, M.D.
Associate Professor of Physiology
Department of Pathophysiology
Faculty of Pediatrics
Charles University
Prague, Czechoslovakia

Michael A. Heymann, M.D., M.B., B.Ch.
Professor of Pediatrics, Physiology, and Obstetrics,
Gynecology and Reproductive Sciences
University of California
San Francisco, California

Julien I.E. Hoffman, M.D., B.Sc.Hons., F.R.C.P., F.A.C.C.
Senior Member, Cardiovascular Research Institute
Professor of Pediatrics and Physiology
University of California
San Francisco, California

Joseph V. Messer, M.D., F.A.C.C.
Professor of Medicine
Rush Medical College
Senior Attending Physician and Director,
Section of Cardiology,
Rush-Presbyterian-St. Luke's Medical Center
Director, Interinstitutional Cardiovascular Center
Chicago, Illinois

Johannes Mlczoch, Dr. Med. Univ., F.C.C.P.
Univ. Dozent fur Innere Medizin
Oberarzt der Kardiologischen Universitatsklinik
Chairman, the Working Group on Pulmonary Circulation
of the European Society of Cardiology
Vienna, Austria

John T. Reeves, M.D.
Professor of Medicine
Associate Director of Cardiovascular Pulmonary
Research Laboratory
University of Colorado Health Sciences Center
Denver, Colorado

Lewis J. Rubin, M.D., F.A.C.P.
Assistant Professor of Internal Medicine
University of Texas Southwestern Medical School
Chief, Pulmonary Section, Dallas V.A. Medical Center
Dallas, Texas

C.A. Wagenvoort, M.D., F.R.C.Path.
Professor of Pathology
University of Amsterdam
Academic Medical Centre
Amsterdam, The Netherlands

John V. Weil, M.D.
Professor of Medicine
Director, Cardiovascular Pulmonary Research Laboratory
University of Colorado Health Sciences Center
Denver, Colorado

E. Kenneth Weir, M.D., M.R.C.P., D.M., F.A.C.C.
Associate Professor of Medicine
University of Minnesota
Director, Cardiac Catheterization Laboratory
Minneapolis V.A. Medical Center
Minneapolis, Minnesota

Foreword

Those who live at the foot of the mountain rightfully picture pulmonary hypertension as a regular feature of normal life at high altitude and as a complication of diseases of the heart, lungs or pulmonary vessels at sea level. They also recognize important differences in the natural history of pulmonary hypertension at sea level and at altitude: as a rule, the pulmonary hypertension at high altitude is mild and tolerated comfortably for a lifetime; in contrast, the pulmonary hypertension that complicates cardiac, respiratory, or pulmonary vascular disease often imposes an intolerable burden on the right ventricle, particularly if chronic respiratory insufficiency coexists with the right ventricular overload (cor pulmonale).

The natural history of most types of pulmonary hypertension is largely a function of the underlying cardiorespiratory or pulmonary vascular disease and its reversibility. The pulmonary hypertension of acquired heart disease is often completely relieved if the cause, such as tight mitral stenosis, is eliminated before irreversible changes have led to pulmonary vascular obstruction. In congenital heart disease, the ability to restore pulmonary arterial pressures toward normal often determines prognosis. Quite different is the evolution of the pulmonary hypertension in disorders of the respiratory apparatus. For example, in chronic obstructive diseases of the airways, mild to moderate degrees of pulmonary hypertension often exist for years without clinical significance unless exaggerated by a bout of acute respiratory illness. Severe structural defects and deformities of the thorax, particularly if associated with dwarfing, often culminate in pulmonary hypertension that is both severe and unremitting. These two roads to pulmonary hypertension by way of chronic respiratory disease differ from that of massive pulmonary embolism in which pulmonary hypertension is often acute in onset and occasionally of such a magnitude as to precipitate immediate ventricular failure and to pose a threat to life.

All the above, which fall within the realm of "secondary pulmonary hypertension," illustrate the importance of the antecedent respiratory disease in the natural history and prognosis of pulmonary hypertension. A different perspective is afforded by primary pulmonary hypertension in which the etiology is obscure, the clinical onset often unexpected and the course often intermediate between that of massive pulmonary thromboembolism on the one hand and chronic cardiorespiratory diseases on the other.

The large literature currently available about the normal and hypertensive pulmonary circulations should not obscure the fact that until about four decades ago the pulmonary circulation of intact animals and humans was virtually inaccessible and its behavior obscure. It was only with the introduction of cardiac catheterization in humans in the 1940s, followed by the standardization of techniques for the determination of pulmonary pressures and blood flow in the 1950s, that the remote pulmonary circulation came within reach for the systematic investigation of regulatory mechanisms in normal and abnormal states and for the testing of therapeutic interventions. Clearly, without cardiac catheterization, the management of congenital and acquired heart disease would still be grim. Also, secondary pulmonary hypertension would remain an enigmatic disorder and primary pulmonary hypertension would be as arcane as in the days of Morgagni.

This year, the Division of Lung Diseases of the National Heart, Lung, and Blood Institute assessed the growth of knowledge about pulmonary hypertension during the past decade. Its inventory failed to provide a clear picture of the epidemiology of pulmonary hypertension. As one basis for uncertainty, it identified the ambiguous or unreliable reporting of underlying diseases, notably of cardiorespiratory disorders leading to secondary pulmonary hypertension. Another reason is the unavailability of reliable, non-invasive methods for the early detection of pulmonary hypertension. Despite these reservations, the data at hand left little doubt about either the prevalence or clinical importance of pulmonary hypertension.

The past decade also witnessed intensive exploration of the effects of hypoxia on the pulmonary circulation. This interest was excited in 1946 by Euler and Liljestrand who surmised from their experiments on the cat that acute hypoxia elicits vasoconstriction and inferred that this is a mechanism by which alveolar blood flow is automatically adjusted to alveolar ventilation. The studies that followed not only substantiated the original premise but also identified hypoxia as the most powerful pulmonary pressor agent in the current armamentarium of vasoconstrictor strategies. In addition to the physiological importance of these observations on hypoxia, the practical prospects for therapeutic intervention in states of hypoventilation and arterial hypoxemia stimulated considerable clinical research. The experimental animal and human studies were greatly enriched by lessons from high altitude. The end result is now a rich bank of information about this one type of pulmonary hypertension. Nonetheless, despite the intense interest and the considerable experimental effort, the intimate mechanisms responsible for hypoxic pulmonary hypertension remain elusive. At present, views are polarized between two schools of investigation, one which postulates direct mechanisms as the basis for pulmonary vasoconstriction during hypoxia and the other advocating indirect mechanisms. The focus on hypoxia has gradually widened to include other regulatory mechanisms, such as acidosis. And, one important byproduct of the continued explorations of hypoxic pulmonary hypertension has been clarification of the control of the pulmonary circulation, including the roles played by nerves, receptors, humoral mediators, electrophysiologic events and the contractile properties of pulmonary smooth muscle. As a result of this ripple effect, the search for the genesis of hypoxic pulmonary hypertension is now being conducted in the broad setting of the overall vasomotor behavior of the pulmonary circulation.

It has been noted above that one handicap to the early detection of pulmonary hypertension as well as to epidemiologic studies is the lack of reliable non-invasive methods to determine pulmonary artery pressure. Several theoretical approaches to non-invasive measurement are being explored. One is the assessment of the closure sound of the pulmonic valve with reference to the level of pulmonary arterial pressure. Another is a measure of right ventricular relaxation time. Ultrasonic techniques are being applied in a variety of ways to obtain estimates of pulmonary arterial pressure. The above list, although not exhaustive, underscores the perceived need of those concerned with pulmonary hypertension for a reliable technique by which pulmonary arterial pressure can be estimated non-invasively.

Although secondary pulmonary hypertension is, by far, more prevalent than primary (unexplained) pulmonary hypertension, the latter is of great theoretical interest. An epidemic of primary pulmonary hypertension, presumably related to the anorexigenic drug, Aminorex, reported from Switzerland, Austria, and Germany in the 1960s, posed the challenging problem of how an agent taken by mouth could selectively evoke pulmonary hypertension. Attempts to reproduce this syndrome in the experimental animal have been a total failure. Much more satisfying has been the experience with Crotalaria spectabilis, a leguminous plant, which does elicit pulmonary hypertension after oral ingestion. Many details of the process, including the role of the liver in metabolizing the critical alkaloid, have been elucidated. Unfortunately, although Crotalaria provides a useful experimental model, it has no direct counterpart in human disease.

The experiences with Aminorex and Crotalaria highlight the scarcity of experimental replicas of human pulmonary hypertension. The most intensively studied has been hypoxic pulmonary hypertension, experimentally induced at sea level and occurring spontaneously in animals and humans at altitude. Sporadic observations have also been made on pulmonary hypertension that follows creation of a shunt between a major systemic artery and restricted segments of the pulmonary vascular bed, embolization of the pulmonary arterial tree, and disorders within the pulmonary parenchyma or airways. The paucity of experimental replicas of the human disorder pinpoints a pressing need for new models of pulmonary hypertension.

A major impetus to the study of pulmonary hypertension was provided in recent years by the advent of effective pharmacologic agents for eliciting vasodilation in the systemic circulation. Inevitably, these have also been tried on the hypertensive pulmonary circulation. Although not consistently effective, the use of these agents is providing a fuller picture of the regulation of the pulmonary circulation. Also, the advent of these agents provided a large impetus for creating a national registry where data concerning primary pulmonary hypertension could be collected in a systematic way for deliberate analysis.

This book reflects the current state of understanding of pulmonary hypertension. All of the topics noted above are considered in the present volume. The accounts are written by experts so that the reader is provided with a comprehensive view of the known and unknown by those actively engaged in clinical investigation. The diagnostic and therapeutic implications of contemporary research are clearly depicted. The essays that comprise this volume constitute a valuable contribution to the literature on pulmonary hypertension by providing a full perspective of the disorder in which lessons from the physiological laboratory and experiences at high altitude are described, analyzed, interpreted and set out as a basis for informed and rational management.

Alfred P. Fishman, M.D.
William Maul Measey Professor of Medicine
Director, Cardiovascular-Pulmonary Division
Department of Medicine
University of Pennsylvania
Philadelphia, Pennsylvania

Introduction

Several books have been written on the physiology and pathology of the pulmonary vasculature, but these have not focused on the clinical diagnosis and treatment of pulmonary hypertension. There has been an enormous recent increase in publications concerning pulmonary hypertension, (nearly 3,000 articles listed in *Index Medicus* during the last 20 years). We feel that a book which distills this mass of knowledge and provides insight into the mechanisms and management of pulmonary hypertension will be helpful. Prior to the introduction of cardiac catheterization, there were no means of measuring pulmonary arterial pressure and consequently, the frequency of pulmonary hypertension and the variety of diseases which could cause it were not appreciated. In addition, the fact that there was no treatment available for most forms of pulmonary hypertension gave rise to clinical pessimism.

Following the advent of right heart catheterization in 1929 and the development of therapeutic options as diverse as vasodilators and heart–lung transplantation, interest in pulmonary hypertension has expanded rapidly. The physicians writing for this book have integrated the most recent information in their fields with current clinical management, to provide a foundation for the investigation and treatment of patients with pulmonary hypertension and future research.

E. KENNETH WEIR, M.D.
JOHN T. REEVES, M.D.

Contents

CONTRIBUTORS v

FOREWORD
Alfred P. Fishman, M.D. vii

INTRODUCTION
E. Kenneth Weir, M.D. and John T. Reeves, M.D. xi

Chapter 1   APPROACH TO THE PATIENT WITH PULMONARY HYPERTENSION
John T. Reeves, M.D. and Bertron M. Groves, M.D. ... 1

Chapter 2   PERSISTENT PULMONARY HYPERTENSION SYNDROMES IN THE NEWBORN
Michael A. Heymann, M.D. and Julien I.E. Hoffman, M.D. 45

Chapter 3   PULMONARY ARTERIAL HYPERTENSION SECONDARY TO CONGENITAL HEART DISEASE
Julien I.E. Hoffman, M.D. and Michael A. Heymann, M.D. 73

Chapter 4   DIAGNOSIS AND MANAGEMENT OF PRIMARY PULMONARY HYPERTENSION
E. Kenneth Weir, M.D. 115

Chapter 5   THROMBOEMBOLIC PULMONARY HYPERTENSION
Joseph V. Messer, M.D. 169

Chapter 6   ACUTE HYPOXIC PULMONARY HYPERTENSION
E. Kenneth Weir, M.D. 251

Chapter 7   PULMONARY HYPERTENSION SECONDARY TO LUNG DISEASE
Lewis J. Rubin, M.D. 291

Chapter 8	PULMONARY HYPERTENSION AND COR PULMONALE IN HYPOVENTILATING PATIENTS *John V. Weil, M.D.* 321	
Chapter 9	DRUG AND DIETARY-INDUCED PULMONARY HYPERTENSION *Johannes Mlczoch, M.D.* 341	
Chapter 10	EXPERIMENTAL MODELS OF PULMONARY HYPERTENSION *John T. Reeves, M.D. and Jan Herget, M.D.* 361	
Chapter 11	LUNG BIOPSIES AND PULMONARY VASCULAR DISEASE *C.A. Wagenvoort, M.D.* 393	
INDEX	438	

CHAPTER 1

APPROACH TO THE PATIENT WITH PULMONARY HYPERTENSION

John T. Reeves and Bertron M. Groves

"Every essence hath its final cause. This is the cause I grope after in the works of nature."
                                    Sir Thomas Browne—Religio Medici.

INTRODUCTION

Much of the pulmonary hypertension observed today is potentially reversible. Further, the physician has available powerful diagnostic tools and new forms of treatment. Yet, for several reasons, pulmonary hypertension remains a clinical problem. Symptoms related to pulmonary hypertension are non-specific and the patients may come to the physician late in the natural history of the disease. Physicians, generally attuned to the diseases of the left heart, are not as aware of the frequency and implications of pulmonary hypertensive disorders. We, the medical community, have relatively recently begun to accumulate experience relating to diagnosis, classification, and therapy so necessary for the care of the pulmonary hypertensive patient. Our knowledge of pulmonary hypertension lags behind that of systemic hypertension. Thus, we have imperfect understanding of the basic mechanisms causing nearly all forms of pulmonary vascular disease. Yet progress is rapidly being made. Physicians and scientists are seeking solutions to these problems to improve the outlook of the pulmonary hypertensive patient. As implied by Sir Thomas Browne, real advance follows the understanding of the basic cause. As we approach the patient with pulmonary hypertensive disease, we will attempt to indicate the state of our knowledge and to point out our areas of ignorance.

DEFINITION

In a broad sense pulmonary hypertension is more than an elevation of pulmonary arterial pressure. Thus, the pulmonary circulation should be considered abnormal when either mean pulmonary arterial pressure, pressure gradient between pulmonary artery and pulmonary arterial wedge or pulmonary vascular resistance exceeds the normal values. Patients having right heart catheterization should be evaluated in terms of all 3 variables. Normal pulmonary hemodynamics vary with age (Table 1). However, in humans, resting mean pulmonary arterial pressure is relatively constant from the early childhood to advanced age. Eighty-four percent of the normal mean values at sea level are expected to be 18 mm Hg or less. The normal left atrial or wedge pressure rises from a value of only a few mm Hg in the newborn to a level of about 8 mm Hg. The pressure gradient from pulmonary artery to vein (as judged by the wedge pressure) ranges between 5 mm Hg for adolescents and young adults to an average of 8 mm Hg in the oldest persons reported. In the majority (84%) of the normal persons between the ages of 6 and 45 years, the normal pressure gradient from pulmonary artery to vein should not exceed 9 mm Hg. Because the resting cardiac output falls throughout life and the pressure gradient tends to increase in the aged, the pulmonary vascular resistance rises from the 6th year onward. But even in the oldest age group, values of resistance calculated by pressure gradient divided by cardiac index should be below 3.6 units.

Thus, we consider that pulmonary hypertension exists when either pulmonary arterial pressure, pressure gradient from artery to vein, or pulmonary vascular resistance is elevated. In the final analysis at our present state of knowledge, the definition is based upon hemodynamic measurement, not upon clinical assessment alone.

INCIDENCE

The incidence of pulmonary hypertension is difficult to assess and we know of no reports directly addressing the problem. One approach

TABLE 1
Normal Hemodynamic Measurements in Man as Related to Post Natal Age.

Age	Minutes 0–30	Hours 1–12	Hours 13–24	Days 1–3	Days 14	Years 6–10	Years 11–14	Years 15–20	Years 20–31	Years 32–45	Years 60–83
P_{PA} (mm Hg)	60 ± 13 (29)	40 ± 10 (33)	32 ± 8 (20)	26 ± 4 (12)	14 (1)	14 ± 3 (15)	13 ± 2 (10)	14 ± 3 (8)	13 ± 4 (39)	14 ± 1 (9)	16 ± 3 (25)
P_W (mm Hg)	—	−2 (2)	−2 (1)	—	0	7 ± 2 (11)	8 ± 3 (8)	8 ± 3 (8)	8 ± 3 (38)	8 ± 4 (9)	8 ± 4 (25)
P (mm Hg)	—	—	—	—	14 (1)	6 ± 2 (11)	5 ± 2 (8)	6 ± 3 (6)	5 ± 2 (38)	6 ± 3 (9)	8 ± 3 (25)
P_{Ao} (mm Hg)	58 ± 12 (29)	54 ± 7 (33)	53 ± 11 (20)	58 ± 7 (12)	—	84 ± 11 (11)	83 ± 6 (7)	90 ± 5 (6)	88 ± 8 (37)	101 ± 16 (4)	102 ± 11 (25)
CI (L/min·m²)	—	—	—	—	—	4.3 ± .9 (15)	3.9 ± .7 (10)	4.2 ± .6 (8)	3.6 ± .7 (38)	3.2 ± .5 (9)	3.1 ± .7 (25)
PVR (units)	—	—	—	—	—	1.4 ± .7 (11)	1.5 ± .6 (8)	1.7 ± 1.0 (6)	1.5 ± .6 (38)	1.8 ± .7 (9)	2.6 ± 1.0 (24)

* Measurements include both males and non-pregnant females and are resting supine values reported in the literature from laboratories at or near sea level. P_{PA} is mean pulmonary arterial pressure; P_W is mean wedge or pulmonary capillary pressure except in the newborns where left atrial pressure was reported; P is $P_{PA} - P_W$; P_{Ao} is mean systemic arterial pressure, C.I. is cardiac index; and PVR is P/CI. In parentheses are the number of measurements. (References 1–12). Values are mean ± one standard deviation.

would be to examine the population being studied for clinical indications in a general cardiac catheterization laboratory, where pulmonary arterial catheterization is routinely done.

We examined the records of 234 consecutive patients regardless of diagnosis who underwent cardiac catheterization for the first time at the University of Colorado Medical Center (Denver) and who had measurements of pulmonary arterial pressure. They were at least 10 days of age, i.e., the youngest patients were those near the earliest time after birth that pressure has normally fallen to a stable life time value, Table 1. The children and adults had similar distributions of pulmonary arterial pressure. The histogram, Figure 1, shows that 105 pa-

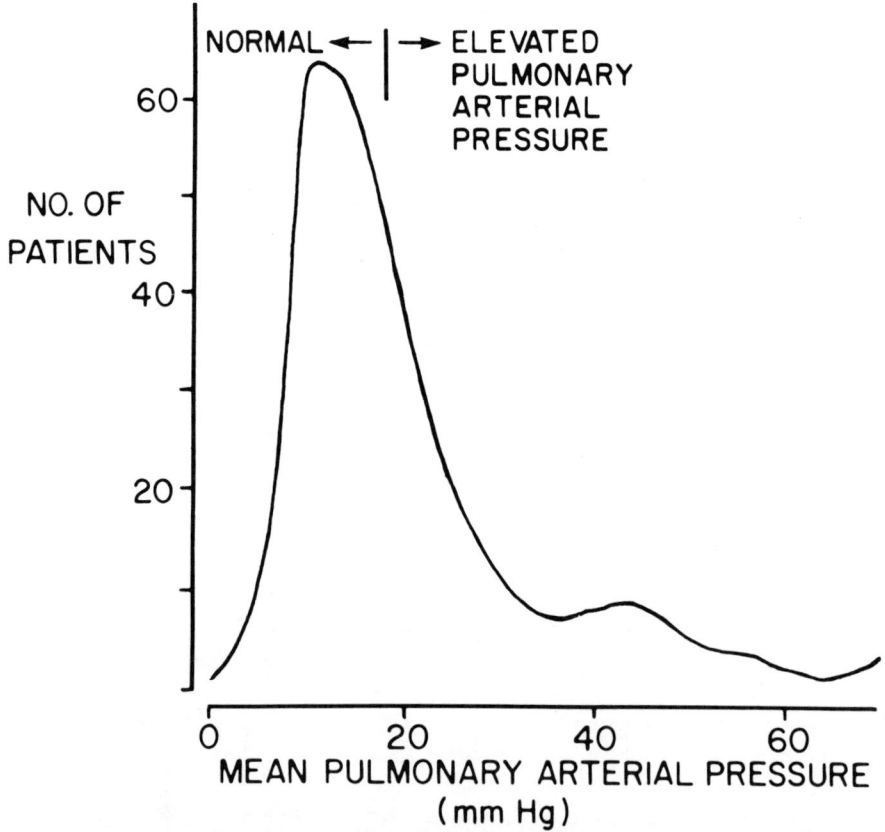

Figure 1. *Histogram of mean pulmonary arterial pressure in 234 consecutive patients coming to heart catheterization in Denver, Colorado (1,600 m). There were 120 adults (aged 21 to 77 yrs.) and 114 children (aged 10 days to 16 yrs.). Pressures above 18 mm Hg are indicated as being abnormal.*

tients, or 45%, had elevated mean pulmonary arterial pressures. Perhaps the surprisingly high incidence of pulmonary hypertension reflects the location of our laboratory and the residence of most of the patients at the modest altitude of 1,600 M.

The 29 adult patients in the cohort having catheterization for valvular heart disease (mostly rheumatic mitral and aortic valve disease and calcific aortic stenosis), had an average pulmonary arterial mean pressure of 30 mm Hg and 20 of them, or 69%, had some elevation of pulmonary arterial pressure. Of the 77 patients coming for coronary heart disease (mostly for coronary arteriography) 64 had measurements of pulmonary arterial pressure. Twenty-eight, or 44%, of the 64 had abnormal pulmonary arterial mean pressure. Because of the low pulmonary blood flows in this group, an even larger percent had abnormally high calculated pulmonary vascular resistance. In the 114 children in the cohort, there were 31 with left-to-right shunts, and 23 of these, 74%, had elevated pulmonary arterial pressures. Thus, some degree of pulmonary hypertension was quite frequent in patients coming for routine, clinical heart catheterization in this laboratory.

CLASSIFICATION OF PULMONARY HYPERTENSION

Paul Wood[13] first classified pulmonary hypertensive disorders according to known pathophysiology: 1) "passive pulmonary hypertension" was that due to obstruction of pulmonary venous outflow as, for example, in mitral stenosis or left ventricular failure; 2) "hyperkinetic pulmonary hypertension" was due to a high flow state as in left-to-right shunts, but without pulmonary vascular disease; 3) "obstructive or obliterative pulmonary hypertension" included those diseases in which vessels were obliterated as in pulmonary embolism or pulmonary parenchymal disease; 4) "vasoconstrictive pulmonary hypertension" was best illustrated by that caused by hypoxia; 5) "reactive pulmonary hypertension," for example, Eisenmenger's syndrome, indicated that some patients with "passive" or "hyperkinetic" hypertension went on to develop very high pulmonary vascular resistance; 6) "primary pulmonary hypertension" constituted a class by itself.

We have chosen a classification oriented by disease categories[14] because a given process may utilize more than one of the pathophysiologic mechanisms described above. For example, chronic lung disease may have hyperkinetic, obstructive, and vasoconstrictive components. Within a disease category, not only the mechanisms of the pulmonary hypertension, but also the morphology of the vascular disease may vary widely. The more common causes of pulmonary hypertension are listed by disease categories in Table 2.

NON-INVASIVE ASSESSMENT

Pulmonary Hypertension Symptoms

Symptoms related to the pulmonary hypertension in any of the diseases mentioned may not develop until the resting pulmonary arterial pressure is approximately 2 or more times normal. Thus symptoms are not a good early indicator of pulmonary hypertensive disorders, yet it is the best we have, for it is symptoms that bring the patient to the physician. There is no symptom which is specific for pulmonary hypertension. The combination of these two facts, i.e., that symptoms do not occur early and that none are specific, results, unfortunately, in many patients coming to diagnosis and therapy late in the natural history of their disease.

The earliest and nearly invariable symptom is *dyspnea*, particularly on exertion, but it is nonspecific and difficult to interpret, e.g., in patients with chronic lung disease the dyspnea may be attributed to airways obstruction, destruction or fibrosis of lung parenchyma with the attendant hypoxemia, or decreased lung compliance. In patients with Eisenmenger's syndrome, dyspnea may be caused by hypoxemia from the right-to-left shunt. In patients with increased venous pressure from left ventricular failure or rheumatic mitral stenosis, fluid filtration into the perivascular spaces stimulates the sensitive "J" receptors, whose afferent traffic up the vagus provides a powerful increase in ventilation. In patients with massive pulmonary embolism, the severe hypoxemia and bronchoconstriction are mechanisms of the distressing dyspnea which occurs. But there is probably more to it, because in patients with primary pulmonary hypertension, or those with recurrent pulmonary embolization in whom none of the above factors need be operative, dyspnea is still the most frequent early symptom and occurs in 95% of 145 reported patients[15] with primary pulmonary hypertension.

In fact, we do not know why the pulmonary hypertensive patient has dyspnea as such a ubiquitous symptom. Stretch receptors are probably present in the main pulmonary artery and could give rise to afferents which cause the sensation of dyspnea. Or it could be that some periph-

TABLE 2
Causes of Pulmonary Hypertension

I. Left ventricular failure
   A. Atherosclerotic heart disease
   B. Hypertensive cardiovascular disease
   C. Aortic valve disease, coarctation of the aorta
   D. Cardiomyopathy
   E. Mitral regurgitation
II. Left atrial hypertension
   A. Mitral stenosis
   B. Left atrial tumor or thrombosis
   C. Cor triatriatum, supravalvar mitral ring
III. Pulmonary venous obstruction
   A. Mediastinal fibrosis
   B. Pulmonary venous thrombosis
IV. Pulmonary parenchymal disease (excluding the newborn period)
   A. Chronic obstructive lung disease
   B. Severe pulmonary fibrosis
      1. Sarcoidosis and other granulomatous lung diseases (many types)
      2. Diffuse interstitial fibrosis (many types)
   C. Acute severe pulmonary injury
      1. Adult respiratory distress syndrome
      2. Severe diffuse pneumonitis
V. Pulmonary artery disease
   A. Primary pulmonary hypertension
   B. Recurrent or massive pulmonary emboli
   C. In situ thrombosis
   D. Vasculitis (Lupus erythematosis, periarteritis, schistosomiasis)
   E. Peripheral pulmonary arterial stenosis
   F. Pulmonary vascular disease resulting from increased blood flow: 1) congenital heart disease with left to right shunt 2) Eisenmenger Syndrome (atrial and ventricular septal defects and patent ductus arteriosus)
   G. Dietary or Drug Induced Pulmonary Hypertension (e.g., Aminorex)
VI. Pulmonary Hypertension in the newborn
   A. Persistence of the fetal circulation
   B. Hyaline membrane disease
   C. Diaphragmatic hernia
   D. Meconium aspiration
VII. Hypoxia and/or hypercapnia
   A. High Altitude Residence
   B. Upper Airway Obstruction, e.g.,
      1. enlarged tonsils, pharyngeal obstruction during sleep
   C. Primary hypoventilation
      1. sleep induced disorders of breathing
      2. obesity-hypoventilation syndrome
      3. primary alveolar hypoventilation

eral mechanism comes into play when cardiac output is insufficient for metabolic requirements, as occurs particularly with exercise in pulmonary hypertensive patients. Tissue hypoxia has been postulated to stimulate respiration[16] and, from a teleological point of view, perhaps the body should have such a mechanism. One group of patients which fails to show dyspnea is, of course, the group with pulmonary hypertension from primary hypoventilation disorders (Chapter 8). In these patients central neurologic mechanisms necessary for hyperventilation or the sensation of dyspnea are presumably inoperative.

Fatigue is likely to reflect impaired oxygen transport due to poor cardiac output and like dyspnea, is not specific for pulmonary hypertension.

Syncope is a symptom which occurs in up to 55% of patients with primary pulmonary hypertension.[15] One expects syncope to occur in any pulmonary hypertensive disorder in which there is sudden reduction of cerebral oxygen transport as might occur: a) when the high pulmonary vascular resistance prevents an increase in cardiac output with exercise; b) with sudden shunting of hypoxemic venous blood into the arterial system in Eisenmenger's syndrome; c) with a sudden decrease in systemic vascular resistance as in (a) or (b) above; d) with spasm of pulmonary arterioles in primary pulmonary hypertension; e) with massive occlusion of the pulmonary arterial bed by embolism; and f) with a sudden abnormality in cardiac rhythm, particularly sudden bradycardia. Syncope has not been attributed to the pulmonary hypertension which occurs in chronic lung disease or disease of the left heart. However, cough-induced syncope may occur in patients with chronic lung disease or in those with primary pulmonary hypertension. Presumably the presence of pulmonary hypertension makes such patients less tolerant of any impairment of venous return or vagally mediated bradycardia.

Anginal like pain occurs in 10 to 50% of patients with pulmonary hypertension regardless of the etiology of the hypertension.[15] Because angina has been described in patients with uncomplicated pulmonary stenosis (where there is right ventricular—without pulmonary—hypertension) the possibility exists that the pain arises from right ventricular ischemia.

Hemoptysis may occur in most forms of pulmonary hypertension. In primary pulmonary hypertension[17] and in patients with left-to-right shunt,[18] there are microvascular aneurysms which form as a result of high pressure being transmitted into the first portion of the pulmonary capillary net. The aneurysms bulge into the alveolar lumen and may rupture, probably causing the hemoptysis. In mitral stenosis, elevated left atrial pressure is reflected in the bronchial venous system. The distended hypertensive submucosal venous plexus is susceptible to irritation and rupture, from forceful coughing which could cause bleeding. In other disorders which lead to pulmonary hypertension, hemoptysis occurs, but is not the result of the hypertensive process. With pulmonary embolism and subsequent lung infarction, the hemoptysis probably reflects the loss of lung capillary integrity. In chronic obstructive lung disease hemoptysis occurs from irritation by cough of inflamed airways.

Hoarseness. The left recurrent laryngeal nerve passes from front to back under the aorta near the attachment of what, during fetal life, was the ductus arteriosus. The nerve is thus between the aorta and the pulmonary artery. High pressure in the pulmonary artery or aneurysmal dilatation in the main or left branches compresses the nerve and may lead to loss of function. In such instances there is paralysis, usually permanent, of the left vocal cord. This complication has been reported in 6 to 8% of persons with long standing severe pulmonary hypertension.[13]

Physical Examination

The physical examination is more specific than the history in indicating the presence of pulmonary hypertension and it complements the history by helping to assign etiology of the pulmonary hypertension, when present. Even so, physical findings are subjective, have a wide normal spectrum, and cannot accurately establish the presence of early, i.e., mild, pulmonary hypertension.

The most quantifiable physical finding in pulmonary hypertension is the increased systemic venous pressure, manifested first as prominence of the *"a"-wave* observed in the jugular venous pulse. The jugular vein has no valve and equilibrates with right ventricular pressure during diastole. A horizontal plane passing through the sternal "angle of Louis" is approximately 5 cm above the atrium and ventricle. A presystolic pulsation in the deep venous system 2 cm vertically above that plane is usually abnormal. If the examiner increases venous return by pushing gently over the abdomen, an abnormal "a" wave should become exaggerated. An abnormal "a" wave points to a stiffened or hypertrophied ventricle expected in pulmonary hypertensive disorders. Presystolic distension of the relatively noncompliant right ventricle produces an audible 4th heart sound (S_4) which increases with inspiration. Emphasis on the "a" wave is justified because observers frequently overlook this simple, quick, and relatively accurate way to quantify the pressure required to fill the right ventricle during atrial systole.

With the onset of right ventricular failure, the right ventricle dilates, producing distortion of the tricuspid valve and regurgitation. On auscultation there is a systolic murmur which increases in intensity during inspiration. When severe, tricuspid regurgitation produces, during systole, a prominent "v" wave in the jugular venous pulse. Thus the jugular venous pulse provides clues as to the presence of pulmonary hypertension and its complications.

A physical finding which is more specific for pulmonary hypertension in adults than in children is that the *pulmonary valvular closure sound* (P_2) increases in pitch and intensity and may become palpable as pulmonary arterial pressure rises. Unfortunately, these changes are subtle in mild pulmonary hypertension and interpretation is complicated by variations in chest wall thicknesses and the amount of lung overlying the pulmonary artery. The pulmonary valve also closes earlier in the ejection period as pulmonary arterial pressure rises, so that the time interval between aortic valve closure and subsequent closure of the pulmonary valve is reduced. The two valves may close together causing a single second heart sound in patients with severe pulmonary hypertension. Assessing the time interval from aortic to pulmonary valve closure is made difficult by the normal delay being short (20–60 msec) and varying with respiration. Interpreting the interval is difficult when there is left ventricular disease, particularly left bundle branch block, which delays aortic valve closure and when right bundle branch block delays pulmonic closure. A systolic ejection click may occur and is thought to reflect sudden distention of the pulmonary arterial wall with rapid pulmonary arterial filling, but it is not specific for pulmonary hypertension. With dilation of the hypertensive main pulmonary artery and the pulmonary valve annulus, a murmur of pulmonary valvular regurgitation occurs. The murmur is a decrescendo diastolic, blowing, murmur heard loudest in the 2nd and 3rd left intercostal spaces, beginning with the loud pulmonary valve closure sound. A 3rd heart sound (S_3) which increases on inspiration is indicative of the right ventricular dysfunction which may occur in pulmonary hypertension.

A sustained *right ventricular lift* is the thrust felt with the palm of the hand placed over the left parasternal region or over the "epigastrium" and indicates forceful activity of the hypertensive right ventricle. An unsustained left parasternal impulse is characteristic of a "volume overloaded" right ventricle as occurs in atrial septal defect or tricuspid valve regurgitation without associated pulmonary hypertension.

Finally, the physical examination may provide important information as to etiology of the pulmonary hypertension, i.e., mitral stenosis, chronic lung disease, congenital heart disease, and thrombophlebitis (which may be associated with embolic pulmonary hypertension).

The Electrocardiogram

The electrocardiogram, by providing evidence of right ventricular hypertrophy, is a time honored, generally available, inexpensive, and universally applied tool in the non-invasive assessment of pulmonary hypertension. Any of the criteria listed in Table 3 we accept as suggesting the presence of right ventricular hypertrophy. The coexistence of right atrial hypertrophy (a symmetrical and peaked P wave greater than 2.5 mm in amplitude in any lead) is consistent with the presence of right ventricular hypertension. The presence of more than one criterion, or a large deviation beyond the normal limit increases the probability of the diagnosis. An illustrative sequence of electrocardiographic changes in progressive pulmonary hypertension is shown in Figure 2.

As can be seen from Table 3, the electrocardiogram is rather specific, in that it gives few false positives. When false positive results occur, they are most frequently seen with right bundle branch block, posterior myocardial infarction, left posterior hemiblock, Wolf-Parkinson-

TABLE 3
Electrocardiographic Criteria of Right Ventricular Hypertrophy

Adult* Criterion	% Sensitivity True Positive	% Missed Diagnosis	% Specificity True Negatives	% False Positive
QRS axis in frontal plane $\geq 110°$	19	81	96	4
04 sec duration R wave in $V_1 > 5$ mm	2	98	99	1
R/S ratio in $V_1 > 1$	6	94	98	2
R/S ratio in $V_6 < 1$	16	84	93	7
S_1, S_2, S_3 pattern	24	76	87	13

In presence of right bundle branch block:
  a. Axis of early (unblocked) forces $> +110°$
  b. R' wave in $V_1 > 15$ mm.

The above criteria can be applied only in the absence of left ventricular posterior hemiblock and "true" posterior infarction.

* In children see References 19, 20, 21.

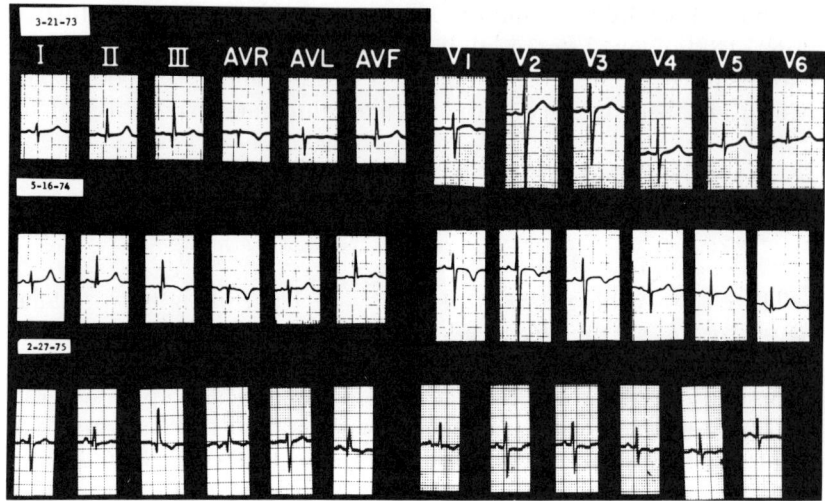

Figure 2. Serial 12 lead electrocardiograms in a 17-year-old girl with primary pulmonary hypertension in 1973. While progressive right ventricular hypertrophy is apparent, clear markers of hypertrophy occurred late. * indicates abnormal values referred to in Table 3. (Courtesy of Dr. R. Pryor.)

	1973	1974	1975
QRS axis in frontal plane	+90°	+90°	+140°
R wave amplitude in V_1	5 mm	5 mm	8 mm*
R/S ratio in V_1	0.5	0.4	4.0*
R/S ratio in V_6	6.0	4.0	1.3
S_1, S_2, S_3 pattern	no	no	no
R wave amplitude in AVR	0.5	1.0	7.0*

White syndrome, or anatomic shifts in position of the heart. The problem with the electrocardiogram is that it is not a very sensitive test for the presence of right ventricular hypertrophy. That is, the electrocardiogram does not detect the presence of right ventricular hypertrophy when the hypertrophy is modest, i.e., early in the natural history of the hypertensive process.

The normal right ventricle has only ¼ to ⅓ the mass of the left ventricle in the adult. Thus, the electrical forces reflecting depolarization of the ventricles primarily represent the left, not the right ventricle. Even doubling the thickness of the right ventricular free wall will not reliably cause an electrocardiographic pattern of right ventricular hypertrophy to appear. Because the electrocardiogram represents electrical activity of cardiac muscle, it is only indirectly related to pressure. Should hypertrophy lag the development of pulmonary hypertension or should there be a pressure gradient across the pulmonary valve, the sensitivity of the electrocardiogram for pulmonary vascular hypertension will be even less. The sensitivity of the electrocardiogram for pulmonary hypertension is less in older than in younger adults, primarily because the QRS axis is more horizontal (leftward) in older subjects and right axis deviation is, therefore, less likely to occur.

The electrocardiogram is most sensitive in predicting pulmonary arterial pressure in the healthy young adult at high altitude.[22] However, even here there is considerable variation. In the 28 school children catheterized in Leadville, Colorado at 10, 150 ft. elevation (3,100 M), 6 had mild pulmonary hypertension missed by the electrocardiographic criteria, but only 1 had a false positive test.

Despite its limitations, when it is placed in the proper perspective, the electrocardiogram is an extremely useful tool. First, when right ventricular hypertrophy is suspected from the electrocardiographic analysis, there is a high probability that pressure is elevated. The physician, thus alerted, must consider whether or not to pursue other non-invasive tests. Our current policy is to utilize rather aggressive readings of the electrocardiogram but to put that reading in context with the history, physical examination, chest roentgenogram, and if indicated, echocardiogram. When the electrocardiogram is normal, pulmonary hypertension, especially of mild or moderate degree, is not ruled out. Again, if other parts of the examination suggest pulmonary hypertension, the physician is justified in pursuing the investigation.

The Chest Roentgenogram

The chest roentgenogram is a standard and extremely useful part of the evaluation of a patient with suspected or known pulmonary hypertension because it permits radiographic evaluation of the chest cage, lungs, pulmonary vessels, heart and diaphragm—lung interface. The chest roentgenogram may provide a clue to the etiology and severity of pulmonary hypertension (Table 4).

The chest roentgenogram as a non-invasive estimate of pulmonary arterial pressure is useful but imperfect.[23-28] The cardiothoracic ratio as a predictor of pulmonary arterial pressure is of limited value because in pulmonary hypertension, even in the absence of left heart disease, it relates more to right atrial and ventricular enlargement from increased right-sided filling pressures, i.e., right heart failure, than to

TABLE 4
Likelihood of Chest Roentgenogram Providing Etiologic Information
in Pulmonary Hypertension

Likely	Unlikely
Chronic obstructive lung disease	Primary pulmonary hypertension
Restrictive lung disease	Large pulmonary emboli (without infiltrate)
	Recurrent pulmonary microembolism
Lung fibrosis or granulomatous disease	
Kyphoscoliosis	Eisenmenger's Syndrome
Congenital heart disease	
Mitral valve disease	
Left ventricular disease	Persistence of fetal circulation
Pulmonary embolic disease (with infiltrate)	Meconium Aspiration
Congenital diaphragmatic hernia	
Hyaline membrane disease	

the level of pulmonary arterial pressure. Assessment of the degree of vascularity in the peripheral lung fields is beset with so many uncertainties (exposure of the film, degree of lung inflation, the problem of distinguishing small pulmonary arteries from veins, airways, and lymphatics) that even experienced radiologists can make only general and tentative evaluation as to the presence of overperfusion as in left-to-right shunts, or of underperfusion as in obliterated or constricted peripheral bed.

The most successful radiographic signs of pulmonary hypertension depend upon measurements relating to diameter of the large pulmonary arteries and reflect primarily the pressure within the arteries. Three radiographic measurements have been evaluated in several forms of pulmonary hypertension: 1) the width of the descending branch of the right pulmonary artery; 2) hilar width, which is the distance from the midline to the left lateral border of the main pulmonary artery, divided by the half the transverse diameter of the chest; and 3) the hilar/thoracic index, which is the horizontal distance on the chest film from the first division of the right main pulmonary artery to the first division of the left main pulmonary artery, divided by the transverse diameter of the thorax. These measurements are indicated in Figure 3.

Of the studies listed, perhaps the size of the pulmonary arteries measured as the hilar/thoracic index provide the best indication of the presence of pulmonary hypertension (Table 5). However, it is not possible to quantitate the level of the pressure. The reasons are probably that vascular distension increases with the duration of the hyper-

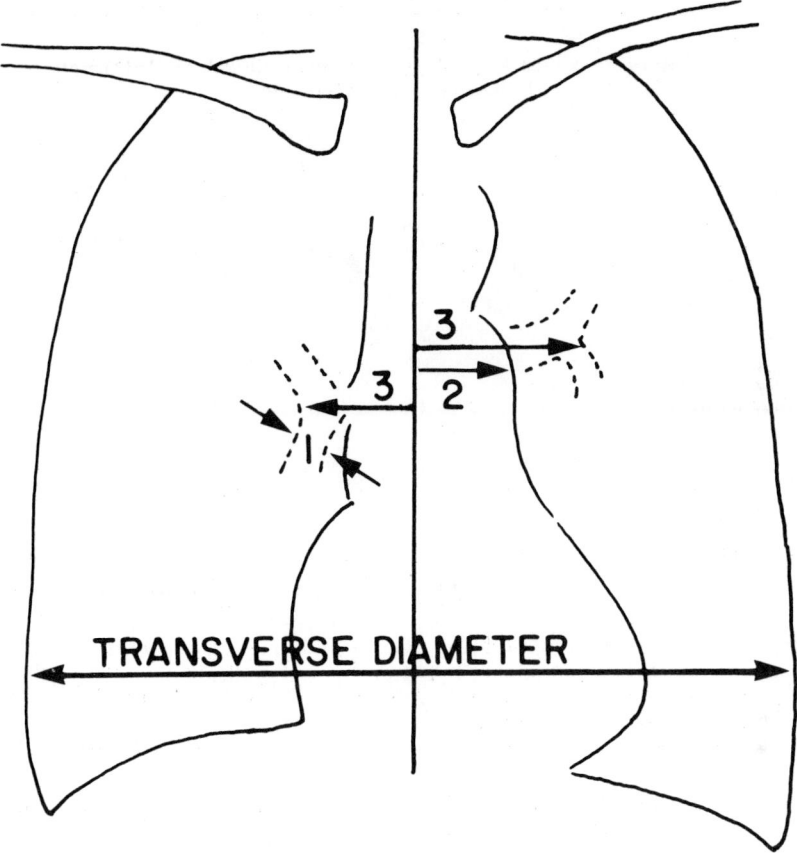

Figure 3. Guide to radiographic measurements of pulmonary hypertension.[28]
1. Width of the descending branch of right pulmonary artery. 2. The hilar width is the measurement labeled 2 divided by ½ transverse thoracic diameter. 3. The hilar thoracic index is the sum of the 2 measurements labeled 3 divided by the transverse thoracic diameter.

tension because there are changes that take place with time within the walls of the large vessels.

Ultrasound

The echocardiogram is useful in assessing pulmonary hypertension even though there is no criterion which universally applies to all patients.[29-35] As discussed in Chapter 7 on chronic lung disease, right

TABLE 5
Usefulness of Chest Radiographic Measurements in Assessing Pulmonary Hypertension

Measurement	Normal value	Measured Value in Pulmonary Hypertension	Reference
Descending right pulmonary artery (mm)	12.1 ± 1.2 S.D. (n = 100) Range 9–16 (n = 1085)	25.1 ± 6.4 S.D. (n = 59)	(24, 25, 27)
Hilar width (%)	28.1 ± 4.5 S.D. (n = 100) range 19–40 (n = 14)	43.7 ± 7.7 S.D. (n = 59) range 25–52 (n = 11)	(23, 27)
Hilar/Thorac Index (%)	34 ± 4 S.D. (n = 150)	44 ± 6 S.D. (n = 59)	(27, 28)

Shown above for 3 radiographic indices of pulmonary hypertension are the normal values when pulmonary hypertension is absent, the measured values in pulmonary hypertension, and the references for the data. Figure 3 indicates how the measurements are made.

---

heart visualization is not possible when a hyperinflated lung covers the anterior surface of the heart. However, when pulmonary hypertension occurs in children or in adults without hyperinflated lungs, the resultant dilation of the right heart and pulmonary artery tends to make the examination easier, not more difficult. When 4 expert observers read 155 echocardiograms without knowing the pulmonary arterial pressures from heart catheterization,[31] the average sensitivity for detecting pulmonary hypertension was only 52%. When they diagnosed pulmonary hypertension, they were right in 85% of the cases. Thus, the echocardiogram is not very sensitive for pulmonary hypertension but it is rather specific. Table 6 indicates measurements which may be helpful in indicating the presence of pulmonary hypertension:

• The pulmonary valve "a" wave occurs when pulmonary diastolic pressure is normal. Apparently right atrial systole generates sufficient energy to cause the pulmonary valve to move toward the open position, even though it may not actually open. When pulmonary diastolic pressure is elevated, as in pulmonary hypertension, the energy im-

TABLE 6
M Mode Echocardiographic Findings in Adults

	Normal	Pulmonary Hypertension	Reference
1) Pulmonary Valve "A" Wave	3–7 mm	0–2 mm	(29)
2) RV End Diastolic Dimension	0.6–2.9 cm	2.2–4.5 cm	(29,32)
3) Thickness of IV septum	5–13 mm	13–19 mm	(34,61)
4) Initial diastolic slope of mitral valve	> 80mm/sec	0–57mm/sec	(35)
5) $\frac{RPEP}{RVET}$	< .30	> .40	(29,35)

parted to the blood is less effective in causing the valve to move and the "a" wave tends to disappear. However, the "a" wave may be present even in severe pulmonary hypertension when the right atrial pressure is high.[29,30]

• Right ventricular diastolic dimension (usually observed in the right ventricular outflow tract) tends to increase as the pulmonary arterial pressure and hence the right ventricular filling volume is greater. In our experience, the largest dimensions we have seen are in patients with pulmonary hypertension plus tricuspid and/or pulmonary regurgitation, or large left-to-right shunt.

• The increase in the interventricular septum thickness is not specific for right ventricular hypertrophy, and can only be interpreted as such when there is no left ventricular hypertrophy. The septum may move paradoxically, showing anterior rather than posterior motion during systole, suggesting hypertrophy of the right ventricle.[63]

• The decreased initial opening velocity of the mitral valve, (reduced mitral valve E–F slope) which is characteristic of mitral stenosis, is seen also in pulmonary hypertension in the absence of mitral valve disease. Possibly the passive left ventricular filling may be prolonged because of increased stiffness of the ventricular septum or by compression of the left ventricular cavity by the bulging septum.

• The right ventricular pre-ejection period (time interval from Q wave on the electrocardiogram to onset of pulmonary valve opening) is increased, presumably because it takes longer for the right ventricle to generate the higher pressures necessary to open the valve in pulmonary hypertension. The right ventricular ejection period (time from opening to closing of pulmonary valve) tends to decrease as pulmonary arterial pressure rises, possibly because the pulmonary valve opening is delayed, and the volume of blood delivered with each stroke into the pulmonary artery is less.

Further, the low compliance in the large arteries and high resistance in the small arteries tend to force early pulmonary valve closure. The ratio of pre-ejection/ejection period should increase with increasing pressure because the numerator gets larger and the denominator gets smaller. Both numerator and denominator shorten to a similar extent with heart rate, so that the ratio is independent of rate. Eighty percent of children with a ratio less than 0.3 had normal pulmonary arterial pressures and 90% of persons with a ratio above 0.4 had mean pulmonary arterial pressures of 25 mm Hg or more.[35] As with many nonspe-

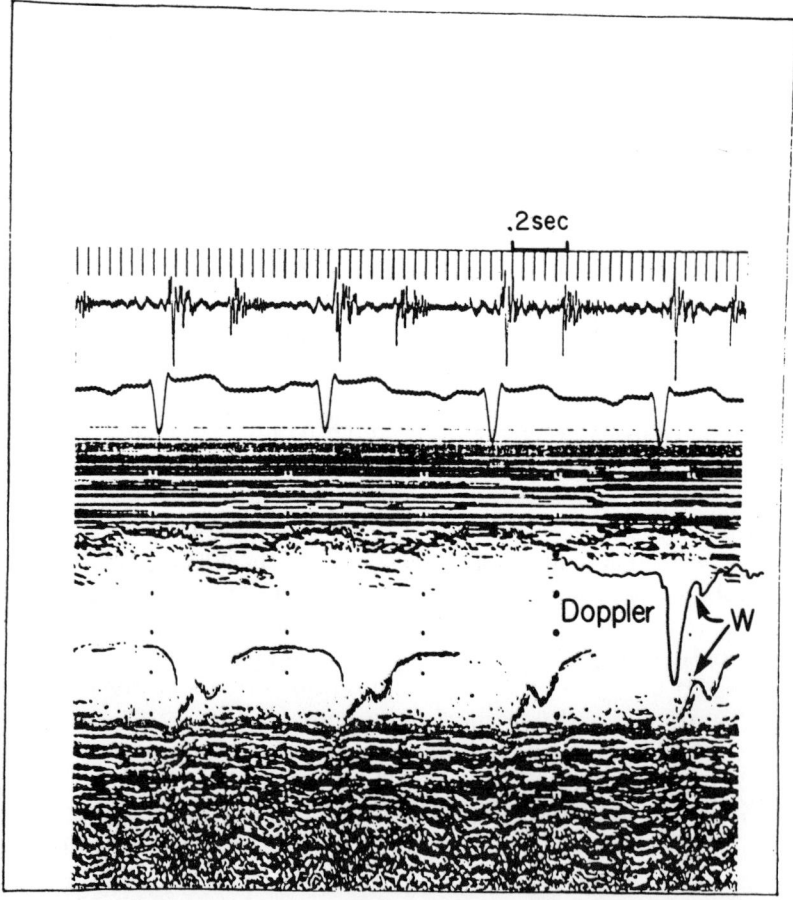

Figure 4. *M-mode echocardiogram in a patient with primary pulmonary hypertension. Shown are the phonocardiogram, and the electrocardiogram above the echo. The "flying W" is indicated in the motion of the pulmonary valve leaflet; superimposed is a Doppler tracing of flow velocity in the main pulmonary artery drawn on the echo to show that flow velocity falls rapidly at the time of the "flying W" in the pulmonary valve. The 1 cm depth calibration points were intensified for reproduction.*

cific tests, this index of pulmonary hypertension is good statistically, but may not be precise for individual patients.

• A mid-systolic notch in the pulmonary valve in some patients with pulmonary hypertension, the "flying W" sign, occurs when the pulmonary valve temporarily moves toward a closed position prior to final closure. In our experience this notch in the pulmonary valve motion occurs simultaneously with a sharp decrease in pulmonary flow in mid-systole. The flow then decreases further for the remainder of systole (Figure 4). We suspect that the sudden decrease in flow and the movement of the valve toward closure indicates the time at which the large pulmonary arteries have reached the limit of their compliance. If so the "flying W" is determined by the relation between vascular compliance and stroke volume and its reported inconstant relation to pressure might be expected.

• Two-dimensional echocardiography is perhaps the best method for estimating right atrial size and encroachment of a dilated right ventricle upon the left ventricular cavity as may occur in right heart failure. Venous injection of saline containing microbubbles while using the 4 chamber view has been useful for detecting right-to-left shunting in pulmonary hypertensive patients.

• The Doppler has considerable promise in the non-invasive assessment of pulmonary hypertension. Flow patterns in the superior and inferior vena cava are useful in indicating tricuspid regurgitation. The Doppler can estimate aortic root flow. Thus, in the absence of intracardiac shunts, and with an echocardiographic estimate of aortic root diameter, the Doppler should estimate pulmonary flow. Reports by Hatle[36] and by Burstin[37] indicate that "right ventricular relaxation time" (pulmonic closure to tricuspid opening) might be particularly useful in estimating pressure. The Doppler is most effective when "looking at" moving targets in the near field, and thus it is particularly well suited for timing of tricuspid and pulmonary valve events.

INVASIVE ASSESSMENT: CARDIAC CATHETERIZATION

Indications

• To determine presence of pulmonary hypertension and to assess its severity when the presence of pulmonary hypertension has been suggested by non-invasive assessment.

TABLE 7

Catheterization May be Essential for Etiological Diagnosis: Etiological Diagnosis at Cardiac Catheterization by Disease Category in Pulmonary Hypertension Patients

Condition	Test Applied	Finding
Congenital heart disease	Step up in O_2 saturation in right heart, H_2 electrode studies in the right heart	Left to right shunt and location of shunt
	Cardiogreen injection in right heart with sampling in systemic artery	Right to left shunt and location of shunt
	Cardiac angiography	
Peripheral pulmonary artery stenoses	Intrapulmonary arterial pressure	Intrapulmonary arterial pressure gradients
	Pulmonary angiograph	Pulmonary arterial branch stenoses
Major pulmonary arterial occlusion by clot, or tumor*	Continuous pressure recording from distal pulmonary artery to main pulmonary artery	Focal pressure gradient in a lobar or larger pulmonary artery, intravascular filling defect or narrowing
	Selective or main pulmonary angiography	
Mitral stenosis Cortriatriatum Supravalvar mitral ring	Simultaneous wedge and left ventricular pressure recording	An elevated wedge pressure and mean mitral valve diastolic pressure gradient > 3 mm Hg at rest, both of which increase with exercise
Mitral regurgitation	Simultaneous wedge and left ventricular pressure recording	Large systolic pressure wave in wedge tracing. Regurgitation of contrast from left ventricular angiogram into the left atrium.
Left ventricular dysfunction or diastolic overload.	Left ventricular pressure Left ventricular angiogram	Left ventricular end diastolic pressure > 15 mm Hg left ventricular contraction abnormality and/or ejection fraction < 50%.

*Ventilation and perfusion lung scans precede catheterization. See Chapter 5.

- To establish etiology, where possible, of the pulmonary hypertension, Tables 7 and 8.
- To determine the potential for acute pulmonary vasodilation or relief of obstruction in certain pulmonary hypertensive disorders, i.e., primary pulmonary hypertension; chronic obstructive lung disease; congenital heart disease; patients with acute or sub-acute pulmonary embolism; or chronic mountain sickness.

The perfect pulmonary vasodilator for use in the catheterization laboratory would be one which is safe and effective in dilating the pulmonary but not the systemic bed, could be infused intravenously

TABLE 8
Catheterization Does Not Establish Etiological Diagnosis

Condition	Procedure Needed to Establish Etiology	Result
Pulmonary parenchymal disease	Chest x-ray	Radiographic abnormality.
	Pulmonary function tests such as spirometry, volumes, compliance, DLCO, A-aO_2 gradient.	Airflow obstruction, pulmonary restriction and/or decreased compliance and diffusion capacity with altered gas exchange
	Bronchoscopy if indicated	See Chapter 7.
Recurrent pulmonary microembolism or micro-arterial thrombosis	Lung biopsy	Eccentric intimal fibrosis, fibrous strands
Pulmonary venous thrombosis or fibrosis	Lung biopsy	Pulmonary venous occlusion and fibrosis.
Primary pulmonary hypertension	Lung biopsy	Pulmonary arterial medial hypertrophy and/or concentric intimal fibrosis see Chapter 4
Pulmonary vasculitis	Clinical and laboratory evidence of collagen vascular disease	
	Lung biopsy	Perivascular inflammation.
Drug induced dietary pulmonary hypertension	History of intake	
Pulmonary hypertension of newborn (see Chapter 2).		

with an immediate effect, and any adverse effect such as systemic hypotension would cease when the infusion was stopped. The use of agents such as prostacyclin,[38] nitroprusside, and acetyl choline are discussed in Chapter 4.

Assessment of the potential for pulmonary vasodilation is usually not recommended in persons with: long-standing right-to-left shunts from pulmonary hypertension (Eisenmenger's syndrome) because the resistance is likely to be fixed. In these patients there is risk of causing selective systemic vasodilation with systemic hypotension and increased right-to-left shunting; in mitral stenosis vasodilators increase cardiac output and heart rate while decreasing pulmonary arteriolar resistance, setting the stage for possible pulmonary edema; and in left ventricular dysfunction, vasodilators are given to unload the systemic circulation rather than to have a direct effect on the lung vessels.

- To assess chronic vasodilator therapy.

Quality Control

Because most catheterization laboratories in the United States are concerned largely with visualization of diseased coronary arteries and abnormal left ventricular function, quality control, appropriately, is focused on radiographic resolving power. For catherization of pulmonary hypertensive patients, however, careful attention must be paid to quality measurements of pressures and flows. Laboratories not willing to provide the necessary quality control should not assume the hemodynamic management of pulmonary hypertensive patients.

Pulmonary Arterial Pressure

The "gold standard" in the assessment of pulmonary hypertension is the direct measurement of pulmonary arterial pressure, but, like the price of gold, the pressure fluctuates. In primary pulmonary hypertension, pressure may vary with the spontaneous variations in vascular tone; in mitral stenosis it varies with heart rate; in Eisenmenger's syndrome it varies with systemic pressure; and in chronic lung disease it varies with oxygenation and with pH. In all forms of pulmonary hypertension pressure varies with intrathoracic pressure and with cardiac output. The physician in charge at catheterization must take the time to monitor the changes when they occur and to assess their cause.

Pulmonary Wedge Pressure

Wedge pressure is the pressure measured through an end hole catheter when the catheter is mechanically "wedged" into a peripheral pulmonary artery. A "balloon-tipped flotation catheter" is "wedged" by inflating the balloon, which then occludes a lobar or segmental branch of the pulmonary artery. The flow is stopped and the pressure measured is that observed in the first downstream vein in which flow is occurring. Thus, conceivably when the catheter is wedged in a small artery, the wedge pressure will be that in a small vein. When a wedge pressure is obtained by inflating a balloon in a lobar artery, one expects the pressure to be that in the left atrium. Measurement of wedge pressure allows not only for the assessment of the downstream pressure but for calculation of the gradient from pulmonary artery to vein, the numerator of the ratio in the pulmonary vascular resistance calculation. The wedge pressure is also one determinant of resistance. For example, when pulmonary venous pressure is elevated for a few minutes or even a few days, the pulmonary vascular resistance is reduced because the pulmonary venules (responsible for one-third of pulmonary vascular resistance)[39] become dilated and the capillaries become fully recruited. But with elevation of pulmonary venous pressure for months or years as in mitral stenosis there is "reactive" pulmonary hypertension. Figure 5 illustrates reactive pulmonary hypertension in mitral stenosis.[40]

To yield a valid wedge pressure, the venous pressure distal to the wedged catheter must exceed alveolar pressure, i.e., West's Zone III lung conditions must exist.[41] If alveolar pressure exceeds venous pressure the vessels of the microcirculation will be collapsed and the catheter will measure alveolar pressure or some pressure other than venous pressure. Thus, a valid wedge pressure is obtained in the dependent portion of the lungs.[42] Criteria for a valid wedge include: a pressure lower than mean pulmonary arterial pressure; a pressure contour which differs from that in pulmonary artery and shows respiratory variations, and in sinus rhythm, the presence of an "a" wave; a catheter tip which on fluoroscopic observation no longer shows motion with each heart beat; and on withdrawal the catheter suddenly "snaps back" with a concomitant return of the contour to that of pulmonary artery. These are guidelines for, but not proof of, a valid wedge pressure. Measurement of a pressure similar in contour and magnitude from another wedge position is supportive evidence of a valid wedge. Withdrawal of arterialized blood from a wedged catheter is also supportive of a valid wedge position.

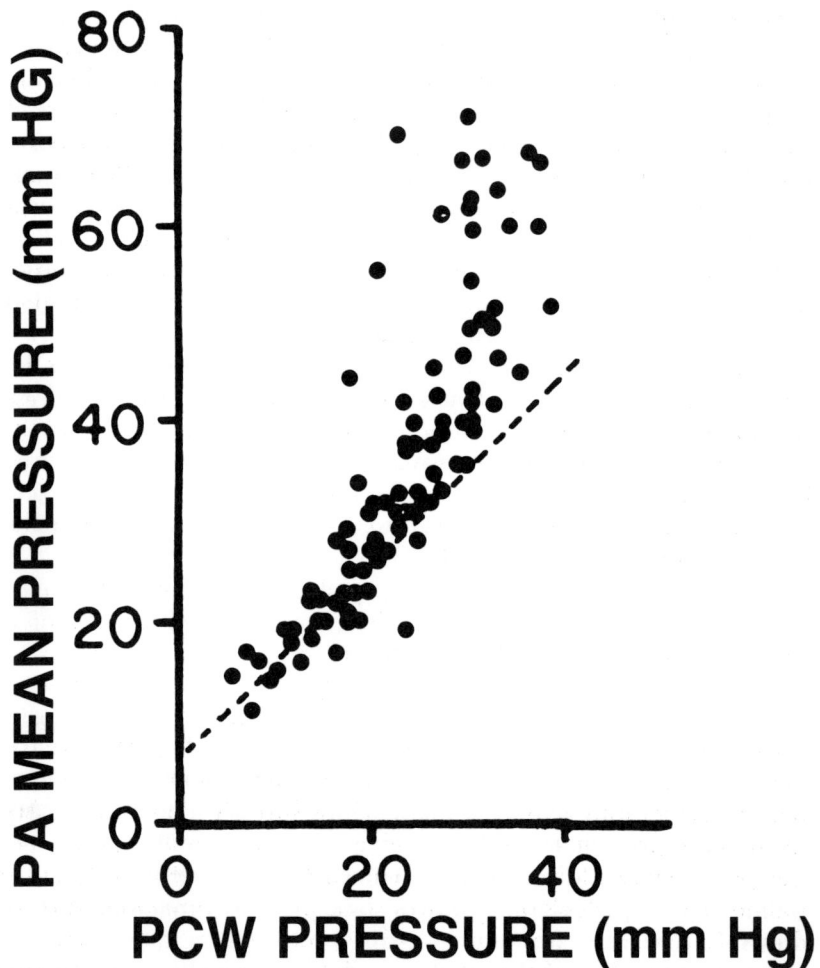

Figure 5. Relation between pulmonary arterial (PA) mean pressure and pulmonary capillary wedge (PCW) mean pressure in 100 patients with mitral stenosis. The dashed line represents the relationship when PA_m pressure rises (to the same extent, to the same amount) as PCW pressure. However, the PA_m pressure in some cases rose higher than the PCW pressure, beginning at 15 to 20 mm Hg, although a few remained on the line of equality despite pressure in excess of this. There were variably elevated PA_m pressures in excess of PCW pressure in the majority of patients whose PCW pressure exceeded 25 mm Hg. (Reproduced with permission from Dexter[41].)

Cardiac Output

Cardiac output measurement is essential for interpreting the pressure and for the determination of resistance. Thermodilution (whereby the cold saline is injected in the right atrium and passes by a temperature sensor in the pulmonary artery) is the methodology used in many laboratories. Each thermodilution cardiac output value should be the average of at least 3 determinations. Values so obtained have agreed well with Fick cardiac output values above 3.5 liters/min in our laboratory.[43] Below 3.5 liters/min, thermodilution overestimates flow by approximately 35%, probably because with low flow there is time for heat loss through cardiac chambers. Thermodilution using right atrial injection is invalidated when there is a right-to-left shunt at the atrial level, as for example, through a patent foramen ovale, a common occurrence in pulmonary hypertension.

Quality control requires that thermodilution measurements be checked against an independent standard for cardiac output. The Fick method, with measurement of both oxygen uptake and oxygen contents for pulmonary arteriovenous difference or an indocyanine green dye (indicator dilution) curve, a variant of the Fick principle, provide near ideal standards as well as a backup for certain instances where the thermodilution method is invalid.

Technique

Risks of cardiac catherization of severe pulmonary hypertensive patients exceed those of other patients coming to the laboratory. Pulmonary arteriography may precipitate sudden death. Pulmonary vasodilators can precipitate life-threatening systemic arterial hypotension. Yet, at present, the diagnosis and management of patients with severe pulmonary hypertension requires multiple catheterization procedures. Care is thus important. Table 9 lists problems encountered by ourselves and others in the catheterization of pulmonary hypertensive patients. It also indicates possible steps to prevent or treat adverse situations.

Our *approach* to adult catheterization is as follows. To avoid altering the patient's hemodynamic status, we usually administer no premedication, preferring to keep the patient well informed before and during the catheterization. We utilize a percutaneous femoral approach for both arterial and venous catheterization. Because there is no incision and the artery and veins are not sacrificed, repeat catheterizations at appropriate intervals can utilize the same femoral technique. The disadvantages of the femoral approach including more difficult catheter placement and the ease with which the catheter tip "flips" out of the pulmonary artery have been largely overcome with the use of a newly

TABLE 9
Problems Encountered during Catheterization of Pulmonary Hypertensive Patients

Problem and Cause	Consequence	Prevention or Treatment
Atrial tachycardia induced by the catheter	Reduced cardiac output and hypotenson if allowed to persist	*Prevention*: use of flow directed catheter; approach from the left arm usually requires less catheter manipulation than approach from the leg; if arrhythmia is recurrent or difficult to control, abandon the procedure *Treatment*: carotid massage, intravenous digitalis, cardioversion if necessary
Sinus bradycardia usually caused by pain or anxiety during catheterization	Reduced cardiac output and hypotension	*Prevention*: insure patient comfort; avoid beta blocking agents *Treatment*: atropine, temporary atrial pacing catheter
Transient right bundle branch block, catheter perforation of the heart; usually caused by a stiff catheter, excess manipulation, or continued catheter monitoring after leaving the catheter laboratory	May lead to impaired right ventricular function; perforation may lead to cardiac tamponade	*Prevention*: utilization of balloon tipped catheter; minimize catheter manipulation; minimize catheter monitoring following the catheterization procedure *Treatment*: appropriate for cardiac tamponade if present
Pulmonary artery catheter repeatedly returns to right ventricle or atrium, usually a consequence of a dilated right heart and tricuspid regurgitation	Impedes progress of diagnostic study, may stimulate premature beats, increase catheter manipulation; catheter cannot pass tricuspid valve because of tricuspid insufficiency	*Prevention*: utilize an approach from the left arm; use guidewire balloon-tipped thermodilution catheter

TABLE 9 *(Continued)*

Idiopathic hypotension or syncope without bradycardia (cause? pulmonary vasospasm, pyrogen reaction, drug idiosyncrasy)	Low cardiac output, shock oliguria	*Prevention*: a systemic arterial catheter for pressure monitoring prior to right heart catheter may give an early warning of hypotension. *Treatment*: ? fluids ? PGI_2 ? Calcium channel blockers
Vasodilator overdose	Hypotension	*Prevention*: use short acting drug for vasodilator challenge; do not administer further vasodilator when systemic systolic pressure decreases 25% or pulmonary arterial pressure begins to rise

* American Edwards model

designed Swan-Ganz® thermodilution catheter (model 93A-821H-7.5F, American Edwards, Santa Anna, California). It has an additional lumen which ends in a *cul de sac* near the tip for a teflon, coated guidewire. By varying the distance from guidewire tip to catheter tip, and the diameter of the guidewire (.028" to .032") the catheter becomes relatively "stiff" or "floppy" on demand. Because the guidewire does not come into contact with blood, it can be left in place for prolonged periods.

After concluding whatever initial investigation is indicated (e.g., a search for shunts), measurements of pulmonary arterial, wedge, and systemic arterial pressures and of thermodilution cardiac output are made. The pressure and flow measurements are repeated about 15 minutes later to provide an index of hemodynamic stability. If acute vasodilation is attempted with one or more agents, we employ first those with brief durations of action, for example, O_2, PGI_2, isoproterenol, each having measurements of pressure and flow before and during administration of the agent. The repeated controls provide a further indication of hemodynamic stability as well as the basis for evaluation of the response to vasodilation. If an agent with longer action, for example, hydralazine or a calcium inhibitor, is to be given, it is the final therapeutic intervention. After assessing the effect, we withdraw the catheter. If indicated, long-term oral therapy is begun while the patient is observed in the hospital, using usual clinical care, including measurements of systemic blood pressure and pulse rate, but without invasive monitoring. (If there is concern about persistent systemic hypotension in the catheterization laboratory, we will leave pulmonary and systemic arterial catheters in place, monitoring pressure and flow in the coronary care unit until the patient is stable.) After an appropriate interval (as short as 1 week in primary pulmonary hypertension), we perform an abbreviated catheterization to measure pressures and flows for the assessment of therapy. Initially we attempted to evaluate by continuous monitoring over 3 days pulmonary and systemic pressures and flows during vasodilator therapy in patients with pulmonary hypertension. After 4 attempts, we have largely abandoned this approach because: 1) the patients found it distressing to be confined to bed in a coronary care unit for several days; 2) in patients the standard balloon-tipped catheter spontaneously prolapsed into the right ventricle (a problem not encountered since we have employed the guidewire-balloon-tipped catheter); 3) and the presence of the catheter may activate cellular or humoral systems in the blood with detriment to the patient. (We know of one young female patient who had a cerebral embolus while being monitored in coronary care unit with a Swan-Ganz catheter. Presumably she had a paradoxical embolus via a patent foramen ovale.) 4) Enforced bed rest and continued catheterization might not provide the proper setting for therapeutic evaluation. A recent report demonstrated that 3 of 11 patients died when catheters were left in place for several days and multiple vasodilators were given.[44] At present we believe it is safer, less distressing to the patient, and may provide more meaningful information to have the patients return for a brief follow-up catheterization after a trial of oral therapy. However, the number of catheterizations should be the fewest possible, consistent with good clinical care.

Evaluation

The assessment of the hemodynamic findings require the physician to answer certain questions:
• Is pulmonary hypertension present? This can usually be answered by applying the criteria given in the section on *Definition*.

- Is pulmonary hypertension impairing cardiovascular function?

—Right ventricular function. Normal values of right atrial pressure measured from mid-chest position in supine subjects are shown in Table 10. Pressures higher than 8 mm Hg would be expected in less than 16% of normal subjects, and when present, suggest impaired right ventricular function. As radionuclide technology becomes more sophisticated,[64] non-invasive right ventricular function measurements should be increasingly useful.

—Oxygen transport to the tissues. Because a main function of the circulation is to transport oxygen, impaired transport indicates impaired function. Oxygen transport depends on oxygen demand, arterial O_2 tension, blood hemoglobin concentrations, cardiac output and its distribution, and the ability of the tissues to extract oxygen from the blood. In the supine resting subject, the net result of all these factors for the body as a whole is the mixed venous oxygen saturation or oxygen tension. For example, the normal resting mixed venous oxygen saturations are shown in Table 10. A value less than 70% indicates that the transport of oxygen via the arteries is less than normal (as a result, e.g., of low cardiac output, hypoxemia, or anemia). Consequently, the tissue demand for oxygen must be met by extraction of oxygen to a lower than normal saturation from blood passing through the capillaries, resulting in reduced venous oxygenation. For the altitude of Denver (1,600 m) and for aged subjects, normal mixed venous saturations tend to be less. Oxygen transport can also be judged by the arteriovenous oxygen difference, the normal value of which is similar at Denver and sea level, but is higher for old men (Table 10).

In assessing the patient, one must be aware that the oxygen transport

TABLE 10
Normal Values of Mean Right Atrial Pressure (P_{RA}), Mixed Venous Oxygen Saturation (SvO_2 and Arterio Venous Oxygen Differences (A-VO_2)

City	P_{RA} (mm Hg)	SO_{O_2} (%)	A-VO_2 ml O_2/L blood
	Young adults, 14–44 yrs., both sexes		
Bern (45)	4.9 ± 1.9 (42)	78.1 ± 3.9 (45)	39.0 ± 5.8 (45)
Denver (46) (1600M)	—	73.1 ± 3.5 (20)	39.8 ± 5.8 (63)
	Healthy men 60–82 years		
Stockholm (10)	6.0 ± 1.6 (9)	72.7 ± 3.0 (19)	44.9 ± 5.5 (19)

Shown are mean ± one standard deviation and in parenthesis, the number of subjects measured.

is altered differently by different etiologies of pulmonary hypertension. For example, in chronic obstructive lung disease, cardiac index, a key factor in oxygen transport, may be rather well maintained in spite of severe pulmonary hypertension (Figure 6). Possibly hypoxemia, hypervolemia, or sympathetic stimulation from hypercapnia, contribute to maintenance of cardiac index. In advanced primary pulmonary hypertension where such factors are not present, cardiac output may be more severely depressed.

• Is vascular reactivity present? Occasionally the physician wishes to know whether lung vessels show excessive vasoconstriction. For example, some persons, particularly children, who develop pulmonary hypertension while residing at high altitude, show exaggerated responses to acute challenges with hypoxic gas mixtures at low altitude.[53] The normal stimulus response curve in man near sea level Figure 7 shows a marked variability, a characteristic of the pulmonary circulation. Some subjects fail to respond and others increase their resistance 6-fold. On the average when the PO_2 is reduced from 100 to 50 mm Hg, the pulmonary vascular resistance doubles.

More commonly one gives an agent to lower an increased pulmo-

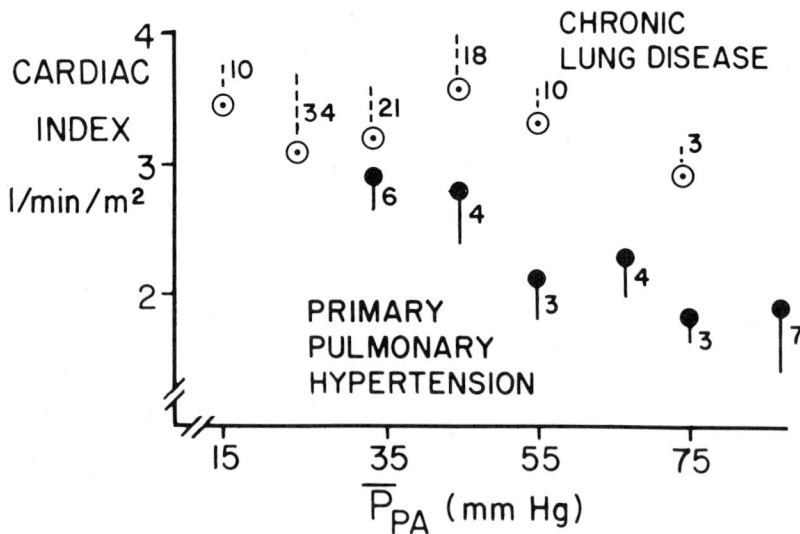

Figure 6. Cardiac index with increasing mean pulmonary arterial pressure in patients with chronic lung disease (open circles)[47–49,51,52] and patients with primary pulmonary hypertension (filled circles)[38,50,56,57] (B. Groves unpublished.) For a given level of pulmonary hypertension, flow tends to be better maintained in the patients with lung disease. Shown are mean values and 1 SEM.

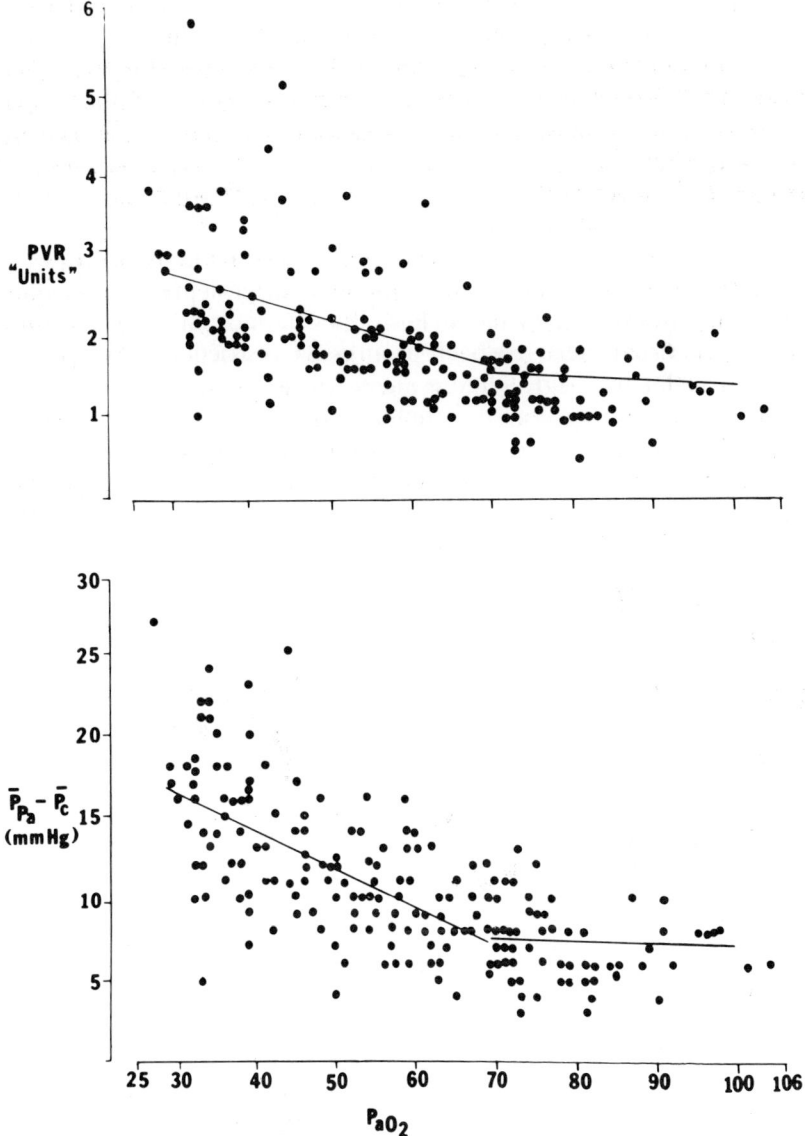

Figure 7. Measurements in 50 patients with normal pulmonary arterial pressures showing the relation of pulmonary vascular resistance (PVR, top) and pulmonary vascular pressure gradient ($\bar{P}_{pa}$, $\bar{P}_c$, bottom) to the arterial oxygen tension (PaO_2) in mm Hg. The patients were undergoing catheterization for coronary artery disease and each had measurement of pressures and flows while breathing air and 3 hypoxic gas mixtures. (FS Daoud and JT Reeves, unpublished.)

nary vascular resistance. If we assume the pulmonary arterial and wedge pressure measurements are each reliable to within ± 5% and the flow to within ± 10%, then we can consider a change in resistance (P/F) to be significant when the change exceeds ± 20%. A fall in resistance is clearly present when there has been a fall in pressure gradient from artery to vein concomitant with a rise in flow. A rise in resistance is clearly present when there has been a rise in pressure gradient concomitant with a fall in flow.

But the problem is often not so simple. When patients having serial catheterizations show a constant pulmonary arterial pressure gradient and a fall in pulmonary blood flow, does the calculated rise in resistance mean that there has been progressive restriction of the pulmonary vascular bed? Or, when patients, given pulmonary vasodilator drugs, show an unchanged pulmonary pressure gradient and a rise in flow, does the calculated fall in resistance indicate some relief of the vascular obstruction? In the normal lung, pressure gradient increases approximately directly with an exercise induced increase in flow (see

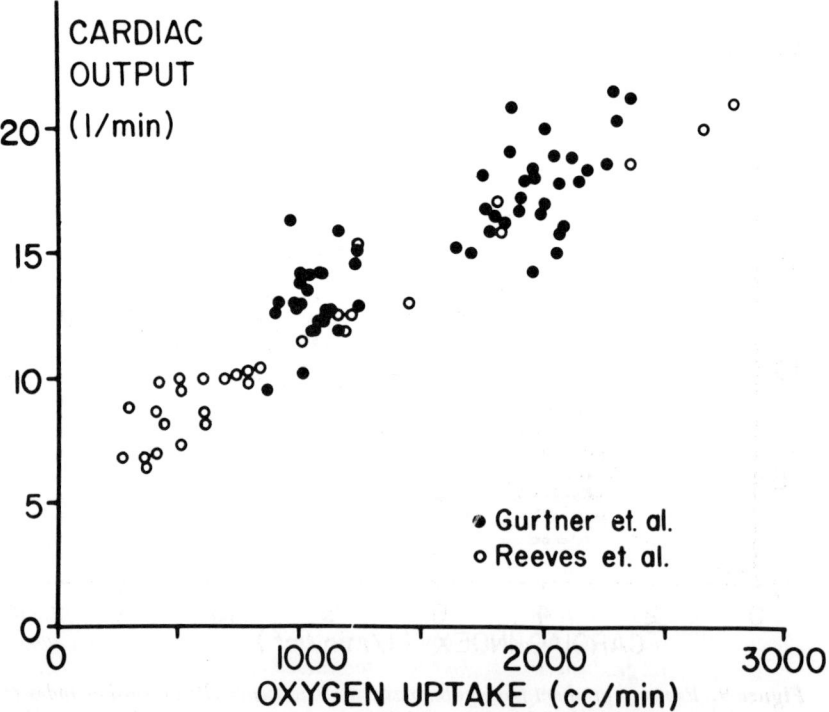

Figure 8. Measurements of cardiac output and oxygen uptake in normal subjects during supine exercise.[45,46]

exercise data, Figure 9, below). From these considerations we think that in the absence of a change of diameter of existing channels, increase in flow must be accompanied by some increase in pressure and the magnitude of the increase will be limited by the recruitment of new channels. In the pulmonary hypertensive lung, an exercise induced increase in flow causes a greater than normal increase in pressure (see exercise data, Figure 10, below). Our present view is that when flow increases, for example, in the absence of a change in pressure gradient, that the calculated fall in pulmonary vascular resistance is consistent with a decrease in the degree of pulmonary vascular obstruction.

The basis for this view is as follows: flow can increase at a constant pressure gradient within the lung vessel system only when there has been a net increase in diameter of existing channels and/or recruitment of new channels. Microvascular recruitment of additional channels in the lung appears to depend on an increased intravascular pressure, not on flow, per se.[54,58] Thus, we consider that an increase in flow with no net change in pressure is most consistent with a net increase in vascular diameter, and hence a decrease in tone in some vascular segment(s).

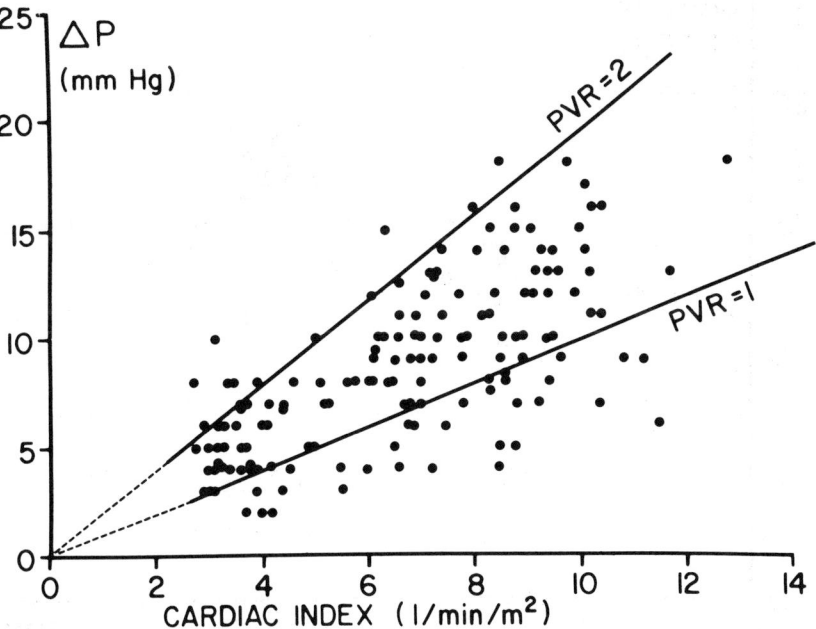

Figure 9. Pressure gradient from pulmonary artery to wedge (P) vs. cardiac index at rest and during exercise in 150 measurements in healthy male and female subjects.[45,55] Most of the data shown lie between isopleths of constant pulmonary vascular resistance having the values of 1 and 2 units.

Exercise Testing during Cardiac Catheterization

Exercise is useful in assessing the limitation of oxygen transport present in patients with pulmonary hypertension. At present this is done largely in the catheterization laboratory. Standards have been developed for normal subjects during supine bicycle exercise, Figure 8,

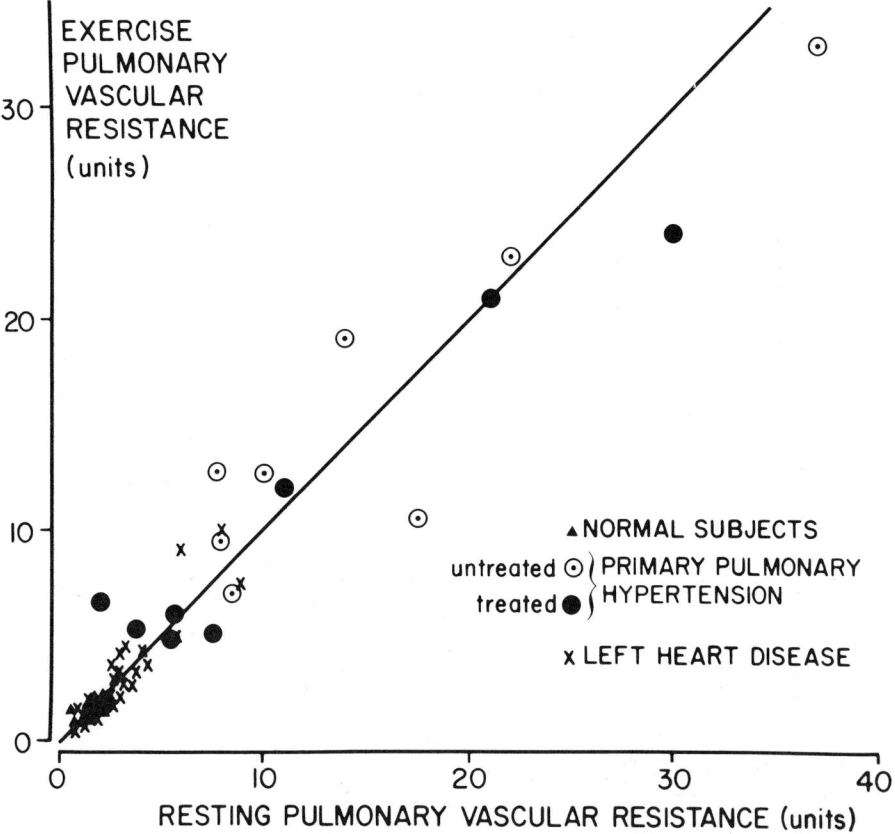

Figure 10a. A comparison of pulmonary vascular resistance measured at rest vs. that during exercise in normal subjects and subjects with various forms of pulmonary hypertension. Normal subjects[55] and patients with primary pulmonary hypertension[50] and with pulmonary hypertension from left heart disease[59,60] tend not to alter pulmonary vascular resistance with exercise, 10a , top. That is, the points fall around the line of identity. Patients with chronic lung disease[47,48] have exercise measurements which lie above the line of identity as seen in 10b, opposite. In them the pulmonary vascular resistance increases with exercise.

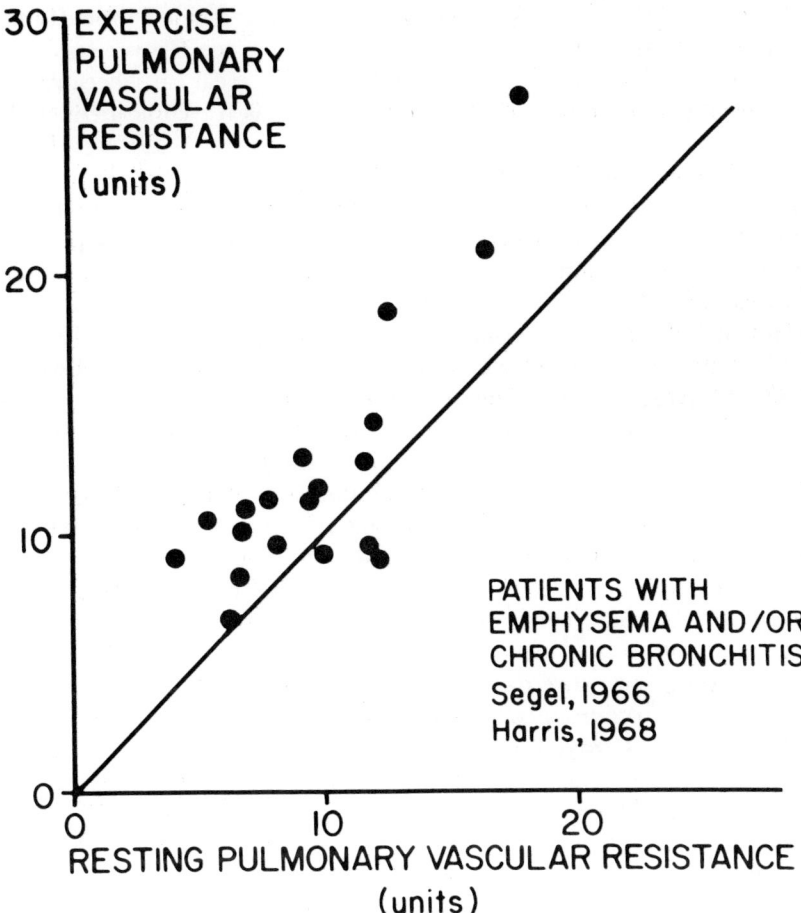

Figure 10b.

where for a given oxygen uptake one can determine whether or not the cardiac output is appropriate. If the output falls below the normal value, then, one may consider that some impairment of flow exists, and pulmonary hypertension is one cause of such impairment.

The normal lung circulation may[59] or may not[47,54,55] show a change in resistance during brief supine exercise, as measured during cardiac catheterization. Measurements relating the pressure gradient (from pulmonary artery to wedge) to the flow, Figure 9, lie along an isopleth of constant resistance. Thus, calculated pulmonary vascular resistance at rest and that during exercise are approximately equivalent for a wide range of exercise intensities (highly trained athletes and healthy, but aged, men constitute special cases; see Grover et al.).[54] Upright exercise (bicycle or treadmill) requires great care, because of the greater risk of systemic hypotension, and is for clinical research only.

In normal subjects, in patients with primary pulmonary hypertension and in pulmonary hypertension secondary to left heart disease, (miral stenosis, aortic insufficiency, left ventricular failure) the pulmonary vascular resistance at rest predicts that during exercise, rather well (Figure 10a). In judging the results of vasodilator therapy in primary pulmonary hypertension, i.e., those patients of Lupi-Herra[50] and Rubin[57] who showed a benefit of vasodilators at rest also showed a benefit during exercise. Patients failing to show a benefit at rest failed also to show a benefit during exercise. Ruskin and Hutter,[62] however, report one patient with primary pulmonary hypertension in whom exercise caused a large increase in pulmonary vascular resistance compared to the resting state. In pulmonary hypertension secondary to chronic lung disease, the exercise pulmonary vascular resistance usually is greater than the resting resistance (Figure 10b). Presumably there is vasoconstriction in part triggered by increased alveolar hypoxia.

The wedge pressure during exercise was not increased in patients with primary pulmonary hypertension, but is modestly increased in normal subjects, moderately increased in those with chronic lung disease and, of course, shows a marked increase in subjects with left heart failure (Table 11). If pulmonary vascular resistance is not much altered by exercise in left heart failure, but the left atrial pressure increases markedly, then the major reasons for performing an exercise test in patients with pulmonary hypertension from left heart failure appear to be to assess left heart function and its effect on pulmonary venous pressure.

Exercise tests require additional time in the catheter laboratory, additional patient discomfort, and are associated therefore with some additional risks. Simply seeing how high the pulmonary arterial pressure goes with exercise provides little clinical information and is not an adequate reason for doing the test. Whether or not the exercise test during catheterization provides a meaningful measure of the patient's exercise capacity remains to be tested. Thus, it behooves each clinician to balance the information to be derived by exercise against the risks involved.

TABLE 11
Mean ± One standard Deviation for Pulmonary Arterial Pressure Ppa (mm Hg), Wedge Pressure Pw (mm Hg), and Cardiac Index CI (L/min × m²) at Rest and During Exercise in Various Conditions

	n	Rest			Exercise		
		P_{PA}	P_W	CI	P_{PA}	P_W	CI
Normals (55)	36	15 ± 2	9 ± 3	4.7 ± .9	23 ± 4*	12 ± 5*	8.3 ± 1.6*
Chronic lung disease (47,48)	19	44 ± 10	12 ± 4	3.4 ± .6	74 ± 8*	18 ± 6*	4.9 ± 1.1*
Primary pulmonary hypertension (50)	9	50 ± 22	10 ± 2	3.2 ± .9	78 ± 25*	11 ± 2	5.1 ± 1.8*
Hydralazine		51 ± 30	10 ± 2	5.2 ± 1.7	69 ± 27*	10 ± 2	7.5 ± 2.4*
Left heart failure (60,61) Before hydralazine	14	33 ± 10	22 ± 9	3.4 ± 8†	48 ± 9*	34 ± 6*	4.7 ± 1.4*†
Hydralazine		31 ± 10	21 ± 9	5.0 ± 1.4†	50 ± 9*	33 ± 6*	6.0 ± 1.8*†

Asterisk (*) indicates that exercise value exceeds that at rest. Plus (†) indicates cardiac output.

INVASIVE ASSESSMENT: LUNG BIOPSY

Open lung biopsy is being employed with increasing frequency to assist in the diagnosis of pulmonary parenchymal disease (see Chapter 7), in pulmonary vascular disease in children with congenital heart disease (Chapter 3), and in primary pulmonary hypertension (Chapter 4). The use of the lung biopsy to establish type and severity of the pulmonary vascular disease is discussed in detail in Chapter 11.

CHRONIC TREATMENT OF PULMONARY HYPERTENSION

Subsequent chapters will discuss treatments available to control primary and secondary causes of pulmonary hypertension. When the therapeutic approach includes an effort to reverse the pulmonary hypertension, the question arises as to how to proceed.

Reversibility

A decision to attempt to reverse the pulmonary hypertension should be based on knowledge that there is a reversible component. That knowledge may arise simply from an understanding of the disease process. For example, in life threatening high altitude pulmonary hypertension, hypoxic pulmonary vasoconstriction is the likely basis of the hypertension, and increasing the ambient oxygen, either by moving the patient to low altitude or giving oxygen, is the appropriate therapy. Also, relief of mitral stenosis will ameliorate (but not abolish) long-standing pulmonary hypertension; and closure of an intracardiac defect with consequent elimination of a large left-to-right shunt will lower pulmonary arterial pressure and flow. Administration of heparin, thrombolytic agents, pulmonary vasodilators, or if necessary, surgical clot removal in acute massive pulmonary embolism provides another example of therapy directed at an obviously reversible cause of pulmonary hypertension.

However, it is often not obvious that the pulmonary hypertension has a reversible component, and the physician wishing to reverse the pulmonary hypertension has three options:

- As discussed above, he may seek evidence of reversibility by administering vasodilators acutely or sub-acutely and measuring the hemodynamic response at cardiac catheterization.
- He may obtain both a histological diagnosis and an assessment by the morphologist of reversibility by having a lung biopsy performed and by having it examined by an expert in vascular pathology (see Chapter 11).
- He may administer a particular therapeutic agent without recourse to the information obtained in either of the above options.

In listing the third option, we are acknowledging our areas of ignorance. For example, it is not known how the pulmonary hemodynamic response to acutely administered vasodilators relates to the chronic response. Also, the experience with lung biopsies in pulmonary hypertension is relatively recent, is limited to a few centers around the world, and interpretation of biopsy material is not a matter of universal agreement. Finally, the clinical evaluation of therapies is itself new.

The third option carries considerable risk for the patient because the spectrum of pulmonary hypertensive disorders includes those with fixed, or irreversible pulmonary hypertension. As discussed in *Noninvasive Assessment*, above, this group includes persons with established Eisenmenger's syndrome, long-standing recurrent pulmonary emboli, and some patients with primary pulmonary hypertension in whom administration of vasodilator drugs may cause life threatening hypoxemia and systemic hypotension. Therefore, there should be either some evidence for potential reversibility, or it should be demonstrated that the drug does not cause significant systemic hypotension, before chronic vasodilator therapy is undertaken. Further, vasodilator therapy is largely experimental and it is urgent that experience gleaned from each patient be recorded with such care as to add to our medical knowledge.

Choice of Agent

The variety of therapeutic agents available, their advantages and disadvantages is given in Chapter 4, and additional considerations are given in Chapters 5 and 7. The pulmonary vasodilator selected may depend heavily on the clinical situation. For example, the surgical management of the post-operative patient following heart valve replacement may require treatment of pulmonary hypertension. Goenen et al.[58] reported in 12 patients, 24 hours after single or multiple valve replacement, nitroglycerine and nitroprusside were more effective in lowering pulmonary vascular resistance than were tolazoline, isoproterenol, or hydralazine. However, they recommended tolazoline and isoproterenol when systemic pressure and cardiac output were low.

SUMMARY

Pulmonary hypertension of some degree occurs in a large proportion of persons with disease of the heart and lungs. In many, the hypertension itself contributes to the morbidity and mortality. Yet, in intervening, to moderate that hypertension, the physician assumes a serious responsibility, because those patients are often fragile and can be easily harmed. The alternative is *no active intervention*, and this is the proper course in persons with irreversible pulmonary hypertension. However, many or even most persons with pulmonary hypertension have in their lung vessels a vasoconstrictive component which is potentially reversible. In these, careful diagnosis, therapy, and continuity of care are indicated. Therapy in pulmonary hypertension is recent and lags far behind the impressive strides made in the control of systemic hypertension. One reason for the lag is obvious. Clinical monitoring for systemic hypertension has been available since Riva-Rici introduced the blood pressure cuff in 1896. The study of the etiologies of the various forms of systemic hypertension, their natural histories, and responses to therapy have all been facilitated by a simple, accurate method for pressure monitoring. Clinical monitoring for pulmonary arterial pressure was not introduced until 1946, and now, as then, requires cardiac catheterization. The vast body of clinical experience on which treatment of systemic hypertension is based, is simply not available in pulmonary hypertension. The rapid accumulation of relevant clinical experience in pulmonary hypertensive disorders and the development of rational management will depend upon advances in: an accurate non-invasive method to monitor pulmonary hemodynamics; an understanding of mechanisms causing pulmonary arterial disease; and the development of new therapies based upon this understanding. We believe these advances will come.

REFERENCES

1. Arcilla RA, et al.: Pulmonary arterial pressures of newborn infants born with early and late clamping of the cord. *Acta Paediat Scand* 1966;55:305.
2. Adams FN, Lind J: Physiologic studies on the cardiovascular status of normal newborn infants (with special reference to the ductus arteriosus). *Pediatrics* 1957;19:431–437.
3. Brotmacher L, Fleming P: Cardiac output and vascular pressures in 10 normal children and adolescents. *Guy Hosp Rep* 1957;106:268–272.
4. Donald KW, et. al: The effect of exercise on the cardiac output and circulatory dynamics of normal subjects. *Clin Sci* 1955;14:37.
5. Doyle JT, Wilson JS, Warren JV: The pulmonary vascular responses to short term hypoxia in human subjects. *Circulation* 1952;5:263.
6. Immanovilides GC, Moss AJ, Duffie ER, Adams FH: Pulmonary arterial pressure changes in newborn infants from birth to 3 days of age. *J Pediatr* 1964;65:327–333.
7. Saling E: Neve untersuchungsergebnisse uber den kreislauf des kindes unmittlebar nach der geburt. *Arch fur Gynakologie* 1960;194:287–306.
8. Alexander JF, Hartley LH, Modelski M, Grover RF: Reduction in stroke volume during exercise in man following ascent to 3100 M altitude. *J Appl Physiol* 1967;23:849–858.
9. Sproul A, Simpson E: Stroke volume and related hemodynamic data in normal children. *Pediatrics* 1964;33:912–917.
10. Granath A, Strandell T: Relationships between cardiac output, stroke volume, and intracardiac pressures at rest and during exercise in supine position, and some anthropometric data in healthy old men. *Acta Med Scand* 1964;176:447.
11. Emergil C, Sobol BJ, Compodonico S, Herbert WH, Mechtaki R: Pulmonary circulation in the aged. *J Appl Physiol* 1967;23:631–640.
12. Daoud FS, Reeves JT:Unpublished.
13. Wood P: *Diseases of the Heart and Circulation.* 2nd ed. Philadelphia: J.P. Lippincott Co., 1956.
14. Zwillich C, Reeves JT: *Pulmonary Hypertension in Conn and Conn. Current Diagnosis.* 5., Philadelphia: W.B. Saunders Co., 1977:294–297.
15. Voelkel NF, Reeves JT: Primary pulmonary hypertension. In: Lenfant C, Moser K, eds. *Pulmonary Vascular Disease,* Vol. 141. New York: Marcel Dekker, 1979.
16. Levine S, Huckabee WE: Ventilatory response to drug-induced hypermetabolism. *J Appl Physiol* 1975;38:827–833.
17. Reeves JT, Noonan JA: Microarteriographic studies of primary pulmonary hypertension. *Arch Pathol* 1973;95:50–55.
18. Reeves JT, Tweedale D, Noonan J, Leathers JE, Quigley MB: Correlations of microradiographic and histological findings in the pulmonary vascular bed. *Circulation* 1966; 34:971–983.
19. Pryor R: The EKG diagnosis of right ventricular enlargement; emphasizing the rightward terminal vector. *Bull Denver Rheumatic Fever Diagnostic Service* 1963;4:9.

20. Pryor R: The diagnostic capabilities and limitations of the electrocardiogram. In: Silverman ME, Silverman BE, eds., *The Heart, Update 1*. New York: McGraw Hill, 1979:13–14.
21. Liebman J, Plonsey R, Gillette PC: *Pediatric Electrocardiography*. Baltimore: Williams and Wilkins, 1982.
22. Pryor R, Weaver WF, Blount SG Jr: Electrocardiographic observation of 493 residents living at high altitude. *Am J Cardiol* 1965;16:494–499.
23. Chen JTT, Behar US, Morris JJ, McIntosh HD, Lester RC: Correlation of roentgen findings with hemodynamic data in pure mitral stenosis. *Am J Roentgenol* 1968;102:280–292.
24. Change CH. The normal roentgenographic measurement of the right descending pulmonary artery in 1,085 cases. *Am J Roentgenol* 1962;87:929–935.
25. Viamonte M, Parks RE, Barrera F: Roentgenographic prediction of pulmonary hypertension in mitral stenosis. *Am J Roentgenol* 1962;87:936–947.
26. Chetty KG, Brown SE, Light RW: Identification of pulmonary hypertension in chronic obstructive pulmonary disease from routine chest radiographs. *Am Rev Resp Dis* 1982;126:388–341.
27. Kanemoto N, Furunya H, Etoh T, Sasamoto H, Matsuyama S: Chest roentgenograms in primary pulmonary hypertension. *Chest* 1979;76:45–49.
28. Lupi E, Dumont C, Tejada VM, Horwitz S, Galland F: A radiological index of pulmonary arterial hypertension. *Chest* 1975;68:28–31.
29. Chang S: *M-mode Echocardiography: Techniques and Interpretation*. Philadelphia: Lea and Febiger, 1981.
30. Acquatella H, Schiller NB, Sharke DN, Chatterjee K: Lack of correlation between echocardiographic pulmonary valve morphology and simultaneous pulmonary arterial pressure. *Am J Cardiol* 1979;43:946.
31. Linhart JW, Joyner CR: *Diagnostic Echocardiography*. St. Louis: C.V. Mosby Co., 1982.
32. Feigenbaum H: *Echocardiography*. Philadelphia:1976. Lea and Febiger.
33. Phillips BJ: *Manual of Echocardiographic Techniques*. Philadelphia: W.B. Saunders, 1980.
34. Goodman DJ, Harison DG, Popp RL: Echocardiographic features of primary pulmonary hypertension. *Am J Cardiol* 1974;23:438–443.
35. Hirschfeld S, Meyer R, Schwarts DC, Korfhagen J, Kaplan S: The echocardiographic assessment of pulmonary artery pressure and pulmonary vascular resistance. *Circulation* 1975;52:642–650.
36. Hatle L, Angelsen BAJ, Tromsdal A: Noninvasive estimation of pulmonary artery systolic pressure with Doppler ultrasound. *Br Heart J* 1981;45:157–165.
37. Burstin L: Determination of pressure in the pulmonary artery by external graphic recordings. *Br Heart J* 1967;29:396–404.
38. Rubin LJ, Groves BM, Reeves JT, Frosolono M, Handel F, Cato AE: Prostacyclin-induced acute pulmonary vasodilation in primary pulmonary hypertension. *Circulation* 1982;66:334–338.
39. Bhatacharia J, Staub NC: Direct measurements of microvascular pressures in the isolated perfused dog lung. *Science* 1980;210:327–328.

40. Dexter L: Pulmonary vascular disease in acquired heart disease. In: Lenfant C, Moser K, eds., *Pulmonary Vascular Disease*, Vol. 14. New York: Marcel Dekker, 1979.
41. West JB: *Respiratory Physiology*. Baltimore: Williams and Wilkins, 1979.
42. Mendel D: *A Practice of Cardiac Catheterization*. 2nd Ed. Oxford: Blackwell Scientific Publications, 1974:275–276.
43. van Grondell A, Ditchey R, Groves BM, Wagner WW Jr, Reeves JT: Thermodilution overestimates cardiac output in the low range. *AM J Physiol* (in press).
44. Hermiller JB, Bambach D, Thompson MJ, Huss P, Fontana ME, Magorien RD, Unverferth DV, Leir CV: Vasodilators and prostaglandin inhibitors in primary pulmonary hypertension. *Ann Int Med* 1982;97:480–489.
45. Gurtner HP, Walser P, Fassler B: Normal values for pulmonary hemodynamics at rest and during exercise in man. *Prog Resp Res* 1975;9:295–315.
46. Reeves JT, Grover RF, Gilley GF, Blount SG Jr: Circulatory changes in man during supine exercise. *J Appl Physiol* 1961;16:279–282.
47. Harris P, Segal N, Bishop JM: The relation between pressure and flow in the pulmonary circulation in normal subjects and in patients with chronic bronchitis and mitral stenosis. *Cardiovasc Res* 1968;2:73–83.
48. Segel N, Bishop JM. The circulation in patients with chronic bronchitis and emphysema at rest and during exercise with special reference to the influence of changes in blood viscosity and blood volume on the pulmonary circulation. *J Clin Invest* 1966;45:1555–1568.
49. Reeves JT, Grover RF: Unpublished data.
50. Lupi-Herra E, Sandoval J, Seoane M, Bialostozky D: The role of hydralazine therapy for pulmonary arterial hypertension of unknown cause. *Circulation* 1982;65:645–650.
51. Rubin LJ, Peter RH: Hemodynamics at rest and during exercise after oral hydralazine in patients with cor pulmonale. *Am J Cardiology* 1981;47:116–122.
52. Ferner MI, Harvey RM, Cathcart RT, Webster CA, Richards DW, Cournand A: Some effects of digoxin upon the heart and circulation in man. *Circulation* 1950;1:161–186.
53. Jones TK, Wiggins JW, Rolfe RR: Symptomatic pulmonary hypertension of high altitude. *Circ Res* 1982;66:48.
54. Grover RF, Wagner WW, McMurtry IF, Reeves JT: Control of the pulmonary circulation. In: *The Handbook of Physiology* (forthcoming).
55. Stanek V, Jebavy P, Horych J, Widimsky J: Central hemodynamics during supine exercise and pulmonary artery occlusion in normal subjects. *Bull Physio Path Resp* 1973;9:1203–1217.
56. Daoud FS, Reeves JT, Kelly DB: Isoproterenol as a potential pulmonary vasodilator in primary pulmonary hypertension. *AM J Cardiol* 1978;42:817–822.
57. Rubin LJ, Peter RH: Oral hydralazine therapy for primary pulmonary hypertension. *N Engl J Med* 1980;302:69–73.
58. Goenen MJ, Leenaert L, Petein M, Pouleur H, Jaumin P, Tremouroux J: The effects of tolazoline, nitroprusside, nitroglycerine, isoproterenol

and hydralazine on pulmonary circulation early after heart valve replacement. *Thor Cardiovasc Surg* 1982;30:253–258.
59. Holmgren A, Jonsson B, Sjostrand T: Circulatory data in normal subjects at rest and during exercise, in recumbent position, with special reference to the stroke volume at different work intensities. *Acta Scand* 1960;49:343–363.
60. Rubin SA, Chatterjee K, Ports TA, Gelberg HJ, Brundage BH, Parmley WW: Influence of short-term oral hydralazine on exercise hemodynamics in patients with severe chronic heart failure. *Am J Cardiol* 1979;44:1183–1189.
61. Greenberg BH, DeMots H, Murphy E, Rahimtoola S: Beneficial effects of hydralazine on rest and exercise hemodynamics in patients with chronic severe aortic insufficiency. *Circulation* 1980;62:49–55.
62. Ruskin JN, Hutter AM: Primary pulmonary hypertension treated with oral phentolamine. *Ann Int Med* 1979;90:772–774.
63. Goodman DJ, Harrison DC, Popp RL: Echocardiographic features of primary pulmonary hypertension. *Am J Cardiol* 1974;33:438–443.
64. Morrison D, Marshall J, Wright AL, Daly M, Henry R: An improved method of right ventricular gated equilibrium blood pool radionuclide ventriculography. *Chest* 1982;82:607–614.

CHAPTER 2

PERSISTENT PULMONARY HYPERTENSION SYNDROMES IN THE NEWBORN

Michael A. Heymann and Julien I.E. Hoffman

INTRODUCTION

The clinical syndrome of persistent pulmonary hypertension in the immediate newborn period, also called persistent fetal circulation syndrome, is characterized by failure of certain parts of the fetal circulation to undergo the normal transition to the postnatal state. It presents shortly after birth with cyanosis and respiratory distress, often severe, in infants who have no evidence of underlying organic disease. The primary abnormality is maintenance of the high pulmonary vascular resistance, normally found in the fetus, with the consequent reduction in pulmonary blood flow and persistence of right-to-left shunting through the ductus arteriosus or foramen ovale, or both. Many factors are responsible for physiologic and physical control of pulmonary vascular resistance and its normal fall after birth; it is likely therefore that the syndrome is caused by alterations in, or failure of, several mechanisms acting in concert rather than a single cause. The resultant syndrome, which generally occurs in otherwise normal full-term infants, leads to severe cardiorespiratory distress regardless of the etiology.

THE FETAL AND NEONATAL CIRCULATIONS

In the fetus gas exchange occurs in the placenta and pulmonary blood flow therefore is very low, supplying only some of the nutritional needs for lung growth and perhaps, as in the adult, subserving some metabolic function. Pulmonary blood flow in near term fetal lambs is only about 35–50 ml/100 g lung tissue, representing about 8–10% of the total (combined left and right ventricular) output of the heart (Figure 1).[1,3] This occurs despite the dominance of the right ventricle which in the fetus ejects about two-thirds of the total cardiac output of 450–500 ml/kg/min.[3] Most of this flow is diverted away from the lungs, through the widely patent ductus arteriosus, to the descending aorta from which the major proportion reaches the placenta for oxygenation. In the younger fetus (at about 0.5 of gestation) only about 3–5% of total cardiac output passes through the lungs. There is a sharp increase at about 0.8 gestation, corresponding temporally with the onset of release of surface active material into lung fluid, and a progressive slow rise thereafter to about 8–10% at term.[2] Pulmonary arterial pressures increase progressively with advancing gestation (Figure 2); at term mean pulmonary arterial pressure is about 50 mm Hg[4] and generally exceeds mean aortic pressure by about 1–2 mm Hg.[5] Pulmonary vascular resistance, relative to the infant or adult, is extremely high early in gestation and falls progressively over the last half of gestation (Figure 2),[6] due most likely to new vessel growth and increase in cross-sectional area.[7]

After birth and the initiation of ventilation, pulmonary vascular resistance falls rapidly, associated with an 8–10-fold increase in pulmonary blood flow. In normal lambs pulmonary arterial pressure falls to near adult levels within 1–2 hours; in the human this takes considerably longer and by 24 hours of age mean pulmonary arterial pressure may only be half the systemic pressure.[8] After the initial rapid fall in pulmonary vascular resistance and pulmonary arterial pressure there is a slow progressive fall, with adult levels reached within 2–6 weeks depending on species.[9,10]

NORMAL MORPHOLOGIC DEVELOPMENT OF THE PULMONARY VASCULATURE

In the fetus and newborn, small pulmonary arteries of all sizes have a thicker muscular wall related to external diameter than do similar arteries in an adult. It is thought that this greater muscularity is at least in part responsible for the vasoreactivity and for the high pulmonary vascular resistance found in the fetus. In fetal lamb lungs that are

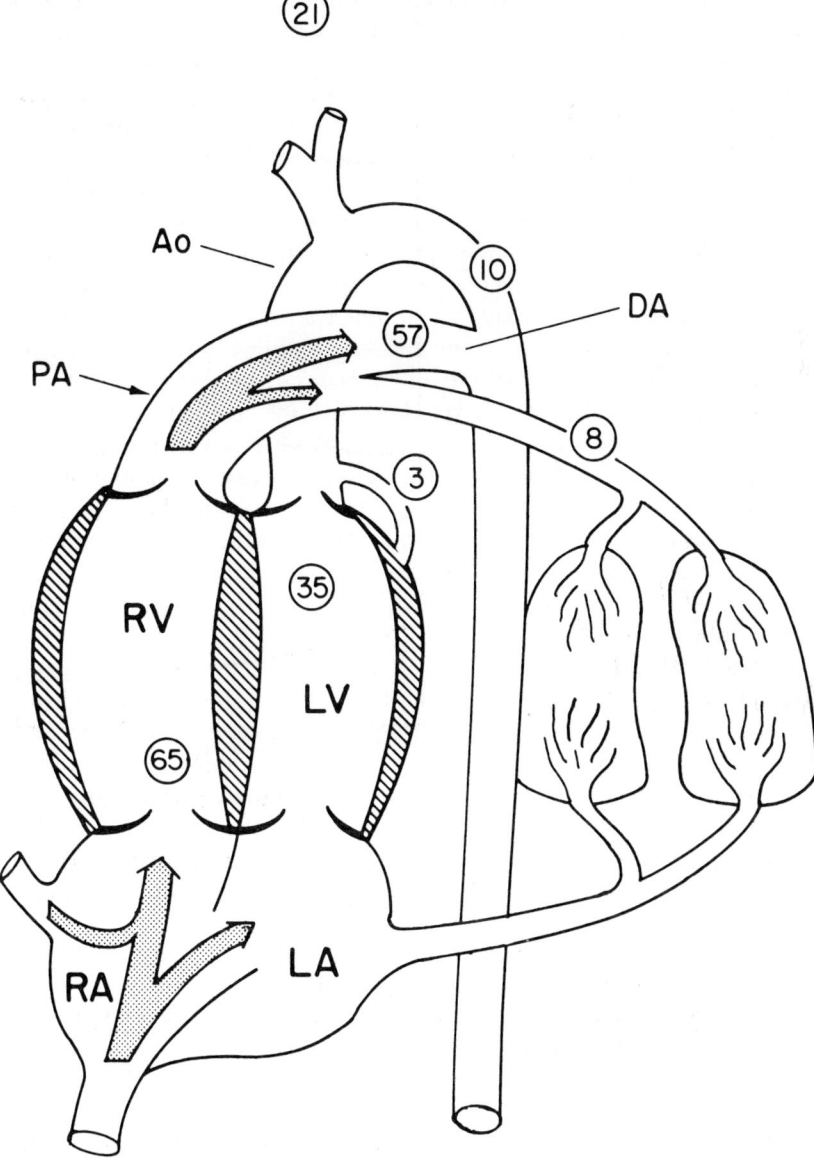

Figure 1. Percentages of combined left and right ventricular outputs ejected by the heart and distributed to major vascular channels in the fetus. Ao = ascending aorta; DA = ductus arteriosus; PA = main pulmonary artery; RV = right ventricle; LV = left ventricle; RA = right atrium; LA = left atrium.

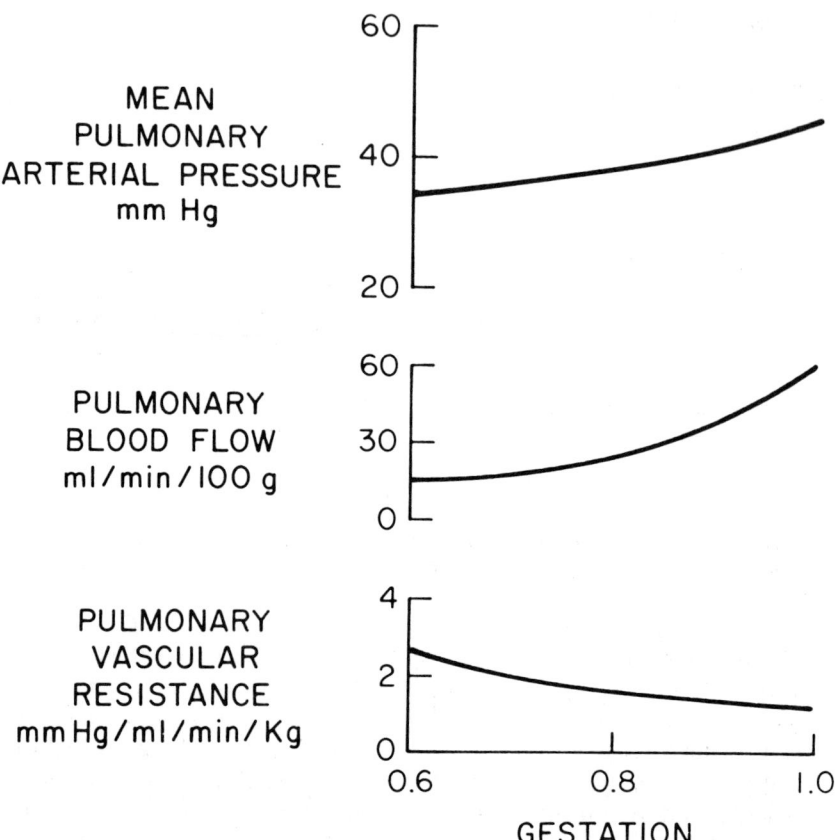

Figure 2. Changes with advancing gestation of pulmonary arterial pressure, pulmonary blood flow, and calculated pulmonary vascular resistance in fetal lambs.

perfusion fixed at pressures similar to those found normally, the medial smooth muscle coat was most prominent in the smallest arteries (fifth and sixth generation arteries; external diameter 20 to 50 μ) and over about the latter half of gestation the muscle thickness remained constant in relationship to external diameter of the artery (Figure 3).[7] Similar observations have been made in human lungs.[11,12]

After birth, particularly within the first 7–10 days, there is a rapid progressive reduction in wall thickness with thinning of muscle and an increase in external diameter.[13–16] More recent studies suggest that at about 15 days there is a short-lived increase in wall thickness followed again by a regression and an increase in external diameter so that by 4–6 weeks the adult medial thickness/external diameter pattern is established.[17]

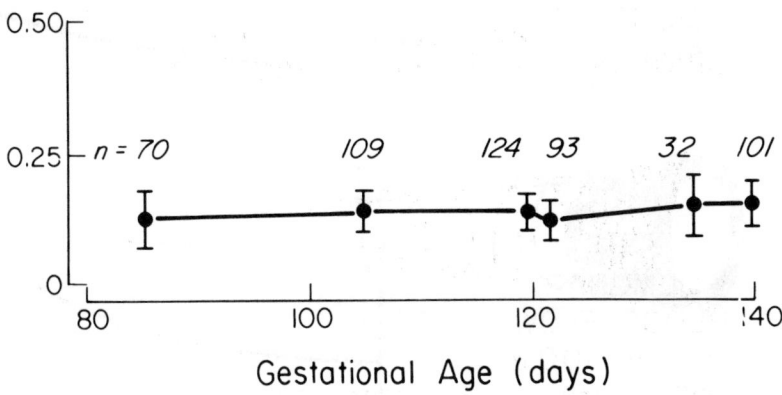

Figure 3. Mean (± SD) values for medial width/external diameter ratio for fifth generation vessels from 6 fetuses. N = number of fifth generation vessels evaluated. (Reproduced with permission of the American Heart Association, Inc.[7])

In any given artery traced peripherally, a level is reached where the completely encircling smooth muscle coat gives way to a region of incomplete muscularization (Figure 4); in these partially muscularized arteries the muscle is arranged in a spiral or helix. The muscle then disappears from the arteries that are still larger than capillaries (non-muscularized arteries).[11] In the non-muscular arteries an incomplete pericyte layer is found within the endothelial basement membrane. In the non-muscular portions of the partially muscular arteries, intermediate cells, i.e., cells intermediate in position and structure between pericytes and mature smooth muscle cells, are found.[18] These cells are precursor smooth muscle cells and under certain conditions, such as hypoxia, they rapidly differentiate into mature smooth muscle cells.[19]

Arteries can be conveniently identified by their relationship to the airways (Figure 4). Preacinar arteries are those proximal to or with the terminal bronchiolus and intra-acinar arteries are those with respiratory bronchioli, alveolar ducts and within the alveolar walls. In the near term fetus, only about half the arteries running with respiratory bronchioli (precapillary) are muscularized or partially muscularized and the alveoli are free of muscular arteries.[12]

During fetal growth in lambs there is a large increase in the number of small arteries, not only in absolute terms but also per unit volume of lung.[7] Halfway through gestation there are about 7,000 arteries per ml of lung; at term this has increased almost tenfold (Figure 5).[7]

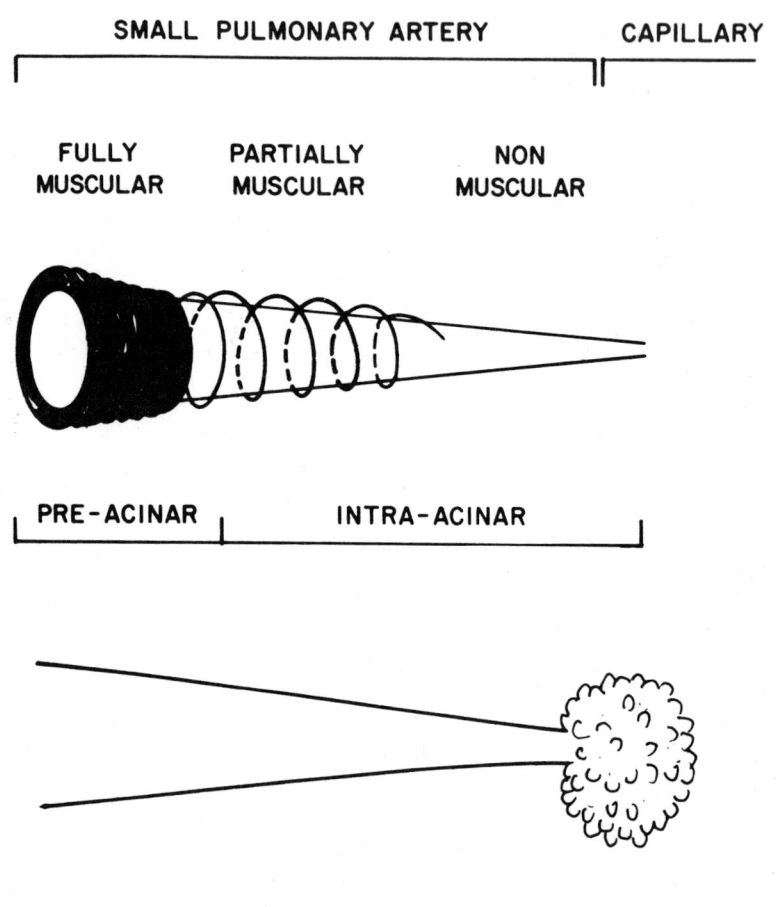

Figure 4. Diagrammatic representation of medial smooth muscle development in the small pulmonary arteries of a normal fetus; vessel relationship to an airway is shown (redrawn after Reid and associates [11,12,14,15,17,20]).

The main preacinar pulmonary arterial branches that accompany the larger airways are developed by 16 weeks gestation in the human[12]; however, the intra-acinar circulation follows more closely alveolar development which occurs late in gestation and perhaps even mainly after birth.[17,20] As alveoli multiply so do arteries, a process generally complete by ten years of age.[14,15]

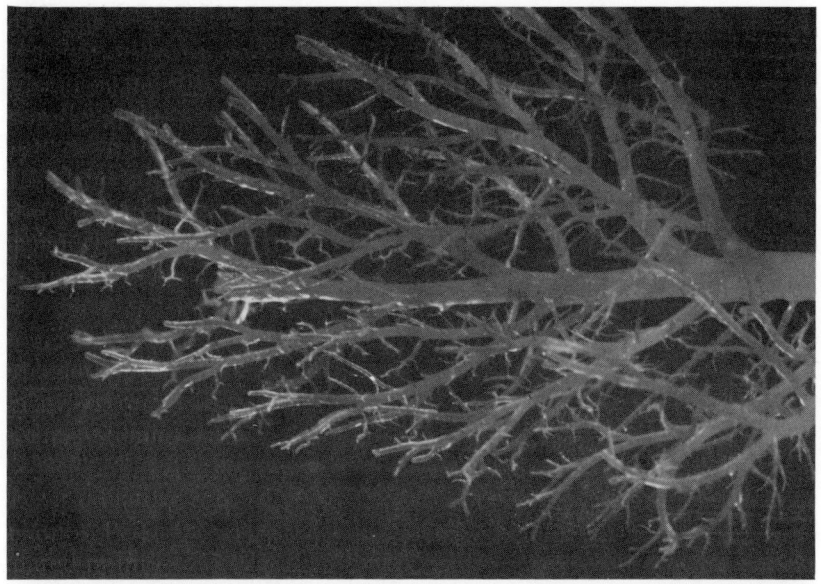

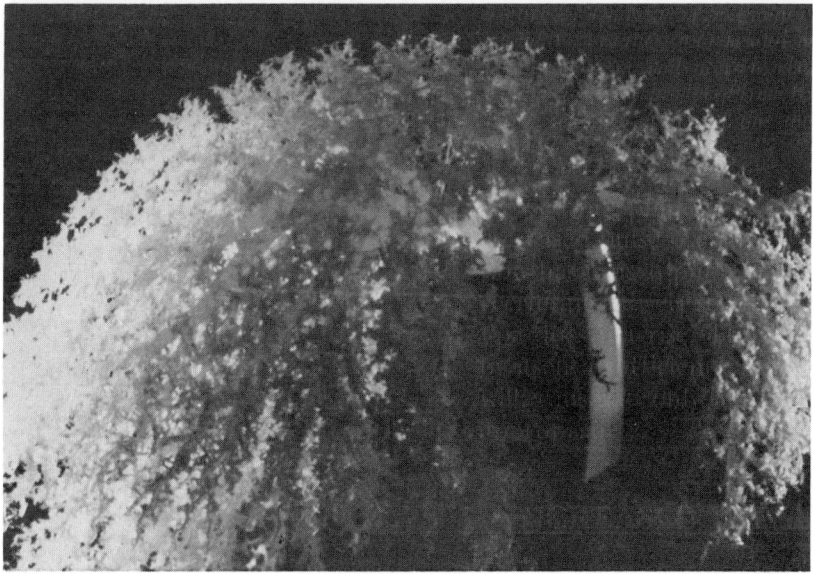

Figure 5. Methylmethacrylate pulmonary arterial casts from (a) a 105-day (0.65) fetal lamb and (b) a 140-day (0.95) fetal lamb. Vessels as small as 20 u are filled. The cast of the 105-day fetus measures 4.5 cm and the cast of the 140-day fetus measures 8.0 cm at their maximum lengths. (Reproduced with permission of the American Heart Association, Inc.[7])

PHYSICS OF FLOW THROUGH THE PULMONARY CIRCULATION IN THE FETUS AND NEWBORN

As outlined in the second and fourth sections of Chapter 3, blood flow through the pulmonary circulation is defined in general terms by the hydraulic equivalent of Ohm's law and by the Poiseuille-Hagen relationship.[21] By applying these relationships, bearing in mind the caveats outlined in Chapter 3, it is apparent that pulmonary vascular resistance is directly related to the viscosity of blood perfusing the lungs and inversely related to the cross-sectional area of the pulmonary vascular bed (radius^4). Increasing viscosity or decreasing vessel radius therefore leads to an elevation of pulmonary vascular resistance. A change in luminal radius is the major factor responsible for maintaining a high pulmonary vascular resistance in the fetus.

By further rearrangement of the Poiseuille equation, pulmonary arterial pressure has the same relationships as resistance to viscosity and cross-sectional area (or radius) and also has a direct relationship to pulmonary venous pressure. Consideration of these factors, particularly viscosity and cross-sectional area of the vascular bed, is important in evaluating the pathophysiology of persistent pulmonary hypertension syndrome in the newborn infant.

FACTORS AFFECTING PULMONARY VASCULAR RESISTANCE IN THE NORMAL FETUS

As described above, in the fetus, the small pulmonary arteries, the resistance vessels, have a thick medial muscular layer and therefore probably vasoconstrict more actively than in the adult. In the fetus, several factors may be responsible for this very active vasoconstriction.

Autonomic Nervous System

In acute studies in exteriorized fetal lambs, bilateral cervical or thoracic sympathectomy had no significant effect on pulmonary vascular resistance.[22] These studies suggested that sympathetic tone likely played little or no role in maintenance of normal resting pulmonary vascular tone. Similarly, in the same study bilateral cervical vagotomy did not affect pulmonary vascular resistance and the parasympathetic nervous system was believed to play no role in maintenance of normal pulmonary vascular tone. Later studies in chronically prepared mature fetal lambs used selective pharmacologic blockade rather than nerve section to study the role of the autonomic nervous system. Alpha-adrenergic blockade with phentolamine and parasympathetic blockade with atropine did not alter resting pulmonary vascular tone.[23] In addition, alpha- and beta-adrenergic and parasympathetic blockade had no effect on the vasoconstrictor response to hypoxemia in mature fetal lambs,[4] thus suggesting that, at least during hypoxemic stress in the fetus, pulmonary vascular changes are not mediated directly by these autonomic nervous pathways. Similar observations have been made in newborn calves with alpha-adrenergic blockade[24]; however, in young lambs beta-adrenergic blockade accentuates hypoxic pulmonary vasoconstriction.[25]

On the other hand, electrical stimulation of the distal end of the cut vagus nerve or the peripheral end of the cut thoracic sympathetic chain in fetal lambs produced pulmonary vasodilatation or vasoconstriction respectively.[22] Pharmacologic receptor stimulation also has a significant effect on vasomotor tone. In perfused fetal lamb lungs or in acute preparations in fetal lambs, acetylcholine produces vasodilatation.[26-28] In intact fetal lambs studied chronically in utero, acetylcholine infused into the pulmonary circulation produced significant vasodilatation close to term but had little or no effect on immature lambs.[4] After ventilation of the lungs the dramatic pulmonary vasodilatation produced by acetylcholine in the fetus was no longer observed.[29] Alpha-adrenergic stimulation by methoxamine[26,27,30] increases pulmonary vascular resistance; and beta-adrenergic stimulation by isoproterenol[27,31] reduces pulmonary vascular resistance.

It appears, therefore, that the autonomic nervous system plays little or no role in normal resting control of the fetal pulmonary vascular resistance, but that when stimulated could alter pulmonary vascular resistance. The increased pulmonary vasomotor tone found in the fetus accentuates the responses to these stimuli. Whether or not these mechanisms are invoked during fetal stress or are involved in perinatal changes is not clear.

Oxygen

Under normal resting conditions in the fetal lamb femoral arterial blood PO_2 is about 22–24 torr and pulmonary arterial blood PO_2 is about 17–20 torr. Since reduction of PO_2 to almost the same levels in newborn animals produces a marked increase in pulmonary vascular resistance,[32–34] it is most likely that the low PO_2 found normally in the fetus is responsible for the pulmonary vasoconstriction. Further reducing fetal PO_2 by inducing maternal hypoxemia [4,35] produces a significant increase in pulmonary vascular resistance (Figure 6) as evidenced either by an increase in pulmonary arterial pressure or fall in pulmonary blood flow.

The mechanisms responsible for the hypoxic vasoconstriction are not clearly established. Both reflex-mediated chemoreceptor stimulation and direct local effects have been considered. Since hypoxia in fetal lambs resulted in significant adrenal secretion of catecholamines,[36] it was considered that norepinephrine may be responsible for the hypoxic pulmonary vasoconstriction. In exteriorized immature fetal lambs bilateral adrenalectomy did not alter the pulmonary vasoconstriction produced by umbilical cord constriction, suggesting that catecholamine release was not involved[27]; however, alpha-adrenergic blockade prevented the pulmonary vasoconstriction induced by asphyxia. Asphyxia-induced pulmonary vasoconstriction, therefore, could have been due either to an extra-adrenal release of catecholamines or to their local release at sympathetic nervous endings. Alternatively, the effects of alpha-adrenergic blockade could have been non-specific. When asphyxia was induced in lamb fetuses in which one lung was perfused either from a reservoir or from a donor twin fetus, pulmonary vasoconstriction developed which was abolished by cutting the sympathetic nerve to the lung. This occurred in mature but not in immature lambs, thereby suggesting that the role of the sympathetic nervous system in producing hypoxic pulmonary vasoconstriction was related to fetal gestation age.[37,38] In more physiologic conditions in chronically instrumented lambs in utero,[4] the fetal pulmonary vasoconstriction produced by maternal hypoxia was not prevented by pharmacologic blockade of alpha- or beta-adrenergic or cholinergic receptor function. Silove and Grover[24] also concluded that the sympathetic nervous system did not contribute to hypoxic vasoconstriction, since pre-treatment of neonatal calves with reserpine did not affect the pulmonary vascular response to hypoxia.

There is strong evidence to indicate that the pulmonary vascular responses to hypoxia are due to direct local effects. In several studies, where one fetal lung was either ventilated to perfused independently in situ without changing the O_2 environment of the other lung, O_2 related vascular changes could be produced in that lung only. These studies thereby showed that resistance changes in the isolated lung were locally mediated.[37–39]

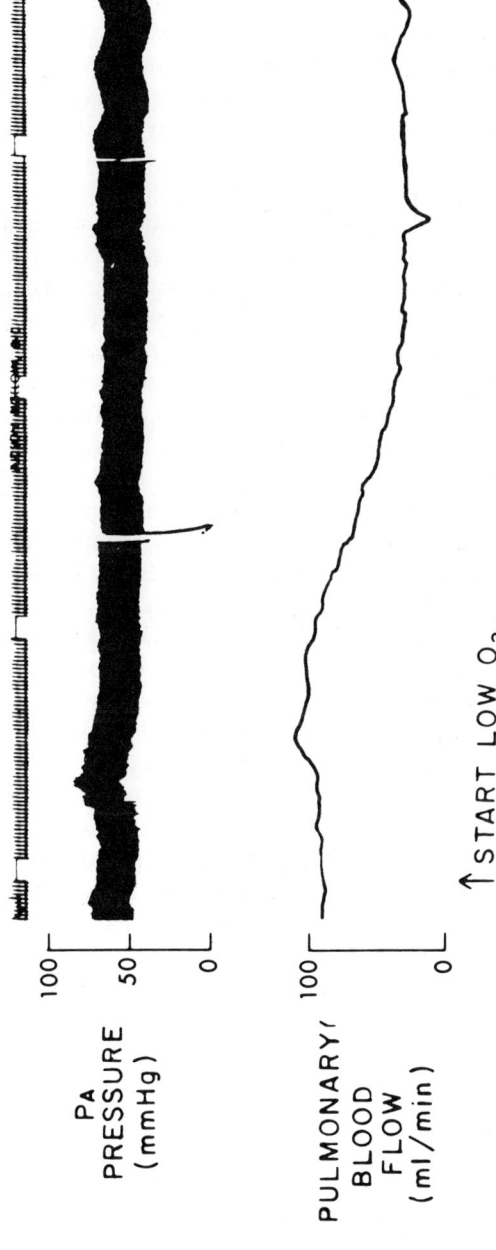

Figure 6. Effects of reducing maternal inspired oxygen concentration on phasic pulmonary arterial (PA) blood pressure and pulmonary blood flow in a fetal lamb in utero.

Oxygen, Vasoactive Substances, and Hormones

Many vasoactive substances have been shown to affect the fetal pulmonary circulation, and some of these substances also have been implicated in pulmonary vascular responses to hypoxia. Whether or not they play a role in the maintenance of the high pulmonary vascular resistance in the fetus is not known. Several studies have suggested that histamine release somehow is involved in the vasoconstrictor response to hypoxia in adults.[40,41] However, in the fetus and newborn, histamine is a pulmonary vasodilator and not a constrictor.[27,42] Similarly angiotensin II has been considered important in the pulmonary vasoconstrictor response to hypoxemia in adults[43] and therefore possibly involved in maintenance of the high pulmonary vascular resistance in the fetus. In the fetus, however, blockade of angiotensin II activity with Saralasin had no effect or pulmonary vascular resistance on the response to further hypoxemia.[44] The role of the various products of the prostaglandin (PG) cascade are also not clear. PGE_1 and E_2 both are modest pulmonary vasodilators[45-47]; PGI_2 is a somewhat more potent vasodilator[48,49] than both PGE_1 and PGE_2. None of these PGs[45-47] are specific for the pulmonary circulation and generally affect the systemic vascular resistance to the same or even a greater degree. It is possible that production and release of these substances may modulate the constrictor effects of, for example, the normally low PO_2, but this has not been established. PGF_2 alpha produces pulmonary vasoconstriction in fetal goats[46] and therefore possibly could play some role in the active production of pulmonary vasoconstriction.

FACTORS RESPONSIBLE FOR IMMEDIATE POSTNATAL PULMONARY VASODILATATION

Physical Factors

Rhythmic ventilation of the lungs with a gas, but not liquid, without changing PO_2, produces a small fall in pulmonary vascular resistance.[22,26,28,29,37] This is likely related to surface tension factors acting at the alveolar air-liquid interface tending to reduce perivascular tissue pressure.[50] Probably more important are the effects of O_2

in the inspired gas and perhaps the release of vasoactive substances by the movement or distention of lung tissue (see below).

Oxygen

Although gaseous expansion or ventilation of the lungs without increasing PO_2 leads to a small fall in pulmonary vascular resistance, a dramatic fall occurs with the addition to the gas of O_2, thereby increasing the PO_2 to which the resistance vessels are exposed.[26,28,39,51] This effect of O_2 has been further substantiated without expanding or ventilating the lungs by exposing fetal lambs to hyperbaric oxygenation.[52,53] It is not known whether the effects of O_2 are directly on the pulmonary vascular smooth muscle or whether a rise in PO_2 results in the release of an intermediary substance which either actively dilates the pulmonary circulation or inhibits vasoconstriction.

Vasoactive Substances and Hormones

Bradykinin, a potent vasoactive peptide, produces marked pulmonary vasodilatation when infused into fetal lambs.[54] Since bradykinin is thought to be released transiently from fetal lungs either following ventilation of the lungs with air or during hyperbaric oxygenation,[53] it is likely that bradykinin plays some role in the immediate postnatal pulmonary circulatory changes. More recent studies further support the possible transient role of bradykinin. One of the functions of pulmonary vascular endothelium is conversion of angiotensin I to the active angiotensin II; this function is performed by angiotensin converting enzyme (ACE) which also serves the function of catabolizing bradykinin to its inactive metabolites.[55] At normal fetal PO_2 pulmonary ACE activity is minimal; however, following exposure to O_2, ACE activity increased markedly.[56] This would result in increased metabolism and thus a reduced circulating concentration of bradykinin as soon as adequate postnatal oxygenation had occurred. A further possible role for angiotensin II or bradykinin has also been suggested since they both induce or stimulate local production of prostacyclin (PGI_2), a pulmonary vasodilating substance.[57]

Since several prostaglandins have been shown to dilate the fetal pulmonary circulation, these agents have received much attention as possible mediators of the postnatal changes. Lung distension or mechanical stimulation of lungs leads to PG production,[57,58] and ventilation of fetal lungs is associated with the net production of PGI_2 by the lungs.[50] If the lungs of fetuses close to term are perfused in situ, inhibition of prostaglandin synthesis by indomethacin attenuates the progressive fall in pulmonary vascular resistance that normally occurs 30 seconds after ventilation is started (Figure 7); the initial rapid fall is unaltered.[60]

Although these studies suggested a possible physiologic role for PGE_2 or PGI_2, further studies in newborn lambs showed that although they indeed produced pulmonary vasodilatation they also caused equal or greater systemic vasodilatation[61]; during hypoxemia the systemic effects were even more pronounced.

More recently PGD_2 has been shown to be a pulmonary vasodilator in perfused fetal lungs.[62] In intact, newly delivered term lambs, PGD_2 produced a fall in pulmonary arterial pressure and calculated pulmo-

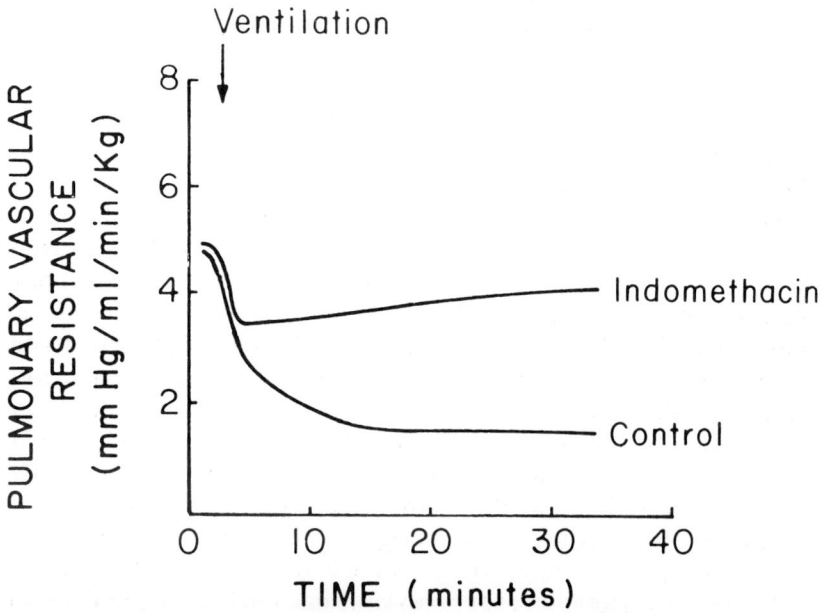

Figure 7. Effects on the fall in pulmonary vascular resistance following ventilation of administration of 2 mg/kg indomethacin shortly before initiation of ventilation in fetal goats. (Redrawn after Leffler, et al.[60])

nary vascular resistance with an increase in pulmonary and systemic blood flows and no change in systemic arterial blood pressure.[34] Beyond about 7–10 days of age this is no longer so and PGD_2 becomes a pulmonary vasoconstrictor,[63] much as the effects of histamine change from dilatation in the fetus and newborn to constriction in the older animal.[42] These specific effects in the newborn suggest a physiologic role for PGD_2 in the immediate perinatal period.

PATHOPHYSIOLOGY OF PERSISTENT PULMONARY HYPERTENSION SYNDROME IN THE NEWBORN

General Features

The pathophysiologic feature common to all infants with this syndrome is failure of the pulmonary vascular resistance to fall normally with the initiation of ventilation. As a result, pulmonary blood flow is restricted and pulmonary arterial pressure remains elevated. Associated with the pulmonary hypertension, right-to-left shunting occurs across the ductus arteriosus (which remains persistently patent in the majority of these infants) and right ventricular end-diastolic pressure is elevated. Consequently, right atrial pressure is increased and right-to-left shunting occurs across the foramen ovale as well. The presence of tricuspid regurgitation will accentuate this. As indicated in the *Physics of Flow through the Pulmonary Circulation in the Fetus and Newborn* section of this chapter, the level of pulmonary vascular resistance is related to several factors, the most important for this situation being viscosity and the cross-sectional area of the pulmonary vascular bed. Conditions which alter these can lead to persistent pulmonary hypertension in the newborn.

Increased Viscosity

Viscosity of blood is related to hematocrit, fibrinogen concentration, and red cell deformability. An increased hematocrit may be found following twin-to-twin or maternal-to-fetal transfusion or delayed cord clamping. Chronic intrauterine hypoxemia is associated with an increased hematocrit, as well as fibrinogen,[64] and infants born to diabetic mothers also may have an elevated hematocrit. Reduced red cell deformability, and therefore a potential increase in pulmonary vascular resistance, is a feature of newborn red cells relative to adult cells and is accentuated by acidemia.

Reduced Cross-sectional Area

Probably the most common cause for reduction in total pulmonary vascular cross-sectional area is failure of the fetal pulmonary circulation to undergo normal postnatal vasodilatation (See *Factors Responsible for Immediate Postnatal Vasodilatation* section). The exact mechanisms responsible for failure of the pulmonary vasculature to dilate are unknown. The most likely common denominator is hypoxemia, which as previously discussed (See sections on *Oxygen* and *Oxygen, Vasoactive Substances, and Hormones*) produces pulmonary vasoconstriction. Why some infants exposed to perinatal asphyxia develop pulmonary hypertension whereas many others, equally stressed in the immediate perinatal period, do not, is unclear. Recent pathologic studies shed some light on this. Morphologic evaluation of the pulmonary vasculature of infants dying with the pulmonary hypertension syndrome have shown clearly that there is excessive pulmonary vascular medial smooth muscle development as well as ontogenetically accelerated distribution of the smooth muscle along the length of the resistance vessels.[17,65-68] The small pulmonary arteries which normally would only be partially muscular or not even muscular at all (Figure 4) are completely muscularized as normally seen in the adult. Perhaps these abnormally developed vessels have an increased constrictor response to low oxygen, either because of the increased muscle mass or because the developmental acceleration is not only structural but also functional. In animal models, chronic intrauterine stress, such as chronic hypoxemia[69] or pulmonary hypertension,[70] is known to produce an increased medial muscle mass in the small pulmonary arteries. Infants exposed to similar intrauterine stresses are perhaps those at high risk for developing pulmonary hypertension.

It is clearly established that inhibitors of prostaglandin synthesis, such as aspirin or indomethacin, constrict the ductus arteriosus in utero,[5] thereby producing pulmonary hypertension and increased pulmonary vascular medial smooth muscle.[71] Use of these agents during pregnancy has been linked to the development of pulmonary hypertension syndrome,[66,72-74] but the association is not clear cut.

CLINICAL SYNDROME AND MANAGEMENT

Clinical Features

The syndrome of persistent pulmonary hypertension of the newborn is characterized by the early onset (generally within 6–12 hours after birth) of cyanosis and tachypnea, often with moderate or even severe respiratory distress, most commonly in full-term but occasionally in premature or postmature infants who are otherwise apparently normal.[75–79] The clinical presentation may be indistinguishable from certain forms of congenital heart disease or primary pulmonary disease such as group B beta hemolytic streptococcal pneumonia. Structural cardiac disease must be excluded very early in the management of these infants and in almost all instances two-dimensional echocardiography with Doppler is all that is required to do this. In the rare instance when clinical, ECG, x-ray, or two-dimensional echocardiographic evaluation is not conclusive, cardiac catheterization is warranted. Without definite bacteriologic evidence to the contrary, treatment of streptococcal pneumonia is initiated until cultures are proven to be sterile. A small group of infants with congenital malformations such as diaphragmatic hernia or chest wall abnormalities have hypoplastic lungs with a decreased pulmonary vascular bed and also may have pulmonary hypertension. This chapter will address only those infants without heart disease, bacterial pneumonia, or structural chest abnormalities.

Infants with true persistent pulmonary hypertension syndrome can be considered in two broad general groups. The first includes those infants with pulmonary hypertension in association with some form of aspiration syndrome. Most commonly this is meconium aspiration; however, aspiration of blood can also lead to the development of pulmonary hypertension. In the second group no obvious intrinsic pulmonary disease is present. The true incidence of the syndrome of persistent pulmonary hypertension in the newborn is unknown but has been estimated to be 1 in 1,454 live births for the non-aspiration group and higher for those infants with aspiration syndromes.[79] The mortality in infants with this syndrome remains high, but no accurate data are available; estimates vary from 20 to 50%, with infants not having aspiration syndromes having a better chance for survival. Many of the clinical features of both groups are similar. In addition to the signs described above, frequently there is a history of a difficult or abnormal labor and delivery, or perinatal asphyxia. Apgar scores are often low and there often is a history of meconium staining of amniotic fluid. Hypoglycemia, hypocalcemia, increased hematocrit, and acidemia are commonly found. A significant number of infants develop a systolic murmur probably due to post-hypoxic myocardial dysfunction with dilatation of either or both ventricles and secondary tricuspid and/or mitral regurgitation.

Right-to-left intrapulmonary or atrial shunting is evidenced by a lower than normal PaO_2 in blood obtained from an artery arising from the ascending aorta (right radial or temporal) (75–80 torr breathing room air) or by a similarly reduced transcutaneous PO_2 measurement on the upper part of the body. Right-to-left atrial shunting may be confirmed by contrast two-dimensional echocardiography done by injecting saline into a lower limb vein and observing the microcavitations entering the left atrium. A further right-to-left shunt through the ductus arteriosus is evidenced by a difference in PaO_2 of greater than 5 torr between blood samples drawn from an artery arising from the ascending aorta and that in the descending aorta (usually sampled via an indwelling umbilical arterial catheter). This difference correlates roughly with the amount of the right-to-left shunt and therefore the degree of pulmonary hypertension when the ductus arteriosus is open and is often more easily demonstrated when the infant is breathing 100% O_2.

The chest x-ray in infants without aspiration syndromes usually shows relatively clear lung fields whereas with aspiration, parenchymal changes are often seen. However, the radiographic appearance of the lungs is quite variable and often the severe degree of hypoxemia is not suggested by the radiographic picture. Cardiomegaly is seen in perhaps half the infants. The electrocardiogram is nonspecific but may show increased right ventricular forces for age (increased R wave height, upright T waves, or Q wave in right precordial leads, right axis deviation).

General Management

Attempts at prevention of persistent pulmonary hypertension should start in utero with good obstetrical management, minimizing intrauterine stress which might lead to the development of an abnormal pulmonary circulation. If perinatal asphyxia should be evident, rapid resuscitation to attenuate any effects of asphyxia is essential. Once the infant has developed respiratory distress, other causes of cyanosis and respiratory distress should be excluded rapidly (as outlined in the *Clinical Features* section above). Careful attention must be paid to maintaining normal blood glucose and calcium concentrations and to assure that the central hematocrit is not above 65%. If it is, it should be reduced by partial exchange transfusion with albuminated saline (4 g salt poor albumin in 84 ml normal saline) or reconstituted fresh frozen plasma. Oxygen consumption should be kept to a minimum by maintaining the infant in a neutral thermal environment.

Ventilation[80,81]

Ventilatory support should be directed toward maintaining the PaO_2 (umbilical arterial) at least above 50 and preferably 70 torr and avoiding acidemia. A plan of support should be initiated to attain these goals. Supplemental oxygen (FIO_2 = 1.0) should first be administered by hood. This alone is usually inadequate and, if so, the infant is intubated and allowed to breathe spontaneously in an FIO_2 of up to 1.0, against an end-expiratory pressure of up to 4–7 cm H_2O. If PaO_2 still cannot be maintained above 50 torr or shows wide swings (+/−10–15 torr), or if $PaCO_2$ is not maintained below 55 – 60 torr and acidemia (pH less than 7.30) develops, assisted mechanical ventilation is necessary.

Since hypoxemia is usually rapidly progressive, the present trend is to start mechanical ventilation (pressure cycled) early. In general, current practice aims at immediate rapid rate ventilation (rates > 100/min) to reduce $PaCO_2$ and increase pH levels (see below), without first ventilating the infant at a slow rate (e.g., 30–40/min) as is more customary with hyaline membrane disease. End expiratory pressures usually are 4–7 cm H_2O. Initial inflating pressures, particularly in infants with aspiration syndromes, may be very high (up to 50 cm H_2O) as compared to those used in infants with other forms of lung disease. When adequate PaO_2 is reached, the peak inspiratory pressure should be reduced as the first change in ventilator settings. In view of the high pressures used, if the infant is breathing spontaneously or struggling against the mechanical ventilator, sedation with morphine is given. Many infants require paralysis with mechanical ventilation at this stage. The development of pneumothorax is less likely to occur with this approach and adequate ventilation is usually easier to accomplish. In general, ventilator rates of between 120 and 150 per minute will be required to achieve the predetermined endpoint which generally attempts to maintain PaO_2 above 70 torr (and if possible even above 100 torr) and $PaCO_2$ below 20–25 torr. Occasionally, in very unstable infants, hand ventilation is the most efficient way of achieving the initial aims.

In most infants who improve with mechanical ventilation an individual "critical" $PaCO_2$ is found, above which PaO_2 starts to fall. Ventilation should maintain $PaCO_2$ just below this point and, where possible, rate rather than inflating pressure should be increased to achieve this. Several important points must be remembered. These infants are extremely labile, and handling of the infant should be kept to an absolute minimum as handling often leads to wide swings in PaO_2. Likewise, it is critical that once stability has been achieved, changes in ventilation be made extremely slowly. Inflating pressure should be reduced by no more than 1 cm H_2O per change and this should be the first change made when peak inspiratory pressure is greater than 35 mm H_2O. Next, FIO_2 can be reduced and this, too, only in very small steps of 1–2%. When rate is reduced this, too, should be by small decrements.

Pharmacologic Intervention

Failure of adequate blood gas response to rapid rate ventilation leads to the next stage in management: the administration of vasodilating agents.[80,82,83] It is not yet clear whether it is appropriate to use dilating agents such as tolazoline before introducing rapid rate ventilation; however, it is our impression that the use of ventilation first is more effective.

A significant problem with the use of vasodilators is that currently no agent specifically affecting the pulmonary circulation is available. All agents used are generalized vasodilators with systemic effects as well.[61] Therefore, with these agents, maintenance of an adequate systemic arterial blood pressure is crucial. To this end, infusion of colloid (e.g., fresh frozen plasma or salt poor albumin) or crystalloids (e.g., Ringer's lactate) have been employed. Unfortunately, large volumes often were required and marked and protracted peripheral edema resulted. To avoid this, systemic vasoconstrictors such as dopamine have been infused either independently or together with small amounts of colloid, to maintain systemic arterial pressure by increasing peripheral vascular resistance or cardiac output.[80]

The most commonly used vasodilator is tolazoline.[80,82,83] It usually is given initially as a trial bolus injection of 1 mg/kg. If a good response occurs, measured by an increase in PaO_2, further amounts may not be required or only 1 or 2 further bolus injections may suffice. However, in most instances, an infusion of 5 mg/kg/hr is started. This dose can be increased, but if no effect is seen with 25 mg/kg/hr it is likely that no response will occur. Experience is quite variable but perhaps 25–30% of infants respond. As with all drugs, complications do occur but are rare and apparently are not dose related; hemorrhage and renal dysfunction have been reported. In some infants the systemic hypotensive effects are dramatic and profound. Other agents such as calcium channel blockers, acetylcholine, nitroprusside, and nitroglycerine have been considered, but no appropriate clinical trials undertaken.

A group of agents with perhaps some promise as pharmacologic pulmonary vasodilators are the prostaglandins. Prostaglandin E_1 (PGE_1) and PGE_2 both produce pulmonary vasodilation but, as previously indicated, the effects are not dramatic and systemic vasodilation also occurs. PGI_2 (prostacyclin) produces quite marked pulmonary vasodilation in animals, more so than either PGE_1 or PGE_2, and this led to the clinical application of PGI_2[84] and even the commencement of clinical trials. Severe hypotension, bradycardia, and death occurred in several of the infants; so the use of this drug is under further review. More recent evidence points to the possibility that in animals PGD_2 may in fact be a fairly specific pulmonary vasodilator with no systemic effects.[34,62,63] These studies need further confirmation before clinical trials with PGD_2 can be considered.

Monitoring

Responses to both rapid ventilation and to the effects of pharmacologic agents are currently monitored by changes in PaO_2 and acid-base status. Indwelling umbilical arterial catheters are used as standard practice in neonatal intensive care and not only allow easy access to arterial blood but also continuous blood pressure monitoring. Radial arterial cannulation may be performed if the umbilical artery cannot be entered. Transcutaneous PO_2 measurement in infants with normal systemic perfusion is a reliable method of obtaining an estimate of PaO_2. Electrodes can be placed both over the upper and lower body, but when an umbilical arterial catheter is in place usually only an upper body electrode is used. Reduction in the differences between upper and lower body PaO_2 indicates reduction in right-to-left shunting across the ductus arteriosus relative to systemic arterial pressure. Direct measurement of pulmonary arterial pressure can be achieved at the bedside by floating an end-hole Swan-Ganz balloon catheter through the right heart chambers under pressure guidance. Although not common or standard practice, in selected instances this gives additional information about the relationship of pulmonary and systemic arterial pressures. This is particularly useful in very sick infants, and allows for tighter titration of doses of pharmacologic agents.

The pathophysiology of persistent pulmonary hypertension syndrome of the newborn remains obscure. Structural morphologic changes in the pulmonary vasculature of infants dying with the syndrome suggest that accelerated maturation and abnormal development of smooth muscle may play a role. Microthrombi also are seen, perhaps pointing to the role of platelets, and perhaps substances released from platelets. Current management is purely supportive and, until more is known about the normal physiologic control of the perinatal pulmonary circulation as well as the pathophysiologic alterations, is likely to remain so. The development of an appropriate animal model of the disease, too, might accelerate our understanding of the pathophysiology and lead to specific therapeutic approaches.

Acknowledgment: Supported in part by USPHS Program Project Grant HL 24056.

REFERENCES

1. Rudolph AM, Heymann MA: The circulation of the fetus in utero. Methods for studying distribution of blood flow, cardiac output and organ blood flow. *Circ Res* 1967;21:163–184.
2. Rudolph AM, Heymann MA: Circulatory changes during growth in the fetal lamb. *Circ Res* 1970;26:289–299.
3. Heymann MA, Creasy RK, Rudolph AM: Quantitation of blood flow patterns in the foetal lamb in utero. In, *Proceedings of the Sir Joseph Barcroft Centenary Symposium. Foetal and Neonatal Physiology.* Cambridge: Cambridge University Press, 1973:129–135.
4. Lewis AB, Heymann MA, Rudolph AM: Gestational changes in pulmonary vascular responses in fetal lambs in utero. *Circ Res* 1976;39:536–541.
5. Heymann MA, Rudolph AM: Effects of acetylsalicylic acid on the ductus arteriosus and circulation in fetal lambs in utero. *Circ Res* 1976;38:418–422.
6. Rudolph AM: Fetal and neonatal pulmonary circulation. *Ann Rev Physiol* 1979;41:383–395.
7. Levin DL, Rudolph AM, Heymann MA, Phibbs RH: Morphological development of the pulmonary vascular bed in fetal lambs. *Circulation* 1976;53:144–151.

8. Moss AJ, Emmanouilides G, Duffie ER Jr: Closure of the ductus arteriosus in the newborn infant. *Pediatrics* 1963;32:25–30.
9. Rudolph AM, Auld PAM, Golinko RJ, Paul MH: Pulmonary vascular adjustments in the neonatal period. *Pediatrics* 1961;28:28–34.
10. Krovetz LJ. Goldbloom J: Normal standards for cardiovascular data II pressure and vascular resistances. *Johns Hopkins Med J* 1972;130:187–195.
11. Reid L: The Pulmonary circulation: Remodelling in growth and disease. *Am Rev Respir Dis* 1979;119:531–546.
12. Hislop A, Reid L: Intra-pulmonary arterial development during fetal life—branching pattern and structure. *J Anat* 1972;113:35–48.
13. Wagenvoort CA, Neufeld HN, Edwards JE: The structure of the pulmonary arterial tree in fetal and early postnatal life. *Lab Invest* 1961;10: 751–761.
14. Davies G, Reid L: Growth of the alveoli and pulmonary arteries in childhood. *Thorax* 1970;25:669–681.
15. Hislop A, Reid L: Pulmonary arterial development during childhood: Branching pattern and structure. *Thorax* 1973;28:129–135.
16. Rendas A, Branthwaite M, Reid L: Growth of the pulmonary circulation in normal pig: Structural analysis and aspects of cardiopulmonary function. *J Appl Physiol* 1978;45:806–817.
17. Reid L: The development of the pulmonary circulation. In, Peckham GJ, Heymann MA, eds. *Cardiovascular Sequelae of Asphyxia in the Newborn. Report of the Eighty-third Ross Conference on Pediatric Research.* Columbus, Ohio, Ross Laboratories, 1982:2–10.
18. Meyrick R, Reid L: Ultrastructural features of the distended pulmonary arteries of the normal rat. *Anat Rec* 1979;193:71–97.
19. Meyrick B, Reid L: The effect of continued hypoxia on rat pulmonary arterial circulation: An ultrastructural study. *Lab Invest* 1978;38:188–200.
20. Reid L: The lung: Its growth and remodelling in health and disease. *Am J Roentgenol* 1977;129:777–788.
21. Prandtl L, Tietjens OG: *Applied Hydro- and Aeromechanics.* New York: Dover Publications, 1957.
22. Colebatch HJH, Dawes GS, Goodwin JW, Nadeau RA: The nervous control of the circulation in the foetal and newly expanded lungs of the lamb. *J Physiol* 1965;178:544–562.
23. Rudolph AM, Heymann MA, Lewis AB: Physiology and pharmacology of the pulmonary circulation in the fetus and newborn. In: Hodson WA, ed. *Lung Biology in Health and Disease. Development of the lung.* New York: Marcel Dekker, 1977:497–523.
24. Silove Ed, Grover RF: Effects of alpha-adrenergic blockade and tissue catecholamine depletion on pulmonary vascular responses to hypoxia. *J Clin Invest* 1968;47:274–285.
25. Lock JE, Olley PM, Coceani F: Enhanced beta-adrenergic receptor responsiveness in the hypoxic neonatal pulmonary circulation. *Am J Physiol* 1981;240:H697–H703.
26. Cassin S, Dawes GS, Mott JC, Ross BB, Strang LB: The vascular resistance of the foetal and newly ventilated lung of the lamb. *J Physiol* 1964;171: 61–79.
27. Cassin S, Dawes GS, Ross BB: Pulmonary blood flow and vascular resistance in immature foetal lambs. *J Physiol* 1964;171:80–89.

28. Dawes GS, Mott JC: The vascular tone of the foetal lung. *J Physiol* 1962; 164:465–477.
29. Dawes GS, Mott JC, Widdicombe JC, Wyatt DG: Changes in the lungs of the newborn lamb. *J Physiol* 1953;121:141–162.
30. Barrett CT, Heymann MA, Rudolph AM: Alpha- and beta-adrenergic function in fetal sheep. *AM J Obstet Gynecol* 1972;112:1114–1121.
31. Smith RW, Morris JA, Assali NS: Effects of chemical mediators on the pulmonary and ductus arteriosus circulation in the fetal lamb. *Am J Obstet Gynecol* 1964;89:252–260.
32. Stahlman M, Shephard F, Gray Jr, Young W: The effects of hypoxia and hypercapnia on the circulation in newborn lambs. *J Pediatr* 1964;65: 1091–1092
33. Rudolph AM, Yuan S: Response of the pulmonary vasculature to hypoxia and H^+ ion concentration changes. *J Clin Invest* 1966;45:399–411.
34. Soifer SJ, Morin FC III, Heymann MA: Prostaglandin D_2 reverses induced pulmonary hypertension in the newborn lamb. *J Pediatr* 1982;100: 458–463.
35. Cohn HE, Sacks EJ, Heymann MA, Rudolph AM: Cardiovascular responses to hypoxemia and acidemia in fetal lambs. *Am J Obstet Gynecol* 1974;120:817–824.
36. Comline RS, Silver M: The release of adrenaline and noradrenaline from the adrenal glands of the foetal sheep. *J Physiol* 1961;156:424–444.
37. Campbell AGM, Cockburn F, Dawes GS, Milligan JE: Pulmonary vasoconstriction in asphyxia during cross-circulation between twin foetal lambs. *J Physiol* 1967;192:111–121.
38. Campbell AGM, Dawes GS, Fishman AP, Hyman AI: Pulmonary vasocontriction and changes in heart rate during asphyxia in immature foetal lambs. *J Physiol* 1967;192:93–110.
39. Cook CD, Drinker PA, Jacobson NH, Levison H, Strang LB: Control of pulmonary blood flow in the foetal and newly born lamb. *J Physiol* 1963; 169:10–29.
40. Hauge A, Melmon KL: Role of histamine in hypoxic pulmonary hypertension in the rat. II. Depletion of histamine, serotonin and catecholamines. *Circ Res* 1968;22:385–392.
41. Hauge A, Staub NC: Prevention of hypoxic vasoconstriction in cat lung by histamine-releasing agent 48/80. *J Appl Physiol* 1969;26:693–699.
42. Goetzman BW, Milstein JM: Pulmonary vascular histamine receptors in newborn and young lambs. *J Appl Physiol* 1980; 49:380–385.
43. Berkov S: Hypoxic pulmonary vasoconstriction in the rat: The necessary role of angiotensin II. *Circ Res* 1974;35:256–261.
44. Hyman A, Heymann MA, Levin DL, Rudolph AM: Angiotensin is not the mediator of hypoxia-induced pulmonary vasoconstriction in fetal lambs. *Circulation* 1975;52:11–132, (Abstract).
45. Cassin S, Tyler TL, Wallis R: The effects of prostaglandin E_1 on fetal pulmonary vascular resistance (38588). *Proc Soc Exp Biol Med* 1975;148: 584–587.
46. Tyler TL, Leffler CW, Cassin S: Effects of prostaglandin precursors, prostaglandins, and prostaglandin metabolites on pulmonary circulation in perinatal goats. *Chest* 1977;71S:271S–273S.

47. Tripp ME, Heymann MA, Rudolph AM: Hemodynamic effects of prostaglandin E_1 on lambs in utero. In: Coceani F, Olley PM, eds. *Advances in Prostaglandin and Thromboxane Research*, Vol. 4. New York: Raven Press, 1978:221–229.
48. Leffler CW, Hessler JR: Pulmonary and systemic vascular effects of exogenous prostaglandin I_2 in fetal lambs. *Eur J Pharmacol* 1979;54:37–42.
49. Cassin S, Winikor I, Tod M, Philips J, Frisinger S, Jordan J, Gibbs C: Effects of prostacyclin on the fetal pulmonary circulation. *Pediatr Pharmacol* 1981;1:197–207.
50. Enhörning G, Adams FH, Norman A; Effect of lung expansion on the fetal lamb circulation. *Acta Paediatr Scand* 1966;55:441–451.
51. Born GVR, Dawes GS, Mott JC: The viability of premature lambs. *J Physiol* 1955;130:191–212.
52. Assali NS, Kirschbaum TM, Dilts PV Jr: Effects of hyperbaric oxygen on uteroplacental and fetal circulation. *Circ Res* 1968;22:573–588.
53. Heymann MA, Rudolph AM, Nies AS, Melmon KL: Bradykinin production associated with oxygenation of the fetal lamb. *Circ Res* 1969;25:521–534.
54. Campbell AGM, Dawes GS, Fishman AP, Hyman AI, Perks AM: The release of a bradykinin-like pulmonary vasodilator substance in foetal and newborn lambs. *J Physiol* 1968;195:83–96.
55. Stalcup SA, Davidson D, Mellins RB: Pulmonary metabolism of vasoactive substances in normal and asphyxiated births. In Peckham GH, Heymann MA, eds. *Cardiovascular Sequelae of Asphyxia in the Newborn. Report of the Eighty-third Ross Conference on Pediatric Research*. Columbus, Ohio, Ross Laboratories, 1982:44–51.
56. Davidson D, Stalcup SA, Mellins RB: Angiotensin converting enzyme activity and its modulation by oxygen tension in the guinea pig fetal-placental unit. *Circ Res* 1981;48:286–291.
57. Gryglewski RJ: The lung as a generator of prostacyclin. *Ciba Found Symp* 1980;78:147–164.
58. Edmonds JF, Berry E, Wyllie JH: Release of prostaglandins by distension of the lungs. *Br J Surg* 1969;56:622–623.
59. Leffler CW, Hessler JR, Terragno NA: Ventilation-induced release of prostaglandin-like material from fetal lungs. *Am J Physiol* 1980;238:H282–286.
60. Leffler CW, Tyler TL, Cassin S: Effect of indomethacin on pulmonary vascular response to ventilation of fetal goats. *Am J Physiol* 1978;234:H346–H351.
61. Tripp ME, Drummond WH, Heymann MA, Rudolph AM: Hemodynamic effects of pulmonary arterial infusion of vasodilators in newborn lambs. *Pediatr Res* 1980;14:1311–1315.
62. Cassin S, Tod M, Philips J, Frisinger J, Jordan J, Gibbs C: Effects of prostaglandin D_2 in perinatal circulation. *Am J Physiol* 1981;240:H755–H760.
63. Soifer SJ, Morin FC, Kaslow DC, Heymann MA: Developmental changes in the effect of PGD_2 on the pulmonary circulation in the newborn lamb. *Pediatr Res* 1982;16:308A (Abst).

64. Pickart LR, Creasy RK, Thaler MM: Polycythemia and hyperfibrinogenemia as factors in experimental intrauterine growth retardation. *Am J Obstet Gynecol* 1976;124:268–271.
65. Haworth SG, Reid L: Persistent fetal circulation: Newly recognized structural features. *J Pediatr* 1976;88:614–620.
66. Levin DL, Fixler DE, Morriss FC, Tyson J: Morphologic analysis of the pulmonary vascular bed in infants exposed in utero to prostaglandin synthetase inhibitors. *J Pediatr* 1978;92:478–483.
67. McKenzie S, Haworth SG: Occlusion of peripheral pulmonary vascular bed in a baby with idiopathic persistent fetal circulation. *Br Heart J* 1981;46:675–678.
68. Murphy JD, Rabinovitch M, Goldstein JD, Reid LM: The structural basis of persistent pulmonary hypertension of the newborn infant. *J Pediatr* 1981;98:962–967.
69. Goldberg SJ, Levy RA, Siassi B, Betten J: The effects of maternal hypoxia and hyperoxia upon the neonatal pulmonary vasculature. *Pediatrics* 1971;48:528–533.
70. Levin DL, Hyman AI, Heymann MA, Rudolph AM: Fetal hypertension and the development of increased pulmonary vascular smooth muscle: A possible mechanism for persistent pulmonary hypertension of the newborn infant. *J Pediatr* 1978;92:265–269.
71. Levin DL, Mills LJ, Weinberg AG: Hemodynamic, pulmonary vascular, and myocardial abnormalities secondary to pharmacologic constriction of the fetal ductus arteriosus. *Circulation* 1979;60:360–364.
72. Manchester D, Margolis HS, Sheldon RE: Possible association between maternal indomethacin therapy and primary pulmonary hypertension of the newborn. *Am J Obstet Gynecol* 1976;126:467–469.
73. Csaba IF, Sulyok E, Ertl T: Relationship of maternal treatment with indomethacin to persistence of fetal circulation syndrome. *J Pediatr* 1978;92:484.
74. Wilkinson AR, Aynsley-Green A, Mitchell MD: Persistent pulmonary hypertension and abnormal PGE levels in preterm infants after maternal treatment with naproxen. *Arch Dis Child* 1979;54:942–945.
75. Gersony WM: Persistence of the fetal circulation: A commentary. *J Pediatr* 1973;82:1103–1106.
76. Levin DL, Heymann MA, Kitterman JA, Gregory GA, Phibbs RH, Rudolph AM: Persistent pulmonary hypertension of the newborn infant. *J Pediatr* 1976;89:626–630.
77. Drummond WH, Peckham GJ, Fox WW: The clinical profile of the newborn with persistent pulmonary hypertension. *Clin Pediatr* 1977;16:335–341.
78. Fox WW, Gewitz MH, Dinwiddie R, Drummond WH, Peckham GJ: Pulmonary hypertension in the perinatal aspiration syndromes. *Pediatrics* 1977;59:205–211.
79. Goetzman BW, Reimenschneider TA: Persistence of the fetal circulation. *Pediatr Rev* 1980;2:37–40.
80. Drummond WH, Gregory GA, Heymann MA, Phibbs RA: The independent effects of hyperventilation, tolazoline, and dopamine on infants with persistent pulmonary hypertension. *J Pediatr* 1981;98:603–611.

81. Fox WW: Arterial blood gas evaluation and mechanical ventilation in the management of persistent pulmonary hypertension of the neonate. In: Peckham GJ, Heymann MA, eds. *Cardiovascular Sequelae of Asphyxia in the Newborn. Report of the Eighty-third Ross Conference on Pediatric Research.* Columbus, Ohio, Ross Laboratories, 1982:102–110.
82. Goetzman BW, Sunshine P, Johnson JD, Wennberg RP, Hackel A, Merten DF, Bartoletti AL, Silverman NH: Neonatal hypoxia and pulmonary vasospasm: Response to tolazoline. *J Pediatr* 1976;89:617–621.
83. Stevenson DK, Kasting DS, Darnall RA Jr, Ariagno RL, Johnson JD, Malachowski N, Beets CL, Sunshine P: Refractory hypoxemia associated with neonatal pulmonary disease: The use and limitations of tolazoline. *J Pediatr* 1979;95:595–599.
84. Lock JE, Olley PM, Coceani F, Swyer PR, Rowe RD: Use of prostacyclin in persistent fetal circulation. *Lancet* 1979;1:1343–1345.

CHAPTER 3

PULMONARY ARTERIAL HYPERTENSION SECONDARY TO CONGENITAL HEART DISEASE

Julien I. E. Hoffman and Michael A. Heymann

DEFINITION

Pulmonary arterial hypertension is defined as a pulmonary arterial pressure above normal, a value that changes during fetal development and in the neonatal period. In the fetal lamb, which in this respect closely resembles the human, pulmonary arterial pressure rises over the second half of gestation [1] and is similar to aortic pressure.[2] At term in humans aortic pressure is about 70/40 (mean 50) mm Hg, and is lower in preterm infants.[3] Pulmonary arterial pressure falls rapidly as the ductus arteriosus closes and pulmonary vasodilation occurs, so that by 24 hours after birth pulmonary arterial pressure is about half of aortic pressure.[4] Thereafter it falls more slowly to reach low adult values by 1 to 4 weeks after birth[1,5,6] (Figures 1 and 2). It may fall a little lower in the next six months to reach its final normal level.[7] The upper limits of normal after about 1 month after birth are generally taken as 25 mm Hg systolic, 13 mm Hg diastolic, and 18 mm Hg mean pulmonary arterial pressure. However, in those who live at high altitude, slightly higher normal values are noted (Figure 2).

Basic Mechanisms

The simplest approach is to consider the hydraulic equivalent of Ohm's law, namely that resistance equals pressure drop divided by

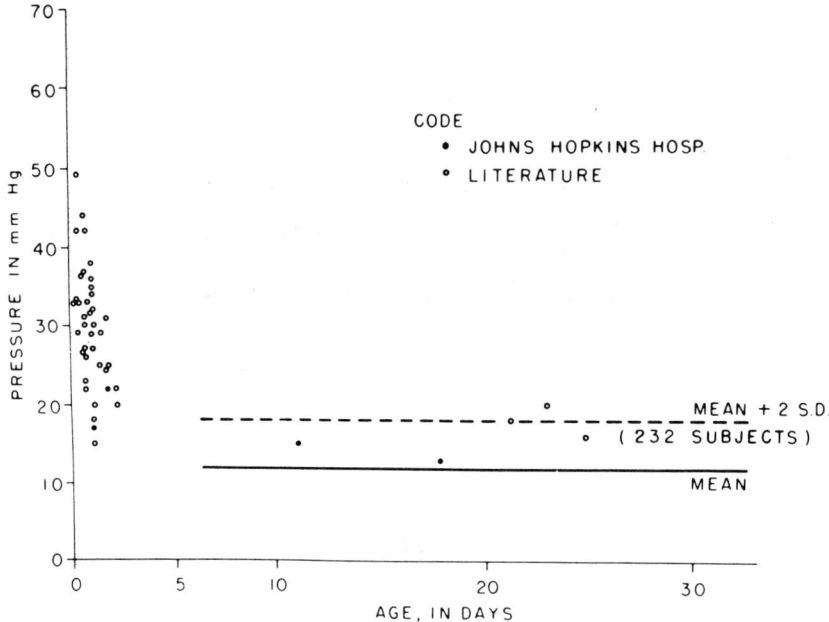

Figure 1. Changes in mean pulmonary arterial pressure during the first month after birth. The mean and 2 S.D. for 232 normal adults is shown for comparison. (Reproduced from Krovetz and Goldbloom, Johns Hopkins Med J, 1972;130:187–195, with permission of the authors and The Johns Hopkins University Press.)

flow. For the pulmonary circulation with resistance R_p and pulmonary blood flow $\dot{Q}_p$ the mean pressure drop is taken from pulmonary artery ($\bar{P}pa$) to pulmonary vein ($\bar{P}pv$). Thus

$$R_p = (\bar{P}pa - \bar{P}pv)/\dot{Q}_p .$$

This can be rearranged to give:

$$\bar{P}pa = \bar{P}pv + R_p \dot{Q}_p .$$

From this, it is clear that an increase in mean pulmonary arterial pressure will occur with increases of pulmonary venous pressure, pulmonary vascular resistance, or pulmonary blood flow. It is important to realize, however, that these factors are not necessarily independent; in particular, pulmonary flow and vascular resistance are often inversely related. In normal people who exercise[8] or in patients with large atrial septal defects, pulmonary blood flow may be much in-

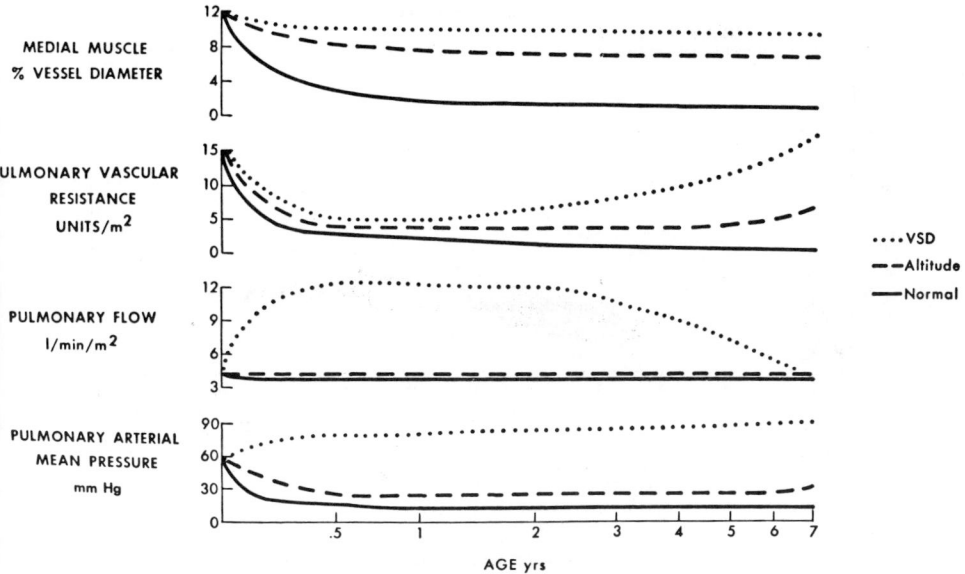

Figure 2. Diagram of postnatal changes in pulmonary arterial mean pressure; flow, vascular resistance, and medial muscle thickness of small arteries. Comparisons are shown among normals at sea level and at altitude, and of children with large ventricular septal defects. (Reproduced from Rudolph A M: Congenital Diseases of the Heart, 1974, with permission of the author and the Year Book Medical Publishers, Inc., Chicago.)

creased but pulmonary arterial pressures are normal except for an increased pulse pressure (Figure 3). The increased pulmonary blood flow has caused pulmonary vascular resistance to fall by dilating and recruiting vessels so that the product $R_p \dot{Q}_p$ does not change and $\overline{P}pa$ does not rise. Thus, an increased pulmonary blood flow is not by itself a sufficient cause for pulmonary arterial hypertension, and will cause it only if pulmonary vascular resistance fails to fall appropriately.

INCREASED PULMONARY VENOUS PRESSURE

Pathophysiology

Whenever pulmonary venous hypertension occurs, there is a rise in mean capillary pressure and pulmonary arterial pressure which causes

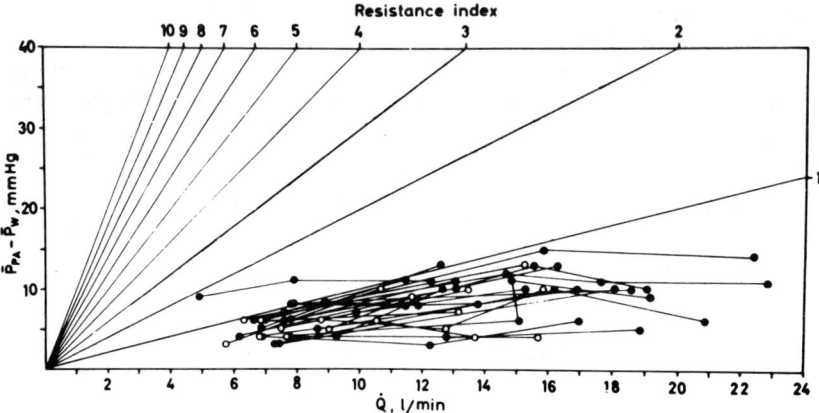

Figure 3. The pressure difference across the lung (Ppa−Ppv) is shown related to cardiac output in supine exercise in healthy young men (●) and women (○). The solid lines are iso-resistance lines. As flow increases, the pressure difference remains almost constant and resistance decreases. (Reproduced from Ekelund and Holmgren, Circ Res 1967;20 (Supp. I):33−43, with permission of the authors and the American Heart Association.)

increased transudation of fluid out of vessels into interstitial spaces. This interstitial fluid lowers lung compliance and causes peribronchial edema that may lead to alveolar hypoxia and pulmonary vasoconstriction.[9,10] Further fluid transudation leads to alveolar flooding[11] that causes more alveolar hypoxia. Because of gravity, when the patient is erect, the excess interstitial fluid is mainly at the lung bases where, in addition to surrounding small airways, it may surround and compress blood vessels.[9,10,12] Therefore, it is common to find some increase in pulmonary vascular resistance when there is pulmonary venous hypertension. A reflex or hormonal cause of pulmonary vasoconstriction has also been postulated but never convincingly demonstrated.

The gravitational effect is responsible for the redistribution of blood flow from bases to apex that was first shown in adults with mitral stenosis[13] but has also been described in children.[14] In acute studies, this redistribution of flow was found only after fluid accumulated in basal alveoli,[15] and the mechanisms of redistribution may in part be related to the associated reduction in basal lung volume.[16] Whatever the mechanism of this redistribution, it tends to minimize pulmonary arterial hypertension by diverting blood from high resistance vessels at the lung bases to newly recruited and dilated vessels in the upper halves of the lungs corresponding to zones I and II. This compensation is denied to infants and small children whose lungs are so small that there may be no zone I and little or no zone II, so that there are no new vessels to recruit.[17] As a result, a given degree of pulmonary venous hypertension tends to produce more pulmonary arterial hypertension in infants than in older children and adults.

Should the pulmonary venous hypertension be prolonged for more than a few months, there may be secondary organic changes in the intima and media of the small pulmonary arteries so that classical organic pulmonary vascular disease may occur.[18,19] This is most likely if pulmonary arterial pressures are markedly elevated by an increase in pulmonary vascular resistance that occurs for one of the reasons discussed above.

Diagnostic Assessment

The diagnosis of pulmonary venous hypertension as a cause of pulmonary arterial hypertension is usually made by finding a raised pulmonary arterial wedge pressure, but sometimes left atrial pressure can be measured directly across a patent foramen ovale or by retrograde catheterization across the mitral valve. Occasionally in children with stenotic anomalous pulmonary venous connections, the high pulmonary venous pressure can be demonstrated by retrograde pulmonary vein catheterization. If the mean pressure drop across the lungs (mean pulmonary arterial pressure minus mean wedge, pulmonary venous or left atrial pressure) is normal, that is, not over about 10–12 mg Hg, or if calculated pulmonary vascular resistance is low, that is, under 3 Wood units/m^2 body surface area, then there is no evidence of added pulmonary vasoconstriction or pulmonary vascular disease. An increased mean pressure drop or pulmonary vascular resistance indicates that pulmonary venous hypertension is not the only mechanism of the pulmonary arterial hypertension even if it is the basic cause of the problem. A fall of pulmonary vascular resistance after breathing 100% oxygen or receiving a vasodilator like tolazoline or acetylcholine indicates that a pulmonary vasoconstrictive component exists, and a similar fall of resistance after diuresis suggests that perivascular edema was probably present.[12,20,21]

Clinical Syndromes

Left Ventricular Failure

The commonest cause of pulmonary venous hypertension in children, as in adults, is left ventricular failure. In young infants, severe coarctation of the aorta and critical aortic stenosis are uncommon but important causes of severe heart failure, pulmonary edema, and pulmonary arterial and venous hypertension.[22] Both of these congenital cardiovascular lesions demonstrate marked right ventricular hypertrophy clinically and on electrocardiography, despite being left-sided obstructive lesions. Critical aortic stenosis in the neonate indicates that the stenosis was probably severe in utero, and suggests that in late fetal life blood might have been diverted from left to right ventricles. The excessive right ventricular load would explain the abnormal right ventricular dominance noted in this lesion in early infancy. Furthermore, both of these lesions, by causing pulmonary venous hypertension and pulmonary edema, usually give rise to marked pulmonary arterial hypertension with resultant right ventricular hypertrophy. A variant presentation in both of these congenital lesions occurs when the high left atrial pressure distends the left atrium and makes the valve of the foramen ovale incompetent. This leads to a left-to-right atrial shunt that is often large and may decompress the left atrium; these infants may have less pulmonary edema than do those with no atrial shunt. The increased right ventricular volume load is added reason for right ventricular dilation and hypertrophy, and the increased pulmonary flow produces clinical and radiographic signs of a left-to-right shunt and contributes to the pulmonary arterial hypertension. Despite having less or no pulmonary edema, these infants are not better off because their left ventricular output is usually very low.

Infants with tight aortic stenosis or coarctation of the aorta are usually critically ill. As non-specific features of biventricular heart failure, they have tachypnea, retractions, tachycardia, hepatomegaly, decreased urine output, and poor skin perfusion. Cardiac output may be so low that characteristic murmurs are absent and the peripheral pulses may be almost impalpable. It is important not to misdiagnose overwhelming sepsis, a metabolic disorder, or some other form of shock because this would delay the surgical treatment that is usually life-saving. The clinical and electrocardiographic signs of pulmonary and right ventricular hypertension, and the radiologic signs of an enlarged heart, pulmonary edema, or increased pulmonary blood flow should lead to the correct diagnosis.

Total Anomalous Pulmonary Venous Connection

An uncommon but important congenital heart lesion causing pulmonary venous hypertension is total anomalous pulmonary venous connection with obstruction to the pulmonary venous channels.[23,24]

About half of these children have supracardiac drainage of the common vein into the superior vena cava, usually by a persistent vertical vein. If there is no obstruction, they have low pulmonary venous pressures and usually resemble uncomplicated secundum atrial septal defects. However, obstruction in the course of the venous drainage is common. It may be due to a stenosis, often where the left innominate vein joins the superior vena cava, or it can be due to compression of the vertical vein between the left bronchus and the pulmonary artery; as pulmonary arterial hypertension gets worse the artery enlarges and compresses the vertical vein more tightly, thus creating a vicious circle. In about 25% of these children the anomalous veins enter the coronary sinus, and there may be a stenosis at the junction. Finally, almost all the other children with this lesion have a long common pulmonary vein that descends through the diaphragm to enter the portal vein. These infants all develop pulmonary venous hypertension, partly because of the resistance to flow offered by the long venous channel but principally because when the ductus venosus closes, all pulmonary venous blood has to traverse the relatively high resistance sinusoids of the liver.

Clinically, most of these children, especially those with infra-diaphragmatic drainage, present in early infancy with tachypnea, cyanosis, and congestive heart failure. They all have florid pulmonary edema and very high, often supra-aortic, pulmonary arterial pressure. Because they have no characteristic cardiac murmurs, they have often been mistakenly diagnosed as some form of lung disease with cor pulmonale. Radiological distinction of pulmonary edema from parenchymal disease is not always easy in neonates, and a high index of suspicion is necessary to pursue the diagnosis. If what is thought to be lung disease is not getting better or is actually getting worse, then an echocardiogram done by someone expert in this field is often helpful; it may show the typically small left atrium, and it may even be possible to see the anomalous common pulmonary vein, or else to fail to find normal pulmonary veins entering the left atrium.[25] Any doubts should be resolved by cardiac catheterization. It is better do do what proves to be an unnecessary cardiac catheterization on an infant with lung disease than to miss a surgically correctable anomaly of the pulmonary veins. Some of these children who have less obstruction initially may present later at 6–12 months of age,[24] but then display the same features. After a few months of age, too, organic pulmonary arterial vascular disease begins to be seen,[26] and this increases the pulmonary vascular resistance further and intensifies the pulmonary arterial hypertension.

Surgical correction of these lesions in infancy carries a mortality of about 10% in the best hands. Those who survive usually do very well, with complete return of pulmonary vascular pressures and resistances to normal. Occasionally in the neonates, however, a fibrotic process at the anastomosis or around the pulmonary veins causes recurrence of the pulmonary edema and necessitates further surgery.

Other Left-Sided Obstructive Lesions

Entirely similar clinico-physiologic events are seen in the rare obstructive lesions of the left atrium—congenital mitral stenosis, supravalvar stenosing mitral ring, and cor triatriatum—as well as in stenotic lesions of one or more pulmonary veins. Finally, some children develop pulmonary venous hypertension and its complications because they have mitral or aortic atresia associated with a foramen ovale that is too small to allow free passage of blood from left to right atrium.

INCREASED PULMONARY VASCULAR RESISTANCE

Pathophysiology

The relationship of pressure (P) and flow (Q) of a Newtonian fluid passing through a straight glass tube is defined by the Poiseuille-Hagen relationship[27]:

$$\text{Resistance} = P/Q = (8/\pi)(l/r^4)(\eta)$$

where l is the length of the tube, r is its internal radius, and η is the viscosity of the fluid. Before applying this formula to the living organism, the differences between physical and biological systems must be evaluated.[28]

• Blood is not a Newtonian fluid. However, at normal hematocrits this makes little difference in practice.[29-31]

• The walls of vessels are not smooth because of the projections of endothelial cells. However, in large pulmonary arteries the relative roughness is negligible, and in small arteries the flow rates are too low for roughness to have much effect.[29]

- Blood vessels branch, curve, and taper. However, the degree of change and the relatively low flow rates make changes due to these effects inconsequential.[29,30]
- Blood flow into the lungs is markedly pulsatile, so that energy is needed to accelerate the blood at each ejection. This pulsatility normally adds about 30% to the pressure needed to perfuse the lungs, that is, 30% higher pressures are needed for pulsatile than steady perfusion.[32,33] However, these inertial energy losses cannot be large, because children with huge pulmonary blood flows due to atrial septal defects usually have normal pulmonary arterial mean pressures.
- Since pulmonary vessels are distensible, changing vascular pressures alters their radii. Therefore, pressure-flow relations are not linear, as in a glass tube, but curvilinear, even if Newtonian fluids are used as the perfusate.[34] Over small pressure differences the relation is almost linear, but ceases to be so over the full range of pressures encountered.
- The lung is made up of many blood vessels in parallel. These vessels are not all open all the time, especially in zone I, and may differ in radii in different lung zones because of gravitational effects and the effects of differing parenchymal elastic retraction on their walls.[35–37]

Despite these divergences from the simple physical system, we can by analogy with the formula for resistance in parallel use the Poiseuille relation, modified by a term k to allow for the numbers of vessels.

$$\text{Resistance} = (8\pi)(l/kr^4)(\eta)$$

This allows us to indicate the 3 main ways in which pulmonary vascular resistance can be changed since l, the vessel length, does not appear to change in disease.
- Altered viscosity, η.
- Altered numbers of vessels, k.
- Altered luminal radius, r.

Changes in Viscosity

Changes in viscosity can be due to changes in plasma viscosity, as in macroglobulinemia; to increased red cell number, as in polycythemia; to increased red cell aggregation, and to increased red cell rigidity,[29,38,39] as may occur in sickle cell disease, iron deficiency anemia, and many other disease states. In congenital heart disease, changes in viscosity are due almost always to polycythemia.

An increase in hematocrit will increase blood viscosity, the exact viscosity being markedly dependent on shear rate[29, 38, 39] (Figure 4). In most organs the resulting effect on organ flows is complicated by the relationship of oxygen supply and demand, and metabolic regulation of vascular tone adjusts flow over a wide range so that oxygen supply is adequate. Pulmonary vessels, however, do not show this metabolic regulation and so act like passive channels. At the flow rates that occur in the lungs, the relation of flow to hematocrit gives a good index of functional viscosity, and pulmonary vascular resistance rises approximately logarithmically with an increase in hematocrit[40-44] (Figure 5). As a rough guide, the pulmonary vascular resistance at a hematocrit of 70% is about twice as high as it would be in the same lung at a hematocrit of 45%. In effect, a hematocrit of 70% doubles the pressure drop across the lung for normal pulmonary blood flows, and explains some of the pulmonary arterial hypertension that is seen in children

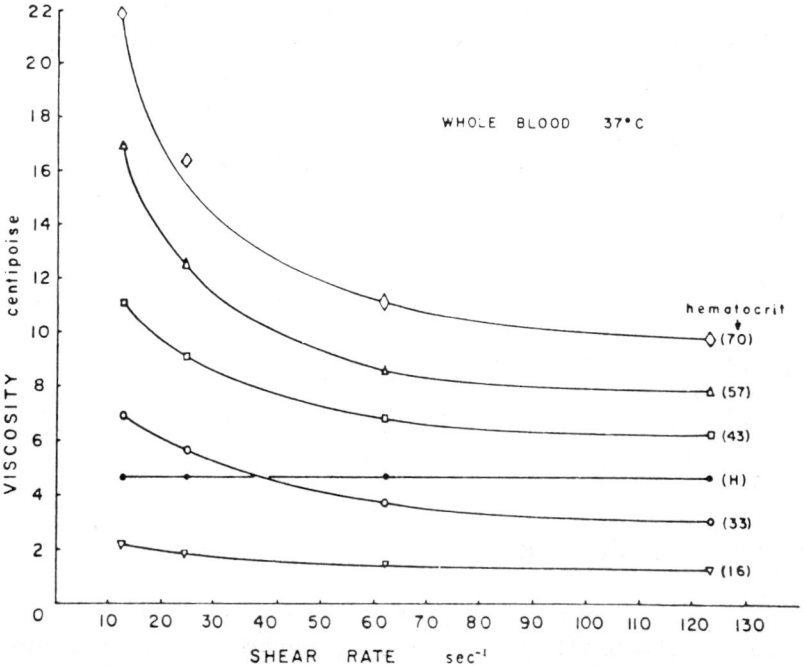

Figure 4. Diagram of relation between shear rate and whole blood viscosity. Viscosity is increased at low shear rates for all hematocrits, but the increase is marked only for hematocrits above normal. The line H is obtained using a Bureau of Standards calibration oil. (Reproduced from Wells and Merrill, J Clin Invest 1962;41:1591-1598 with permission of the authors and the American Society for Clinical Investigation.)

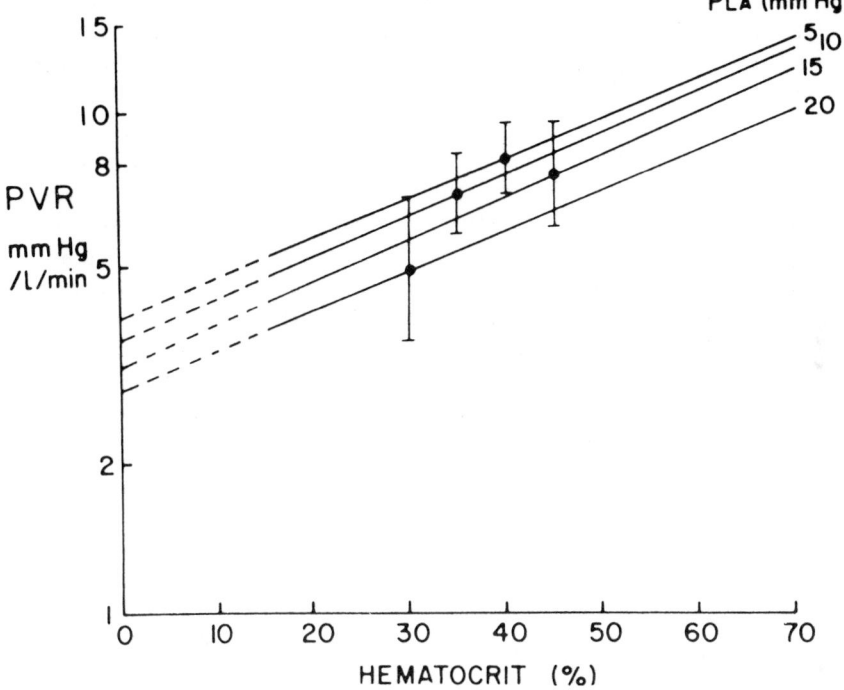

Figure 5. Relation of pulmonary vascular resistance (PVR) to hematocrit in the lungs of anesthetized dogs at 4 different left atrial pressures (Pla). Vertical bars represent one standard error from regression. Dashed lines are extrapolated from the data. Note that PVR is a logarithmic scale. (Reproduced from Agarwal, Paltoo and Palmer: J Appl Physiol 1970:29:866–871, with permission of the authors and the American Physiological Society.)

with high hematocrits and normal or increased pulmonary blood flows, for example, in complete transposition of the great arteries. Obviously, polycythemic children with decreased pulmonary blood flow, as in tetralogy of Fallot, may have an increased pulmonary vascular resistance due to the increased viscosity but normal or low pulmonary arterial pressures because of the low pulmonary blood flow.

Changes in Numbers of Vessels

Recruitment

A modest decrease in numbers of vessels will at first be compensated for by recruitment and dilation of the remaining vessels so that at rest there may be no pulmonary arterial hypertension. To bring out the effect of the missing vessels, it would be necessary to calculate the pulmonary vascular resistance during maximal exercise. In adult animals and man, about 75% of the lung vessels can be removed before resting pulmonary arterial pressure rises more than a few mm Hg[45–48]; with exercise, though, pulmonary arterial pressure will rise with less of the lung removed. This vascular reserve is absent in newborn infants for two reasons: first, they have no zone I and little zone II, so that recruitment of new vessels is limited or absent, and second, they have a raised pulmonary vascular resistance due to medial thickening that limits vasodilation. This may explain why pneumonectomy in newborn animals does cause pulmonary arterial hypertension[49,50] and why pulmonary arterial hypertension is common in children with one congenitaly absent pulmonary artery or in whom one pulmonary artery arises from the aorta.[51,52]

Reduction in Number of Intra-acinar Pulmonary Arteries

Pulmonary vessels can also be lost if they are occluded by emboli, although this is not a feature of congenital heart disease per se, or thrombi (to be discussed below), and their numbers may not increase at a normal rate in certain forms of congenital heart disease. The main pulmonary arterial branches that accompany the major airways form at about 16 weeks of gestation in the human fetus.[53] Subsequently, growth of vessels accompanies growth of peripheral acini, a continuous growth process that is complete by 8–10 years of age.[54,55] As new acini form they acquire new intra-acinar arteries, and as expected, the proportion of intra-acinar arteries to alveoli remains constant as the lung grows.[54,55] This proportionality between small intra-acinar arteries and alveoli is disturbed in many congenital heart lesions, and in particular there is a deficiency in the numbers of intra-acinar arteries (a reduced arterial: alveolar ratio) in lesions like pulmonary atresia,[56] experimental coarctation of the aorta in fetal lambs,[57] and especially in lesions with large left-to-right shunts like ventricular septal defects, atrioventricular (endocardial cushion) defects, and some instances of complete transposition of the great arteries.[58–60] In those patients with the highest pulmonary vascular resistance, the normal arterial: alveolar ratio of 1:10 was reduced to 1:30; in other words, 2 out of 3 intra-acinar arteries had not developed (or possibly had disappeared). Since these changes may take place in fetal life or within the first year after birth, the decreased vascular bed accentuates the chances of developing pulmonary arterial hypertension by making recruitment of vessels even less likely than it would have been.

Anomalies of Main Pulmonary Arteries

Finally, the total numbers of lung vessels perfused from the pulmonary artery may be reduced if one lung is hypoplastic, if there is only one pulmonary artery, or if one pulmonary artery originates from the aorta. There may be some differences in effects on pulmonary arterial pressure and resistance depending on which pulmonary artery is absent. Normally the right lung receives about 55% of the right ventricular output, so that one might conceive of a greater flow overload on the left lung if the right pulmonary artery is missing, than on the right lung if the left pulmonary artery is missing. However, the presence of associated lesions and the possibility of a compensatory increase in the vascular bed of the normally perfused lung make it impossible to decide if indeed there is a difference when one or the other pulmonary artery is missing.

Decreased Luminal Radius

The effects of decreased radius will obviously depend on how much decrease there is and how many vessels are affected. As with decrease in vessel number, moderate vascular changes will not alter resting pulmonary arterial pressure but will reduce the maximal vascular reserve. The major causes of decreased vascular radius are external compression, vasoconstriction, thickening of the wall, and partial thrombotic occlusion of vessels.

External Compression and Vasoconstriction

External compression of vessels can occur with marked lung inflation,[61] but in congenital heart disease is most likely due to pulmonary edema secondary to pulmonary venous hypertension.[11,12,15] Pulmonary vasoconstriction can experimentally be caused by a number of neurogenic or hormonal stimuli,[17] but there is no good evidence that any of these factors operate in people with congenital heart disease. On the other hand, alveolar hypoxia and acidemia are potent constrictors of pulmonary vessels and do occur in patients with congenital heart lesions. Metabolic acidemia is a serious consequence of severe hypoxemia that occurs in many infants with cyanotic heart disease, and the resulting increase in pulmonary vascular resistance further impedes pulmonary blood flow. Since, however, in the majority of these cyanotic heart lesions pulmonary flow is already low, significant pulmonary arterial hypertension is uncommon. However, alveolar hypoxia and pulmonary vasoconstriction do occur in congenital heart diseases if there is pulmonary edema, or if airways are compressed by an enlarged left atrium, or pulmonary artery[62] (Figure 6), or by vascular rings, or a

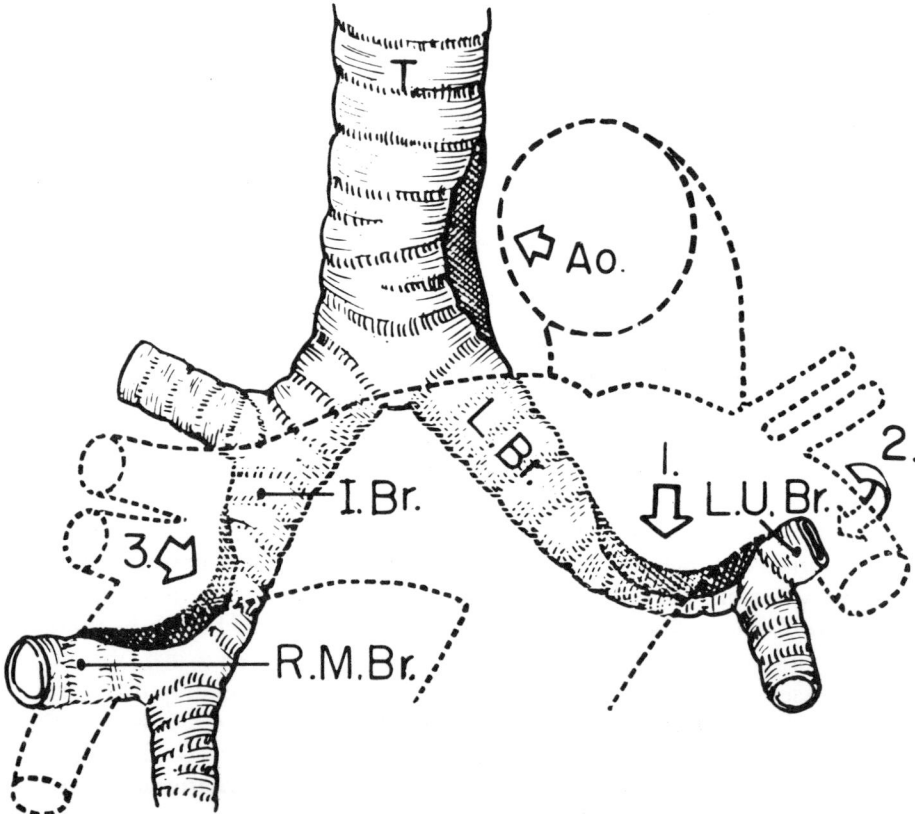

Figure 6. Common sites of compression of tracheobronchial tree by distended pulmonary arteries. 1) The superior aspect of the left bronchus (L.Br) where it is crossed by the left pulmonary artery. 2) The posterior aspect of the left upper bronchus (L.U.Br) where the left pulmonary artery hooks around it. 3) The intermediate bronchus (I.Br) and right middle bronchus (R.M.Br) where they are crossed by the artery to the right lower lobe. (Reproduced from Stanger, Lucas and Edwards: Pediatrics 1969;43:760–769 with permission of the authors and the American Academy of Pediatrics.

pulmonary artery sling.[63,64] Pulmonary edema and local alveolar hypoxia are thus the most likely causes of extrinsic pulmonary vascular narrowing in congenital heart disease.

If patients live at high altitude—and a large proportion of the world's population lives more than 1,500 meters above sea level—then the resulting alveolar hypoxia will add to the pulmonary vasoconstriction and pulmonary hypertension.

Thickening of the Vessel Wall

This is an important cause of pulmonary arterial hypertension and a raised pulmonary vascular resistance in congenital heart disease.[65] The thicker wall in any given sized artery will narrow the lumen, and the thickening can affect the medial muscle or the intima; in addition, thrombi attached to the intima also thicken the wall and further narrow the lumen.

An increased mass of the medial muscle is found whenever there is any pulmonary arterial hypertension, and represents the response of muscle to increased isometric or isotonic work. It is therefore found whenever there is pulmonary arterial hypertension due to a large communication between the ventricles or between aorta and pulmonary artery,[60,66] to pulmonary venous obstruction,[18,19,26] or to complete transposition of the great arteries with or without associated defects.[67,73] Certain lesions with high pulmonary blood flows but normal pulmonary arterial mean pressures (atrial septal defects, some simple transposition of the great arteries, some total anomalous venous connection) may also have more than the normal amount of pulmonary arterial smooth muscle manifested mainly by extension of the muscle more distally than expected for age.[54,60] Although in these lesions pulmonary arterial mean pressure may be normal, the increased pulse pressure is associated with both a higher pulmonary arterial systolic pressure and more distension of the vessel wall, and both of these are stimuli to increased muscle mass. It may be difficult to assess the increased cross-sectional muscle mass because the vessels are dilated.[74] To allow for this problem, special methods are needed to identify the increased amount of muscle. Some investigators have related the cross-sectional area of medial muscle to the cross-sectional area of the adjacent lung parenchyma[66,74] or to the estimated total length of the internal elastic lamina;[71] others have related medial wall thickness to age and the type of associated airway.[54,60]

Most of the increased muscle mass is due to hyperplasia rather than to hypertrophy. The new muscle cells are probably formed locally from mesenchymal cells.[75]

One of the most important causes of pulmonary arterial hypertension in congenital heart disease is intimal hyperplasia which, in its advanced stages, may prevent successful surgery of the defects and eventually kill the patient. Six stages of pulmonary vascular disease from muscular hypertrophy to advanced intimal and medial disease were described first by Heath and Edwards,[18,76] although some of these findings were described earlier by Dammann and Ferencz.[77] Muscular hypertrophy of small pulmonary arteries, as described above, is grade I (Figure 7a). Grade II vascular disease is manifested by medial hypertrophy and intimal hyperplasia varying from minimal thickening to thickening that almost occludes the vessel (Figure 7b). In grade III, these intimal cells are replaced by hyalinized, collagenous tissue in what often resembles a concentric "onion-skin" lesion in the artery (Figure 7c). Late grade III lesions may be associated with luminal thrombosis and recanalization. Grade IV is characterized by plexiform lesions, locally dilated segments of an artery with a thin wall showing tissue damage, and with the lumen filled with cellular septa, between which are capillary-like channels. These lesions usually occur just after the artery has branched off from its parent vessel. There may also be clusters of thin-walled dilated arteries with patent lumina (angiomatoid lesions); these lesions also occur near the origin of the arterial branch (Figure 7d). In grade V, there is extensive fibrosis of the media and intima of the small arteries, which appear as rigid dilated tubes. The various dilation lesions of grade IV are still present, and the very fragile vessels often rupture. As a result, small foci of hemosiderosis are characteristic of this stage. Finally, grade VI is an acute arteritis with fibrinoid necrosis (Figure 7e).

There is some disagreement about the order of appearance of the last 3 grades. Some experiments have shown that fibrinoid necrosis may follow acute pulmonary vasoconstriction and hypertension, with a subsequent inflammatory reaction.[18,19] The plexiform lesions of grade IV appear to develop in areas that have undergone fibrinoid necrosis; they may, therefore, indicate a state of proliferative repair.[78,79] The timing and pathogenesis of grade V lesions are unknown. In general, grades IV to VI overlap and represent advanced disease.

The cells that occur in the hyperplastic intima of grade II lesions come from the media, and may be seen crossing the internal elastic lamina and have features of smooth muscle. Whether they come from muscle cells or other mesenchymal cells is unknown.[75,80]

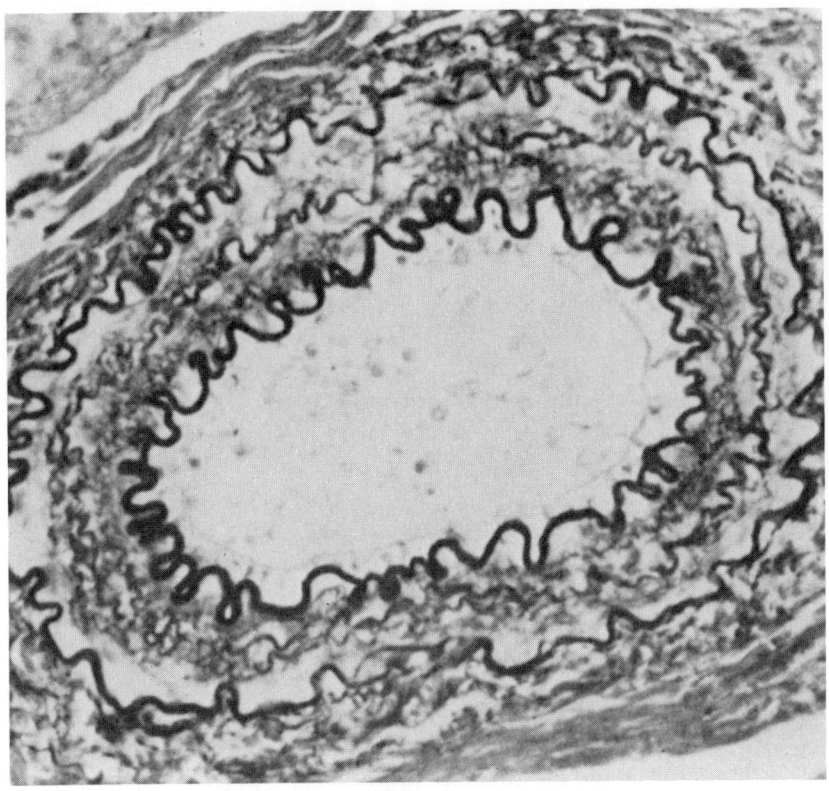

Figure 7a.

Figure 7. *Histological features of pulmonary vascular disease. a. Grade I.   The thick media is shown between the well outlined internal and external elastic laminae. There is no intimal thickening. (× 250) b. Grade II.   The media is thick, and the lumen is partly occluded by cellular intimal proliferation. (× 250) c. Grade III.   Almost total occlusion of lumen by fibroelastic relatively acellular tissue. (× 150) d. Grade V.   Arrow shows a thin walled, dilated branch of a muscular pulmonary artery with some cellular proliferation, which is one type of plexiform lesion. To the right is the angiomatoid lesion which has come from the same artery. (× 100) e. Grade VI.   Acute necrotizing arteritis with rings of fibrin in the media and an infiltration with neutrophils. (× 100) (All reproduced from Wagenvoort, Heath and Edwards:* Pathology of the Pulmonary Vasculature, 1964, *with permission of the authors and Charles C Thomas, Publisher, Springfield, Illinois.)*

The first person to indicate a possible mechanism of these intimal changes was Fry in 1968.[81] He developed methods for measuring shearing forces made by blood moving past the (stationary) endothelium, and then studied the acute effects of increased shearing forces obtained by constricting the abdominal aorta in the dog. When shear-

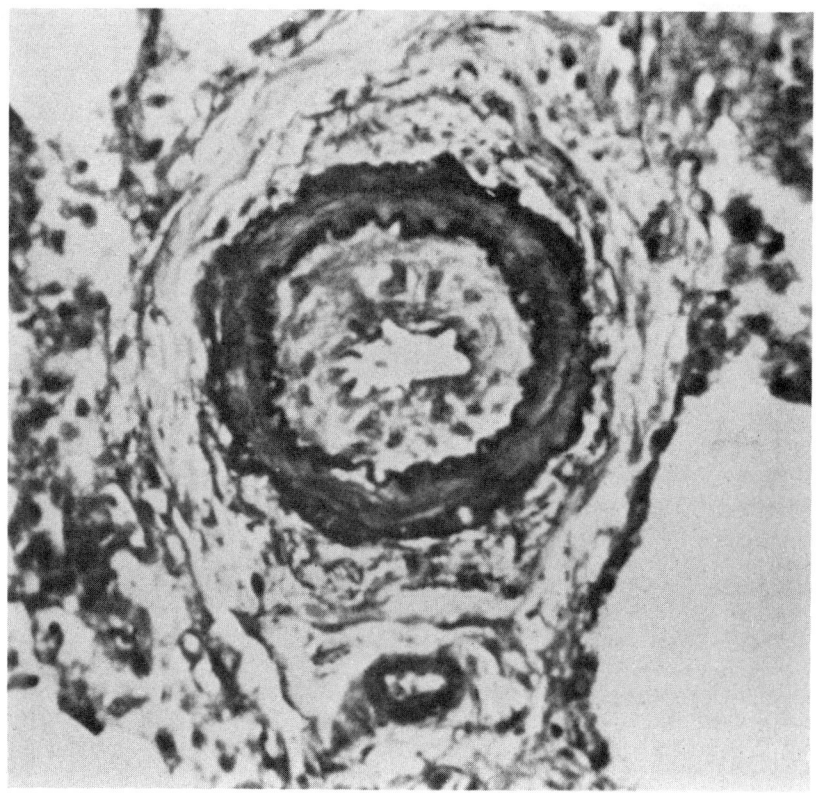

Figure 7b.

ing forces were more than 3 times the normal value, there was endothelial damage. Endothelial cells were sometimes stripped away from the intima, or remained in place but were necrotic, or else looked normal on light microscopy but were abnormally permeable to lipoproteins.

The link between these acute studies and the hyperplastic intimal changes found after many years in patients has not been defined, but studies of atherogenesis in systemic arteries suggest a plausible sequence of events. Endothelial injury, as might be caused by excessive shear forces, causes local platelet adherence and activation; the platelets may be attracted by exposed basement membrane or products liberated by damaged cells, and the endothelial damage reduces local prostacyclin (PGI_2) production which normally acts to prevent platelet adhesion. Once the platelets adhere and degranulate, they release many substances: ADP promotes more platelet aggregation; phospho-

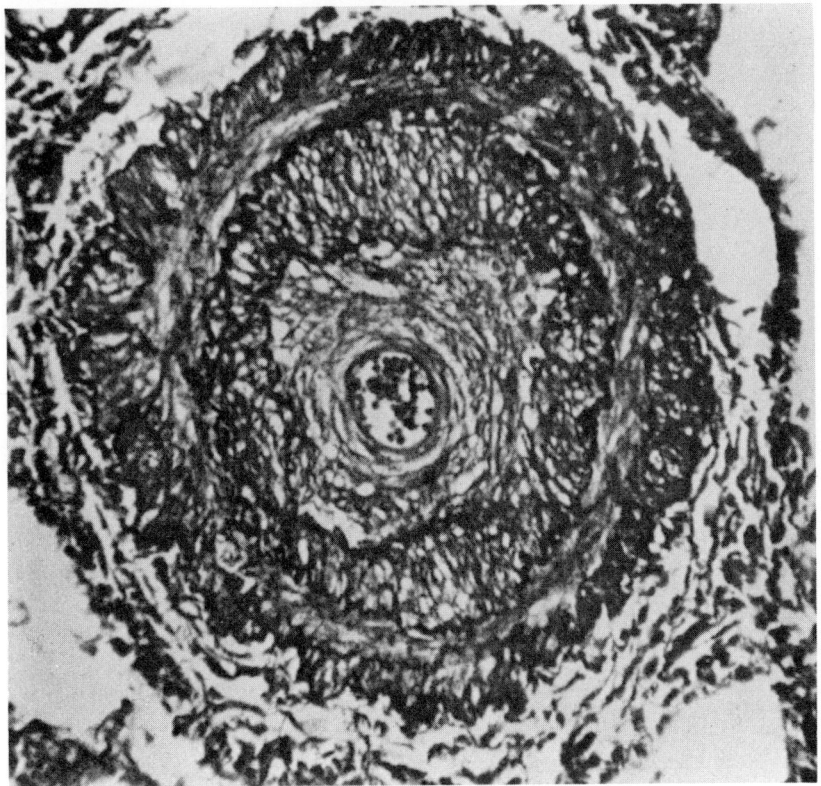

Figure 7c.

lipase A_2 in the vessel and platelet membranes is activated to release arachidonic acid with resultant formation of thromboxane A_2 which causes more persistent platelet aggregation; and a partly characterized mitogenic factor is liberated, and this evokes a proliferative response of smooth muscle cells which migrate into the intima.[82-88] In systemic vessels these lesions are followed by deposition of cholesterol which does occur in hypertensive pulmonary arteries but at a slower rate and to a lesser extent.

Thrombotic narrowing or occlusion of small pulmonary arteries may be secondary to these events or it may, perhaps, have other origins in certain patients in whom the typical factors that cause endothelial damage are absent.[89] Whether there is an independent hypercoagulable state to cause these microthrombi is still disputed.[90-92]

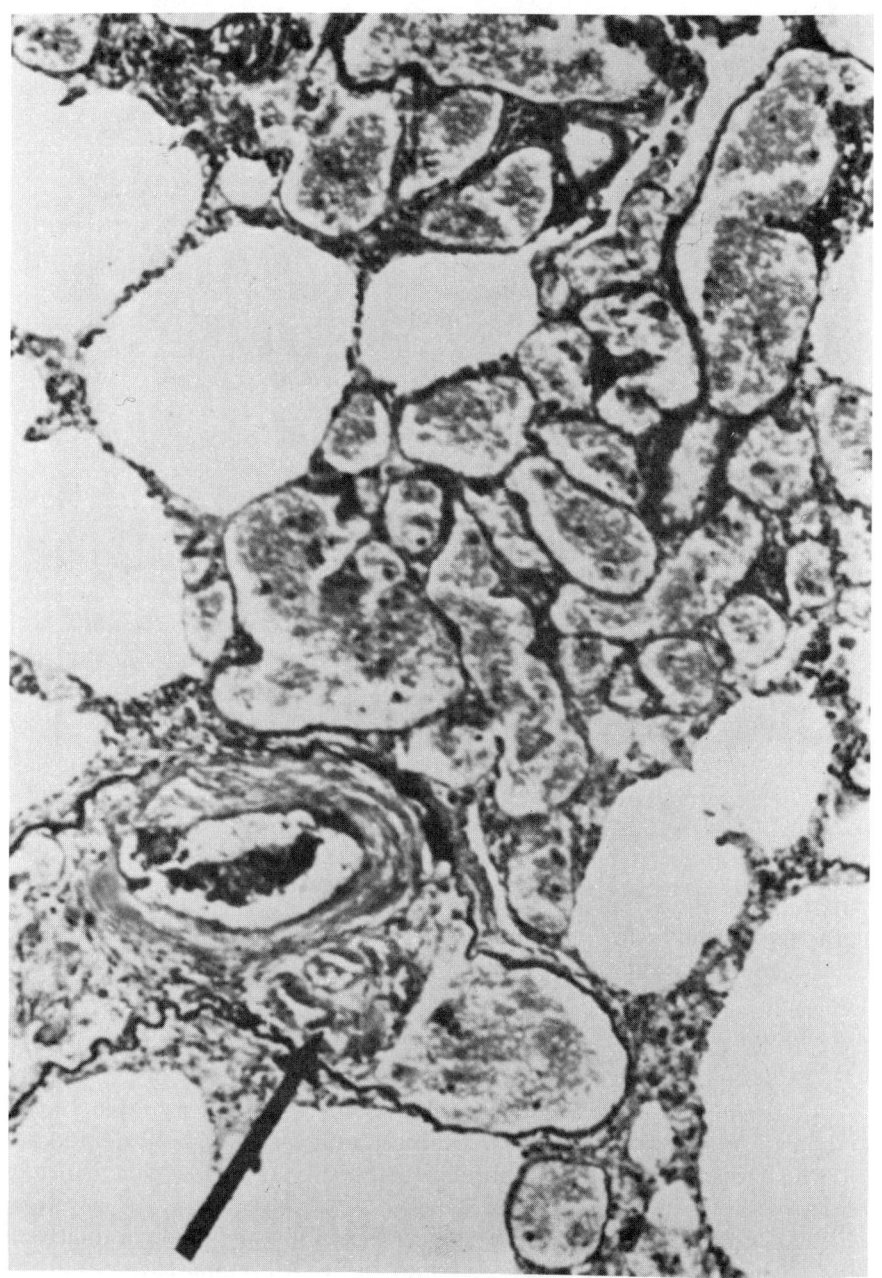

Figure 7d.

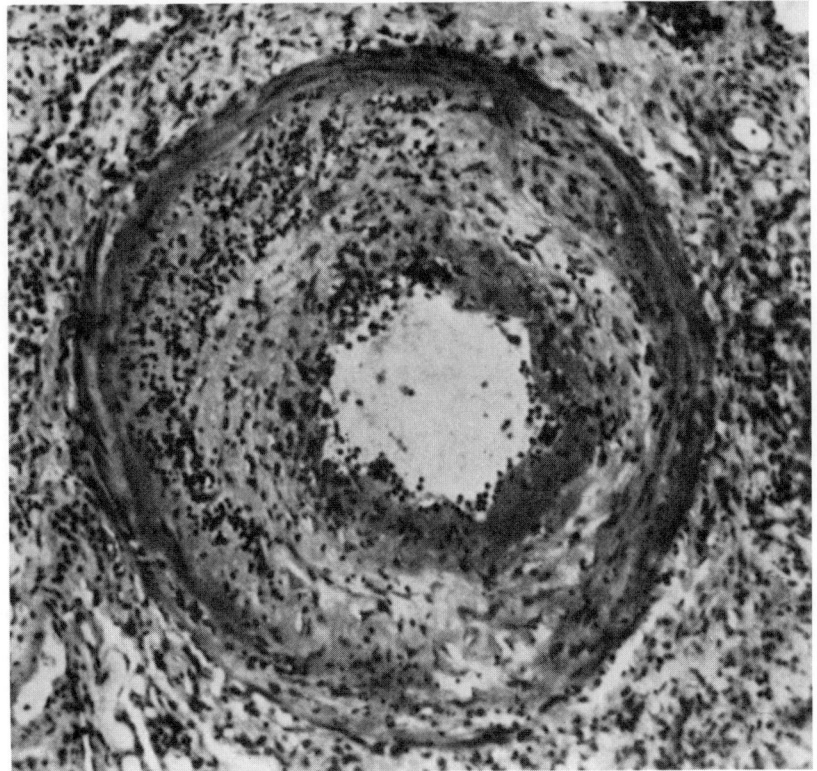

Figure 7e.

Diagnostic Assessment

Assessing the effects of an increased blood viscosity in polycythemia can be done simply by determining the hematocrit and estimating from graphs what proportion of the increased pulmonary arterial pressure might be due to polycythemia (Figure 5).

Judgment that there is extravascular compression, for example, by edema fluid, is made readily by the clinical setting, although the degree to which this contributes to pulmonary arterial hypertension is difficult to assess.

Evaluating vasoconstriction usually goes hand in hand with evaluating vessel number and the degree and cause of luminal narrowing, since these mechanisms frequently co-exist. When medial thickening (grade I pulmonary vascular disease) is present, there is usually some tone, possibly increased, in the smooth muscle; whether this is an example of myogenic tone[93] or not is unknown. It is often possible to reduce this tone by giving the patient 100% oxygen to breathe or by injecting acetylcholine or tolazoline into the pulmonary artery. By measuring pressures and flows before and after giving these agents, it is possible to determine if there has been a fall in pulmonary vascular resistance. If the decrease in resistance is dramatic, for example, from 12 to 3 units/m^2, then it is likely that there is relatively little intimal damage and that most of the increased resistance is purely vasoconstrictive or muscular in origin. However, with less impressive changes of resistance there are numerous pitfalls in this assessment, not the least of which is the accuracy of calculating pulmonary flows if they are increased so that arteriovenous oxygen differences across the lung are small. Other difficulties of interpretation have been described elsewhere.[28] It is important to appreciate that even with no intimal disease and complete muscular relaxation, the pulmonary vascular resistance will not be completely normal because the thickened medial muscle by its bulk will still narrow the lumen.

Estimating vessel number and the extent of intimal damage is best made by biopsy examination of the lung[60]; it is even possible to examine frozen sections taken at the time of surgery to aid in deciding whether to proceed with surgical correction of a defect.[94] Fortunately, the changes of vessel number and distal extension of muscle and muscle thickness are evenly distributed in all lung lobes.[95] Apart from biopsy, assessment of pulmonary vascular disease can be made semiquantitatively[96] or quantitatively[97] by wedged angiography; the angiogram correlates quite well with what is found on light microscopy of a biopsy (Figure 8). The wedged angiogram is best done with magnification, and if care is taken to follow the descriptions given[96,97] causes no significant complications.

An important issue is presented when assessing the pulmonary vascular resistance in patients with one pulmonary artery. Since the total flow now goes through one lung, the interpretation of a given value for pulmonary vascular resistance must of necessity be changed. This point has been put forward by Mair et al.[98] in evaluating patients with a truncus arteriosus and one pulmonary artery. They gave as an example a patient with a truncus arteriosus and 2 pulmonary arteries, and a fixed pulmonary vascular resistance equal to 20 units/m^2 in each

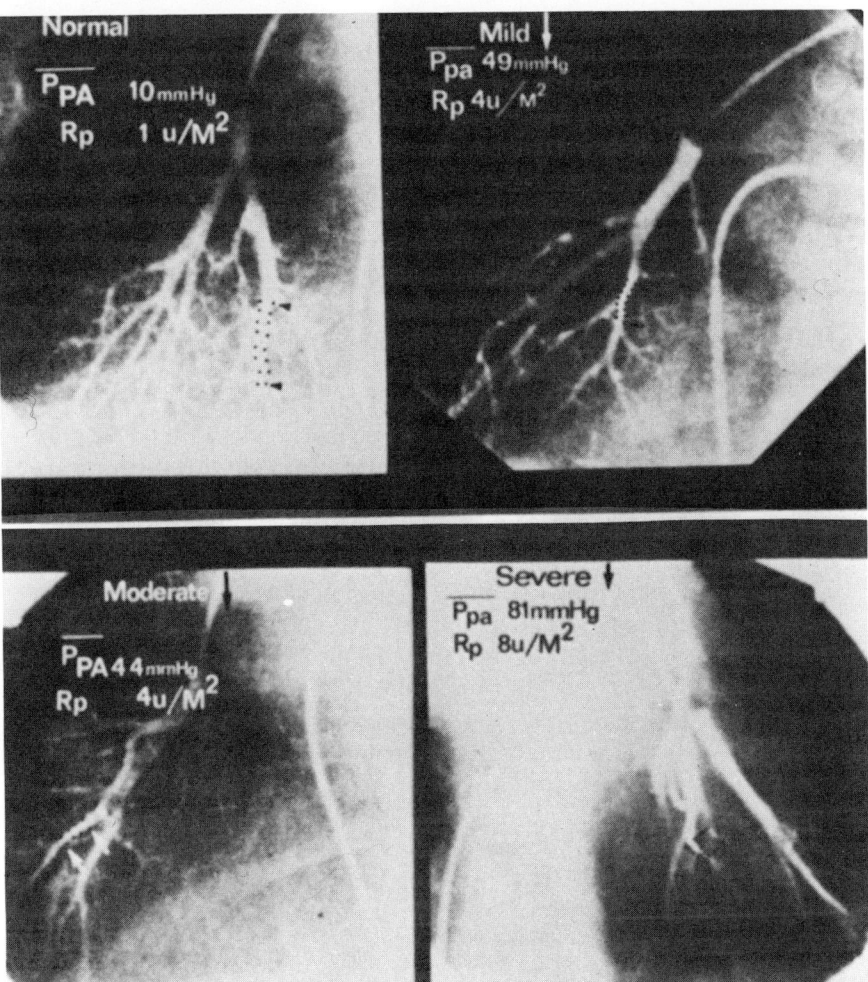

Figure 8. Wedge pulmonary angiograms from 4 patients with pulmonary vascular resistances ranging from normal to very high and angiographic appearances ranging from normal to severely abnormal. The arrows indicate luminal diameters of 2.5 mm (upper arrow) and 1.5 mm (lower arrow). These arrows move closer to each other as the vascular disease gets worse, indicating more rapid tapering of the small arteries with vascular disease. In addition, as vascular disease increases there are fewer small vessels seen, and the background haze due to filling of very small vessels gets less and then disappears. (Reproduced from Rabinovitch, Keane, Fellows, Castenada, Reid: Circulation 1981;63:152−164 with permission of the authors and the American Heart Association.

artery. Then the total pulmonary vascular resistance (R) would be calculated as:

$$1/R_T = 1/R_L + 1/R_R,$$

where R_L and R_R are the resistances in the left and right pulmonary arteries respectively. Therefore,

$$1/R_T = 1/20 + 1/20 = 1/10, \text{ and } R_T = 10 \text{ units/m}^2.$$

If now one pulmonary artery were ligated, then

$$1/R_T = 1/R_L = 1/20 \text{ and } R_T = 20 \text{ units/m}^2$$

In this circumstance, the histological correlate would be that for a resistance value of 10 units/m^2, not the more severe disease implied by a resistance of 20 units/m^2.[98,99] They therefore recommended that the pulmonary vascular resistance in the normally supplied lung should be assessed by dividing the calculated pulmonary vascular resistance by 2. As they pointed out, this argument is oversimplified because it does not allow for resistances that are not fixed, but their biopsy findings and surgical results in this group support their approach. It is important to note, however, that this assessment at a point in time does not imply that there is no danger in forcing total pulmonary flow through one lung.

Clinical Syndromes

Effects of Polycythemia

Any of the cyanotic heart diseases can cause severe polycythemia, which contributes not only to an elevated pulmonary vascular resistance and arterial pressure but may also accelerate the onset of organic pulmonary vascular disease. In addition, thrombo-embolic episodes as have been described in tetralogy of Fallot[100] or complete transposition of the great arteries[67,89] will reduce vascular radius and number, and can cause markedly increased pulmonary vascular resistance and pulmonary arterial hypertension.

Effects of Left Atrial and Pulmonary Arterial Hypertension

Lesions causing pulmonary venous hypertension (see above) may produce pulmonary edema which, by direct vascular compression or causing alveolar hypoxia, may raise pulmonary vascular resistance and further increase pulmonary arterial pressure. These two components may also contribute to the pulmonary arterial hypertension that occurs in patients with large left-to-right shunts. Finally, the enlarged left atrium and pulmonary artery that are characteristic of children with large left-to-right shunts may cause airway compression and alveolar hypoxia.[62] The extreme example of this is found in children who have the syndrome of tetralogy of Fallot with an absent pulmonary valve. As an associated lesion they have massively dilated right and left pulmonary arteries which compress bronchi, cause serious pulmonary problems, and incidentally cause pulmonary arterial hypertension from the combined effects of hypoxic pulmonary vasoconstriction plus the left-to-right shunt through the ventricular septal defect.

Absence or Aortic Origin of One Pulmonary Artery

Early in development, when the human fetus is about 6 mm long, 3 paired aortic arches (the third, fourth, and sixth) connect the trunco-aortic sac at the base of the heart to the paired dorsal aortae. From the middle of the sixth arches 2 primitive pulmonary arteries arise (Figure 9). If development continues normally, then the trunco-aortic sac separates into ascending aorta and main pulmonary artery; the proximal parts of the sixth arches arise from this main pulmonary artery and convey blood to the true primitive pulmonary arteries; and the distal part of each sixth arch becomes the ductus arteriosus which normally disappears on the right side.

Absence of one pulmonary artery will occur if the proximal part of a sixth arch does not form or disappears; the pulmonary artery will then be attached to the ductus arteriosus, and when this closes there will be no attachment of the intrapulmonary artery to aorta or main pulmonary artery. That lung will be nourished only by multiple small bronchial arteries. The origin of one pulmonary artery from the aorta might occur if the division of the trunco-aortic sac is abnormal so that the proximal part of one-sixth arch becomes attached to ascending

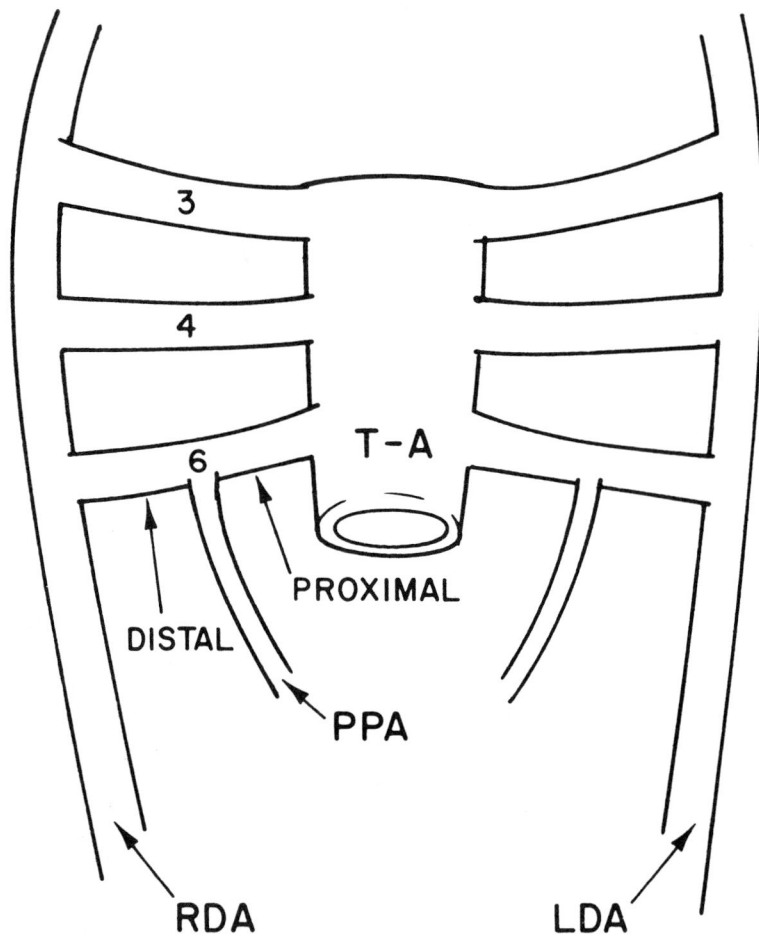

Figure 9. Diagram of development of main pulmonary arteries. The 3 major aortic arches (3, 4, 6) come off the trunco-aortic sac (T-A) and join the right and left dorsal aortae (RDA, LDA). From the 6th arch on each side the primitive pulmonary artery (PPA) enters the embryonic lung. The proximal parts of the 6th arch become the main pulmonary arteries, and the distal parts become the ductus arteriosi.

aorta rather than to main pulmonary artery. Growth patterns and migration of vessels often carry the origin of this aberrant pulmonary artery away from the ascending aorta. Finally, it is possible for this aberrant pulmonary artery to regress, thereby giving another mechanism for absence of one pulmonary artery.[51,64,101]

Absence of one pulmonary artery may occur as an isolated congenital vascular lesion, or may be associated with tetralogy of Fallot, truncus arteriosus, or occasionally other lesions. It is usually the left pulmonary artery that is absent when there are other lesions. In the absence of other lesions, the absent pulmonary artery is usually on the side opposite to the aortic arch.[51]

If there were no associated cardiac lesions, Pool et al.[51] found that 19% of the patients had pulmonary arterial hypertension. On the other hand, when there was an increased pulmonary blood flow in addition, then 88% had pulmonary arterial hypertension. Evidently perfusion of one lung with the total cardiac output is near the limit of what the newborn infant can tolerate without incurring permanent vascular damage; any added stress from a left-to-right shunt usually exceeds the threshold for causing pulmonary hypertension.

Origin of one pulmonary artery from the aorta has a similar effect. The lung with a normally attached pulmonary artery receives about twice the normal flow and can develop pulmonary arterial changes and organic pulmonary vascular disease. The lung receiving its blood supply from the aorta can also be damaged, but is frequently protected by a stenosis at the aortic origin of the abnormal pulmonary artery.[52]

There are variants of this single pulmonary artery theme. In complete transposition of the great arteries, the obliquity of the pulmonary artery often results in preferential flow into the right pulmonary artery. As Muster et al.[102] have shown, this distribution can lead to failure of development and even obliteration of the arteries to the left lung so that perfusion is exclusively to the right lung (Figure 10). This obviously increases the risk of pulmonary vascular disease in that lung, particularly since this risk is always present in any form of complete transposition of the great arteries.[67,73] A similar maldistribution is at times seen in patients with a truncus arteriosus, where it may contribute to pulmonary vascular disease. Preferential distribution may also occur after a Waterston anastomosis (aorto-right pulmonary artery anastomosis) is done for pulmonary or tricuspid atresia. Kinking of the pulmonary artery may direct all flow into the right pulmonary artery, which becomes hypertensive and develops vascular disease whereas the left pulmonary artery, cut off from almost all flow, becomes hypoplastic and unsuitable for further surgical repair.

INCREASED PULMONARY BLOOD FLOW

Pathophysiology

As mentioned above, increased pulmonary blood flow per se is not a sufficient cause for pulmonary arterial hypertension, as indicated by

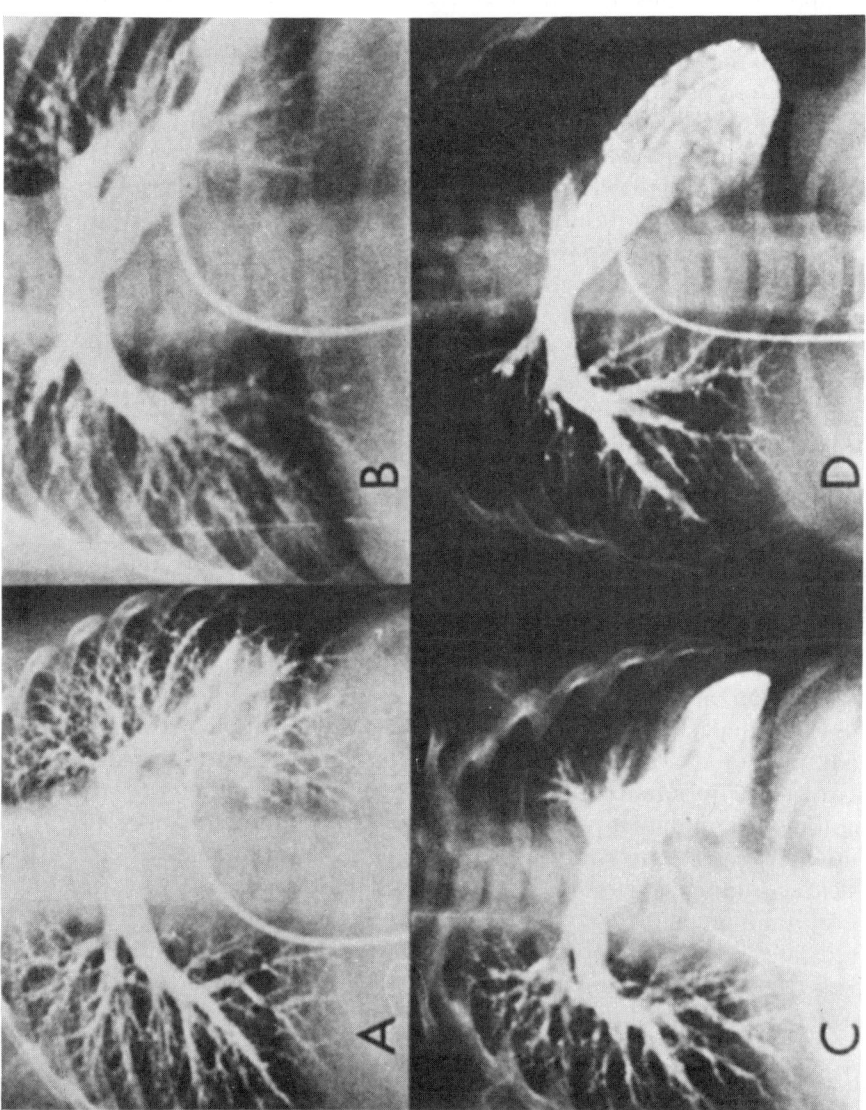

Figure 10. Pulmonary angiograms showing variable degrees of maldistribution of flow to each lung in 4 patients with d-transposition of the great arteries. Evolution from pattern in panel A to panel D has also been observed in the same patient. (Reproduced from Muster, Paul, van Grondelle, Conway,: Am J Cardiol 1976;38:352–361 with permission of the authors and the American Journal of Cardiology.)

the normal pulmonary arterial mean pressures noted in people with huge pulmonary blood flows due to exercise or atrial septal defects. The added factor necessary is usually an elevated pulmonary vascular resistance, even if this is not obvious. The classical example of high flow pulmonary arterial hypertension is found in patients with large ventricular septal defects. Because there is a large communication between the ventricles, the pulmonary arterial systolic pressure will be high, even systemic. There is thus medial hypertrophy of the small pulmonary arteries which is manifestly abnormal by 2 months after birth.[66] This medial hypertrophy narrows the lumen and increases pulmonary vascular resistance above what would be expected for the high flow. In other words, what is abnormal is the failure of pulmonary vascular resistance to fall to very low levels—below 1 unit/m^2; this failure indicates that there is a vascular abnormality.

The pulmonary vascular resistance in these patients and those with patent ductus arteriosus is not fixed at birth, but probably declines from the high fetal level, much as occurs in the normal infant but probably at a slower rate[1] (Figure 2). For this reason pulmonary blood flow may not be high immediately after birth; indeed, there may be no murmur detected when the child is in the newborn nursery. As pulmonary vascular resistance falls over the next few months the pulmonary flow increases. This growing left ventricular volume load, added to the child's increasing activity and the "physiologic" postnatal fall of hemoglobin, eventually causes overt congestive heart failure. In term infants, heart failure usually becomes manifest between 6 and 12 weeks after birth. In preterm infants, however, congestive heart failure comes on early, often within the first week after birth. Whether this early onset represents a high pulmonary blood flow due to decreased reactivity of the immature pulmonary vessels,[103] decreased distensibility of the immature ventricle,[104] abnormal pulmonary water exchange or a combination of these is uncertain.

In term infants, then, the pulmonary blood flow rises only after pulmonary vascular resistance falls; the increase in flow thus depends on the fall in pulmonary vascular resistance, so that the left-to-right shunt of a ventricular septal defect or patent ductus arteriosus has been termed a *dependent* shunt.[1] By contrast, many children with atrioventricular (endocardial cushion) defects have left ventricular to right atrial shunts. The amount of shunting here depends only on the size of the left ventricular to right atrial communication since the shunt is from a high pressure to a low pressure chamber. The shunt is thus independent of pulmonary vascular resistance and is termed an *independent* or *obligatory* shunt.[1] A similar obligatory shunt occurs with a large arteriovenous fistula in the head, liver, or occasionally the extremities; in these, the huge venous return coupled with the normally high neonatal pulmonary vascular resistance maintains a high pulmonary arterial pressure.

If the large pulmonary blood flow and high pressure are maintained for several months, the intimal changes of grade II begin and gradually progress. In addition, as mentioned above, failure of normal numbers of intra-acinar arteries to develop adds to the increase in pulmonary vascular resistance. The timing of onset of these changes and their rate of progression are variable. Nevertheless, substantial increases of pulmonary vascular resistance are common by 1 year after birth, and by 2 years after birth the pulmonary vascular changes have often progressed so far as to be irreversible and to preclude successful surgery.[105,106] The combination of systemic pressures and very high blood flows in the pulmonary artery is particularly dangerous, but anyone with pulmonary arterial pressures more than 50% of systemic pressures and flows more than twice normal is at risk of developing pulmonary vascular disease.

Sometimes pulmonary vascular disease is accelerated in these shunt lesions. Newfeld et al.[69] observed that infants with complete transposition of the great arteries and a large ventricular septal defect or patent ductus arteriosus developed advanced pulmonary vascular disease if the shunt was not reduced by closure of the defect or banding the pulmonary artery by 4 months of age. Our own personal experience here has shown accelerated pulmonary vascular disease to be common in infants over 4 months of age with a truncus arteriosus. The explanation for this accelerated change is unknown but may reflect in part the added shear stress due to raised hematocrit.

By contrast, pulmonary vascular disease is characteristically delayed in patients with large atrial septal defects; it rarely occurs under 20 years of age. The likely explanation for the late onset of a raised pulmonary vascular resistance and pulmonary arterial hypertension in these patients is that although these are dependent shunts the shunt is between 2 low pressure chambers. Given a large inter-atrial communication, the direction and amount of shunting depend upon the relative distensibility of the two ventricles since most of the shunt takes place in diastole. At birth the 2 ventricles have similar wall thicknesses and thus probably have similar distensibilities; little atrial shunting will occur. As pulmonary vascular resistance and arterial pressure fall normally postnatally, the left ventricle gradually becomes thicker than the right ventricle, and presumably becomes less distensible than the right ventricle. A left-to-right atrial shunt develops and progressively enlarges as the right ventricle becomes more and more distensible. In this way the atrial shunt develops only after pulmonary arterial pressure and resistance have fallen to low levels, so that in effect the falling pulmonary arterial pressure draws the shunt across the atrial septum. This is why pulmonary vascular resistance is abnormally low in atrial septal defects and why the small pulmonary arteries are relatively dilated.[74] However, as pointed out above, the total medial mass may be increased and there is early distal extension of muscle.[60] Even though pulmonary blood flow may be torrential, the velocity of flow through these dilated vessels is much lower than it would be for the same flow in a ventricular septal defect in which the vessels are narrowed by medial hypertrophy. The shear stress on the endothelium is thus much lower in atrial than in ventricular septal defects, and the rate of intimal damage is therefore much reduced.

Another possible factor in the delayed onset of pulmonary vascular disease when there is a secundum atrial septal defect is that the left atrial and pulmonary venous pressures are low. With a large ventricular septal defect, however, left atrial pressure is usually high; this pressure elevation adds to the pulmonary hypertension, thereby accelerating the onset and course of the pulmonary vascular disease.

Diagnostic Assessment

As pointed out, the calculated pulmonary vascular resistance may appear to be normal when there is a large ventricular septal defect. Frequently the resistance figure is $2-3$ units/m^2, under normal upper limits. However, these limits are for normal flows, and should probably be under 1 unit/m^2 at high flows. An even easier way to decide if pulmonary vascular resistance is increased is to examine the pressure drop across the lung; any mean pressure drop over about $10-12$ mm Hg indicates an increased pulmonary vascular resistance.

Once an increased vascular resistance is diagnosed it must be evaluated to find out if it is due to hypoxic vasoconstriction, muscular hypertrophy, or intimal change. This has been discussed above, but it is worth re-emphasizing that the assessment of the extent of each of these causes of a raised pulmonary vascular resistance is difficult. It is made by a combination of response of the resistance to 100% oxygen or to vasodilators, by wedged angiography or, in the last resort, by open biopsy examination of lung tissue.

Clinical Syndromes

Any child with a large left-to-right shunt and pulmonary arterial hypertension is at risk of developing pulmonary vascular disease. This includes large ventricular septal defect, large patent ductus arteriosus, atrioventricular (cushion) defect, truncus arteriosus, tricuspid atresia with transposition or a large ventricular septal defect, and transposition of the great arteries with a large ventricular septal defect or patent ductus arteriosus. Some of these may develop accelerated vascular disease, as mentioned above. On the other hand, patients with large pulmonary blood flows but low pressures, as with atrial septal defects or a few ventricular septal defects, may develop pulmonary vascular disease after a lag of 20 or more years. That the pulmonary vascular disease is not an independent lesion is shown by the fact that it can be prevented by early closure of the defect or banding of the pulmonary artery.[69,107]

In infants with large left-to-right shunts, congestive heart failure is usually manageable with medical treatment. Some lesions like a patent ductus arteriosus are suitable for early surgery since the operation is simple and safe. Other lesions like truncus arteriosus warrant repair in the first 6 months after birth to reduce the risk of developing severe pulmonary vascular disease as well as to improve the infant's health. On the other hand, ventricular septal defects may warrant more conservative management because of the relatively high incidence of spontaneous closure or diminution in size of the defect.[107] If conservative management is chosen and the usual medical regimen of digoxin and diuretics seems ineffective, manipulation of the balance between pulmonary and systemic vascular resistances has been advocated. The infusion of sodium nitroprusside during the cardiac catheterization of infants with large ventricular septal defects was shown to increase the pulmonary-to-systemic flow ratio because of a decrease in systemic flow[108]; there was a modest fall of pulmonary arterial pressure and pulmonary vascular resistance. Because this acute effect was not what is wanted clinically, the same investigators studied the effects of hydralazine in a similar group of infants.[109] With this agent systemic flow increased and pulmonary flows, pressures, and vascular resistances were unchanged. The improved systemic flow might well be expected to improve growth and organ function of these infants, but the stress on the pulmonary vascular bed is not altered. A different approach was used by Lister and colleagues.[110] They made measurements at cardiac catheterization of 9 infants with large ventricular septal defects before and after an isovolemic exchange transfusion that raised average hemoglobin concentrations from 9.9 to 14.6 g/dl and average hematocrits from 30 to 45%. Systemic and pulmonary vascular resistances rose, and systemic and pulmonary flows as well as the left-to-right shunt decreased. Systemic oxygen transport (the product of systemic flow and arterial oxygen content) increased after the transfusion. All these effects would be expected to reduce congestive heart failure and ventricular volume overloads, with consequent clinical improvement. Once again, pulmonary vascular stresses remain elevated as long as the defect remains large.

If conservative therapy is followed, it is essential to realize that both a decrease in size of the defect and a rise in pulmonary vascular resistance will at first produce the same results. Because both reduce the left ventricular volume load, the heart becomes smaller and less active, and radiologic and echocardiographic signs of a large shunt regress. Clinical signs of congestive heart failure decrease: less tachypnea and tachycardia, less hepatomegaly, lesser need for medication, better appetite and growth. In theory these two causes of improvement could be differentiated by the fact that in a closing defect pulmonary arterial pressure will fall, so that pulmonic closure will not be so loud and right ventricular hypertrophy will eventually regress. It should be emphasized, however, that these changes cannot be detected early. The intensity of pulmonic closure is difficult to quantitate, and regression of right ventricular hypertrophy lags by many months the fall of pulmonary arterial pressure, particularly because there may still be a right ventricular volume load. It may be possible by careful echocardiography to determine if the defect is getting smaller. In general, though, the only way to make sure that pulmonary vascular disease is not developing is to recatheterize the patient. An unnecessary cardiac catheterization is far preferable to missing pulmonary vascular disease while it is still treatable.

An important variation on the theme of large ventricular septal defects occurs at high altitude because of the pulmonary vasoconstriction secondary to the alveolar hypoxia. The increased pulmonary vascular resistance might be expected to decrease the amount of left-to-right shunting and thus to produce less severe congestive heart failure. This is indeed what happens. A comparison of infants with large ventricular septal defects in Denver and Houston[111] showed that the average pulmonary to systemic (Qp:Qs) flow ratio was 3.0 in Houston and 2.0 in Denver, and that with tolazoline injection the average Qp:Qs in Denver rose to 2.9. This physiologic improvement, however, is not translated into permanent cure, and if the large defect persists there is as great a tendency for pulmonary vascular disease to occur at high altitude as at sea level.

Since ventricular septal defects are the commonest congenital heart lesions, it is worth discussing what happens to pulmonary vascular disease and pulmonary arterial hypertension after surgical closure of large defects. As expected, the pulmonary arterial pressure falls at first in proportion to the reduction of pulmonary blood flow, and so the fall is more marked in those with large than with small left-to-right shunts and in those with mild than severe pulmonary vascular disease.[112] If there is a marked fall in pulmonary arterial pressure post-operatively there may be some regression of pulmonary vascular disease.[113] There is little doubt that the thickened medial muscle can regress to normal, but whether intimal changes return to normal is hard to prove. Not only is it impossible to follow the course of any given arterial lesion, but since there is considerable lung growth for the first 5 years of life, serial biopsies after surgical closure, done for example at 1 to 2 years of age, might show fewer abnormal vessels because of "dilution" by newly developed normal vessels. The largest clinical follow-up to date has been reported from Hammersmith Hospital in London.[114,115] Almost all the patients surviving surgery were well and asymptomatic. Most of them had some pulmonary arterial hypertension at rest when studied about a year after surgical closure of the defect, and 5 out of 15 restudied some years later had had a significant rise in resting pulmonary arterial pressure. In all, the pulmonary arterial pressures rose with exercise. Evidently in these patients there was residual pulmonary vascular disease that could sometimes be slowly progressive and that prevented recruitment of new vessels with exercise. What we do not know from this study is if the residual increase in pulmonary vascular resistance was due to persistent intimal scarring, a deficiency of vessels, or both. The ages at which these patients had their defects closed varied from 3 to 12 years, and during normal development two-thirds of the final number of intra-acinar arteries are present by 18 months of age and most of the rest form by 5 years of age.[54,55] Thus the earlier the surgical closure of these defects the better the prospects for a relatively normal pulmonary vasculature in adult life.

If the pulmonary vascular disease is very advanced, then surgical closure of the defect is contra-indicated. No good controlled studies have been or will be done on this subject, but two instructive publications from the Mayo Clinic confirm what has been almost everyone's personal experience.[106,116] Out of 13 patients with severe pulmonary vascular disease who had surgical closure of a large ventricular septal defect, 9 (71%) had died within a year. By contrast, 58 patients whose pulmonary vascular disease was considered too severe to permit surgery were usually gainfully employed and well, although restricted, into the third or even fourth decades. Closing the defect in the face of severe fixed pulmonary vascular disease does not lower pulmonary arterial pressure because there will be little or no decrease in pulmonary flow. With the closed defect and a fixed high pulmonary vascular resistance, two serious consequences take place. Any increased venous return, as with exercise, causes acute right ventricular hypertension because the increased return cannot be ejected instantly as would happen in normal people. Second, any fall in systemic blood pressure due, for example, to exercise or bradycardia, will decrease coronary perfusion of the thick walled right ventricle. Either of these events may cause acute right ventricular failure, arrhythmias, and sudden death. Thus clinical emphasis must be placed on early detection of pulmonary vascular disease so that surgery can be done and the progression of vascular disease can be halted. If that is not possible then care must be taken in selecting older patients for surgery to avoid the disastrous consequences of closing a defect in the face of irreversible vascular disease.

There are still, unfortunately, patients with various congenital heart lesions who have irreversible pulmonary vascular disease. They all have right-to-left shunts through the defects (or, if they have transposition of the great arteries, greatly reduced mixing of pulmonary and systemic venous blood) and consequently are very cyanotic and polycythemic. No specific treatment is available for the vascular disease, but some ways of reducing morbidity have been advocated. Because the increased viscosity of polycythemia is an added impediment to flow through the high resistance pulmonary vessels, there are those who advocate periodic phlebotomy. In other types of cyanotic patients with polycythemia, decreasing the hematocrit to about 60% but keeping blood volume constant has improved systemic oxygen delivery to tissues.[117] This effect has not been formally studied in patients with pulmonary vascular disease, but anecdotal information suggests that it is worth trying. Furthermore, reducing the blood viscosity may help to reduce the risk of thromboses that can occur in many organs. If periodic phlebotomy is embarked upon, it is important to make sure that the blood loss does not cause iron deficiency anemia. Not only does the anemia reduce the oxygen carrying capacity of the blood but iron deficiency makes red cells more rigid and so increases blood viscosity. The simplest method of ruling out iron deficiency anemia is to examine hematocrit and hemoglobin concentration. Normally the hematocrit is 3 times the hemoglobin concentration, as befits a normal mean hemoglobin concentration of 33%. If, for example, the hematocrit is 60%, but the hemoglobin is only 15 g/dl, the 4:1 ratio suggests a hypochromic anemia that is likely to be due to iron deficiency.

A troublesome complication that some of these patients have is hemoptysis. This might result from local thrombotic episodes in the lung or could be related to the abnormal thin-walled vessels that are noted in advanced pulmonary vascular disease. Agents that prevent platelet aggregation (acetylsalicylic acid, indomethacin, dipyridamole) or that prevent blood clotting (coumadin) have been used. Once again, there is anecdotal evidence of their effectiveness in preventing recurrent hemoptysis, but no adequate clinical trials have been done.

Acknowledgment: Supported in part by USPHS Program Project Grant HL 24056.

REFERENCES

1. Rudolph AM: The changes in the circulation after birth. Their importance in congenital heart disease. *Circulation* 1970;41:343–359.
2. Heymann MA, Rudolph AM: Effects of acetylsalicylic acid on the ductus arteriosus and circulation in fetal lambs in utero. *Circ Res* 1976;38: 418–422.
3. Kitterman JA, Phibbs RH, Tooley WH: Aortic blood pressure in normal newborn infants during the first 12 hours of life. *Pediatrics* 1969;44: 959–968.
4. Moss AJ, Emmanouilides G, Duffie ER Jr: Closure of the ductus arteriosus in the newborn infant. *Pediatrics* 1963;32:25–30.
5. Rudolph AM, Auld PAM, Golinko RJ, Paul MH: Pulmonary vascular adjustments in the neonatal period. *Pediatrics* 1961;28:28–34.
6. Krovetz LJ, Goldbloom J: Normal standards for cardiovascular data II pressure and vascular resistances. *Johns Hopkins Med J* 1972;130: 187–195.
7. Lucas RV Jr, St. Geme JW Jr, Anderson RC, Adams P Jr, Ferguson DJ: Maturation of the pulmonary vascular bed: A physiologic and anatomic correlation in infants and children. *Am J Dis Child* 1961;101: 467–475.
8. Ekelund LG, Holmgren A: Central hemodynamics during exercise. *Circ Res* 1967;20(Supp I):33–43.
9. Hoff JC, Agarawal JB, Gardiner AJS, Palmer WH, Macklem PT: Distribution of airway resistance with developing pulmonary edema in dogs. *J Appl Physiol* 1972;32:20–24.
10. Iliff LD, Greene RE, Hughes JMB: Effect of interstitial edema on distribution of ventilation and perfusion in isolated lung. *J Appl Physiol* 1972; 33:462–467.
11. Staub NC, Nagano H, Pearce ML: Pulmonary edema in dogs, especially the sequence of fluid accumulation in the lungs. *J Appl Physiol* 1967;22: 227–240.

12. West JB, Dollery CT, Heard BE: Increased pulmonary vascular resistance in the dependent zone of the isolated dog lung caused by perivascular edema. *Circ Res* 1965;17:191−206.
13. Dollery CT, West JB: Regional uptake of radioactive oxygen carbon monoxide and carbon dioxide in the lungs of patients with mitral stenosis. *Circ Res* 1960;8:765−771.
14. Friedman WF, Braunwald E, Morrow AG: Alterations in regional pulmonary blood flow in patients with congenital heart disease studied by radioisotope scanning. *Circulation* 1968;37:747−758.
15. Ritchie BC, Schauberger G, Staub NC: Inadequacy of perivascular edema hypothesis to account for distribution of pulmonary blood flow in lung edema. *Circ Res* 1969;24:807−814.
16. Muir AL, Hall DL, Despas P, Hogg JC: Distribution of blood flow in the lungs in acute pulmonary edema in dogs. *J Appl Physiol* 1972;33: 763−709.
17. Hoffman JIE: The normal pulmonary circulation. In: Scarpelli EM, Auld PAM, Eds. *Pulmonary Physiology in the Fetus, Newborn and Child.* Philadelphia: Lea and Febiger, 1975:259−272.
18. Wagenvoort CA, Heath D, Edwards JE: *The Pathology of the Pulmonary Vasculature.* Springfield, Illinois: Charles C. Thomas, 1964:146−212.
19. Wagenvoort CA, Wagenvoort N: Pulmonary vascular bed: Normal anatomy and responses to disease. In: Moser KM, ed. *Pulmonary Vascular Diseases.* New York: Marcell Dekker, 1979:1−109.
20. Lal S, Murtagh JG, Pollock AM, Fletcher E, Binnion PF: Acute haemodynamic effects of frusemide in patients with normal and raised left atrial pressures. *Br Heart J* 1969;31:711−717.
21. Bland RD, McMillan DD, Bressack MA: Decreased pulmonary transvascular fluid filtration in awake newborn lambs after intravenous furosemide. *J Clin Invest* 1978;62:601−609.
22. Heyman MA: Left-to-right Shunts. In: Rudolph AM, Hoffman JIE, eds. *Pediatrics.* New York: Appleton-Century-Crofts, 1982:1281−1297.
23. Paul MH. Right-to-left Shunts. In: Rudolph AM Hoffman JIE, ed. *Pediatrics.* New York: Appleton-Century-Crofts, 1982:1316−1341.
24. Gersony WM: Presentation, diagnosis and natural history of total anomalous pulmonary venous drainage. In: Godman MJ, Marquis RM, eds. *Paediatric Cardiology, Vol. 2, Heart Disease in the Newborn.* Edinburgh: Churchill Livingstone, 1979:463−473.
25. Snider AR, Silverman NH, Turley K, Ebert PA: Evaluation of infradiaphragmatic total anomalous pulmonary venous connection with two-dimensional echocardiography. *Circulation* 1982;66:1129−1132.
26. Newfeld EA, Wilson A, Paul MH, Reisch JS: Pulmonary vascular disease in total anomalous venous drainage. *Circulation* 1980;61:103−109.
27. Prandtl L. Tietjens OG: *Applied Hydro- and Aeromechanics.* New York: Dover Publications, Inc., 1957.
28. Hoffman JIE: Diagnosis and treatment of pulmonary vascular disease. In: Bergsma D, Blumenthal S, eds. *Congenital Cardiac Defects—Recent Advances: Birth Defects.* Original Article Series, 1972;8:9−18.
29. Whitmore RL: *Rheology of the Circulation.* London: Pergamon Press, 1968.

30. Caro CG: Mechanics of the pulmonary circulation. In: Caro CG ed. *Advances in Respiratory Physiology.* London: Edwin Arnold, 1966: 255–296.
31. Benis AM, Usami S, Chien S: Effect of hematocrit and inertial losses on pressure-flow relations in the isolated hindpaw of the dog. *Circ Res* 1970;27:1047–1068.
32. Bergel DH, Milnor WR: Pulmonary vascular impedance in the dog. *Circ Res* 1965;16:401–415.
33. Milnor WR, Conti CR, Lewis KB, O'Rourke MF: Pulmonary arterial pulse wave velocity and impedance in man. *Circ Res* 1969;25:637–649.
34. Roos A: Poiseuille's law and its limitations in vascular systems. *Med Thorac* 1962;19:224–238.
35. West JB, Dollery CT, Naimark A: Distribution of blood flow in isolated lung: Relation to vascular and alveolar pressures. *J Appl Physiol* 1964;19:713–724.
36. Permutt S, Howell JBL, Proctor DF, Riley RL: Effect of lung inflation on static pressure-volume characteristics of pulmonary vessels. *J Appl Physiol* 1961;16:64–70.
37. Glazier JB, Hughes JMB, Maloney JE, West JB: Measurements of capillary dimensions and blood volume in rapidly frozen lungs. *J Appl Physiol* 1969;26:65–76.
38. Dintenfass L: *Rheology of Blood in Diagnostic and Preventive Medicine.* London: Butterworths, 1976.
39. Wells RE, Merrill EW: Influence of flow properties of blood upon viscosity–hematocrit relationships. *J Clin Invest* 1962;41:1591–1598.
40. Murray JF, Karp RB, Nadel JA: Viscosity effects on pressure-flow relations and vascular resistance in dogs' lungs. *J Appl Physiol* 1969;27:336–341.
41. Agarwal JB, Paltoo R, Palmer WH: Relative viscosity of blood at varying hematocrits in pulmonary circulation. *J Appl Physiol* 1970;29:866–871.
42. Benis AM, Tavares P, Mortara F, Lockhart A: Effect of hematocrit on pressure-flow relations for perfused isolated lobes of the canine lung. *Pflueger's Arch* 1970;314:347–360.
43. Bucens D, Pain MCF: Influence of hematocrit, blood gas tensions, and pH on pressure-flow relations in the isolated canine lung. *Circ Res* 1975;37:588–596.
44. Surjadhana A. Rouleau J, Boerboom L, Hoffman JIE: Myocardial blood flow and its distribution in anesthetized polycythemic dogs. *Circ Res* 1978;43:619–631.
45. Lategola MT: Pressure-flow relationships in the dog lung during acute, sub-total pulmonary vascular occlusion. *Am J Physiol* 1958;192:613–619.
46. Burrows B, Harrison RW, Adams WE, Humphreys EM, Long ET, Reimann AF: The post-pneumonectomy state. *Am J Med* 1960;28:281–297.
47. Downing SE, Pusel SE, Vidone RA, Brandt HM, Liebow AA: Studies on pulmonary hypertension with special reference to pressure-flow relationships in chronically distended and undistended lobes. *Med Thorac* 1962;19:268–282.
48. Harris PC, Heath D: *The Human Pulmonary Circulation: Its Form and Function in Health and Disease.* Edinburgh: Churchill Livingstone, 1977.

49. Rudolph AM, Neuhauser EBD, Golinko RJ, Auld PAM: Effects of pneumonectomy on pulmonary circulation in adult and young animals. *Circ Res* 1961;9:856–861.
50. Pool PE, Averill KH, Vogel JHK: Effect of ligation of left pulmonary artery at birth on maturation of pulmonary vascular bed. *Med Thorac* 1962;19:362–369.
51. Pool PE, Vogel JHK, Blount SG Jr: Congenital unilateral absence of a pulmonary artery. The importance of flow in pulmonary hypertension. *Am J Cardiol* 1962;10:706–732.
52. Caudill DR, Helmsworth JA, Daoud G, Kaplan S: Anomalous origin of left pulmonary artery from ascending aorta. *J Thorac Cardiovas Surg* 1969;57:493–506.
53. Hislop A, Reid L: Intra-pulmonary arterial development during fetal life—branching pattern and structure. *J Anat* 1972;113:35–48.
54. Hislop A, Reid LM: Pulmonary arterial development during childhood: Branching pattern and structure. *Thorax* 1973;28:129–135.
55. Davies G, Reid L: Growth of the alveoli and pulmonary arteries in childhood. *Thorax* 1970;25:669–681.
56. Haworth SG, Reid L: Quantitative structural study of pulmonary circulation in the newborn with pulmonary atresia. *Thorax* 1977;129–133.
57. Levin DL, Mills LJ, Parkey M: Morphologic development of the pulmonary vascular bed in experimental coarctation of the aorta. *Circulation* 1979;60:349–354.
58. Hislop A, Haworth SG, Shinebourne EA, Reid L: Quantitative structural analysis of pulmonary vessels in isolated ventricular septal defect in infancy. *Br Heart J* 1975;37:1014–1021.
59. Haworth SG, Sauer V, Buhlmeyer K, Reid L: Development of the pulmonary circulation in ventricular septal defect: A quantitative structural study. *Am J Cardiol* 1977;40:781–788.
60. Rabinovitch M, Haworth SG, Castaneda AR, Nadas AS, Reid LM: Lung biopsy in congenital heart disease: A morphometric approach to pulmonary vascular disease. *Circulation* 1978;58:1107–1122.
61. Roos A, Thomas LJ Jr, Nagel EL, Prommas DC: Pulmonary vascular resistance as determined by lung inflation and vascular pressures. *J Appl Physiol* 1961;16:77–84.
62. Stanger P, Lucas RV Jr, Edwards JE: Anatomic factors causing respiratory distress in acyanotic congenital cardiac disease. *Pediatrics* 1969;43:760–769.
63. Hendren WH, Kim SH: Pediatric thoracic surgery. In: Scarpelli EM, Auld PAM, Goldman, HS, eds. *Pulmonary Disease of the Fetus, Newborn and Child*. Philadelphia: Lea and Febiger, 1978:166–234.
64. Stewart JR, Kincaid OW, Edwards JE: *An Atlas of Vascular Rings and Related Malformations of the Aortic Arch System*. Springfield, Illinois: Charles C. Thomas, 1964.
65. Hoffman JIE, Rudolph AM, Heymann MA; Pulmonary vascular disease with congenital heart lesions. Pathologic features and causes. *Circulation* 1981;64:873–877.
66. Wagenvoort CA, Neufeld HN, DuShane JW, Edwards JE: The pulmonary arterial tree in ventricular septal defect. A quantitative study of anatomic features in fetuses, infants and children. *Circulation* 1961;23:740–748.

67. Ferencz C: Transposition of the great vessels. Pathophysiologic considerations based on a study of the lungs. *Circulation* 1966;33:232–241.
68. Wagenvoort CA, Nanta J, van der Schaar PG, Weeda HWH, Wagenvoort N: The pulmonary vasculature in complete transposition of the great vessels, judged from lung biopsies. *Circulation* 1968;38:746–454.
69. Newfeld EA, Paul MH, Muster AJ, Idriss FS: Pulmonary vascular disease in complete transposition of the great arteries; A study of 200 patients. *Am J Cardiol* 1974;34:75–82.
70. Lakier JB, Stangr P, Heymann MA, Hoffman JIE, Rudolph AM: Early onset of pulmonary vascular obstruction in patients with aortopulmonary transposition and intact ventricular septum. *Circulation* 1976;54:805–809.
71. Yamaki S, Tezuka F: Quantitative analysis of pulmonary vascular disease in complete transposition of the great arteries. *Circulation* 1976;54:805–809.
72. Waldman JD, Paul MN, Newfeld EA, Muster AJ, Idriss FS: Transposition of the great arteries with intact ventricular septum and patent ductus arteriosus. *Am J Cardiol* 1977;39:232–238.
73. Newfeld EA, Paul MH, Muster AJ, Idriss FS: Pulmonary vascular disease in transposition of the great vessels and intact ventricular septum. *Circulation* 1979;59:525–530.
74. Wagenvoort CA, Neufeld HN, DuShane JW, Edwards JE: The pulmonary arterial tree in atrial septal defect. A quantitative study of anatomic features in fetuses, infants and children. *Circulation* 1961;23:733–739.
75. Wissler RW: The arterial medial cell, smooth muscle or multi-functional mesenchyme? *Circulation* 1967;36:1–4.
76. Heath D, Edwards JE: The pathology of hypertensive pulmonary vascular disease. A description of six grades of changes in the pulmonary arteries with special reference to congenital cardiac septal defects. *Circulation* 1958;18:533–547.
77. Dammann JF Jr, Ferencz C: The significance of the pulmonary vascular bed in congenital heart disease. III. Defects between the ventricles or great vessels in which both increased pressure and blood flow may act upon the lungs and in which there is a common ejectile force. *Am Heart J* 1956;52:210–231.
78. Wagenvoort CA: The morphology of certain vascular lesions in pulmonary hypertension. *J Pathol Bacteriol* 1959;78:503–511.
79. Wagenvoort CA, Wagenvoort N, Dijk HJ: Effect of fulvine on pulmonary arteries and veins of the rat. *Thorax* 1974;29:522–529.
80. Stemerman MB: Vascular intimal components: Precursors of thrombosis. *Prog Hemost Thromb* 1974;2:1–47.
81. Fry DL: Acute vascular endothelial changes associated with increased blood velocity gradients. *Circ Res* 1968;22:165–197.
82. Friedman M, Byrs SO: Experimental thrombo-atherosclerosis. *J Clin Invest* 1961;40:1139–1152.
83. Williams AW, Montgomery GL: Chemical injury of arteries. *J Pathol Bacteriol* 1969;77:63–69.
84. Ross R, Glomsett J, Kariya B, Harker L: A platelet-dependent serum factor that stimulates the proliferation of arterial smooth muscle cells in vitro. *Poc Natl Acad Sci* 1974;72:1207–1210.

85. Ross R, Glomsett JA: The pathogenesis of atherosclerosis. *N Engl J Med* 1976;295:369–377 and 420–425.
86. Harker LA, Ross R, Slichter J, Scott CR: Homocysteine-induced arteriosclerosis. The role of endothelial cell injury and platelet response in its genesis. *J Clin Invest* 1976;58:731–741.
87. Friedman RJ, Burns ER: Role of platelets in the proliferative response of the injured artery. *Prog Hemost Thromb* 1978;4:249–278.
88. Gerrard JM, White JG: Prostaglandins and thromboxanes: "Middlemen" modulating platelet function in hemostasis and thrombosis. *Prog Hemost Thromb* 1978;4:87–125.
89. Berman W Jr, Whitman V, Pierce WS, Waldhausen JA: The development of pulmonary vascular obstructive disease after successful mustard operation in early infancy. *Circulation* 1978;58:181–185.
90. Komp DM, Sparrow AW: Polycythemia in cyanotic heart disease—a study of altered coagulation. *J Pediatr* 1970;76:231–236.
91. Ihenacho HNC, Breeze GR, Fletcher DJ, Stuart J: Consumption coagulopathy in congenital heart disease. *Lancet* 1973;1:231–234.
92. Waldman JD, Czapek EE, Paul MH, Schwartz AD, Levin DL, Schindler S: Shortened platelet survival in cyanotic heart disease. *J Pediatr* 1975;87:77–79.
93. Sheperd JT: Bayliss response in the umbilical artery. *Fed Proc* 1968;27:1408–1409.
94. Rabinovitch M, Castaneda AR, Reid L: Lung biopsy with frozen section as a diagnostic aid in patients with congenital heart defects. *Am J Cardiol* 1981;47:77–84.
95. Haworth SG, Reid L: A morphometric study of regional variation in lung structure in infants with pulmonary hypertension and congenital cardiac defect. *Br Heart J* 1978;40:825–831.
96. Nihill MR, McNamara DG: Magnification pulmonary wedge angiography in the evaluation of children with congenital heart disease and pulmonary hypertension. *Circulation* 1978;58:1094–1106.
97. Rabinovitch M, Keane JF, Fellows KE, Castaneda AR, Reid L: Quantitative analysis of the pulmonary wedge angiogram in congenital heart defects. Correlation with hemodynamic data and morphometric findings in lung biopsy tissue. *Circulation* 1981;63:152–164.
98. Mair DD, Ritter DG, Danielson GK, Wallace RB, McGoon DC: Truncus arteriosus with unilateral absence of a pulmonary artery. Criteria for operability and surgical results. *Circulation* 1977;55:641–647.
99. Mair DD, Ritter DG, Davis GD, Wallace RB, Danielson GK, McGoon DC: Selection of patients with truncus arteriosus for surgical correction: Anatomic and hemodynamic considerations. *Circulation* 1974;49:144–151.
100. Rich AR: A hitherto unrecognized tendency to the development of widespread pulmonary vascular obstruction in patients with congenital pulmonary stenosis (tetralogy of Fallot). *Johns Hopkins Med J* 1948;82:389–401.
101. Cucci CE, Doyle EF, Lewis EW Jr: Absence of a primary division of the pulmonary trunk. An ontogenetic theory. *Circulation* 1964;29:124–131.
102. Muster AJ, Paul MH, van Grondelle A, Conway JJ: Asymmetric distribution of the pulmonary blood flow between the right and left lungs in d-transposition of the great arteries. *Am J Cardiol* 1976;38:352–361.

103. Lewis AB, Heymann MA, Rudolph AM: Gestational changes in pulmonary vascular responses in fetal lambs in utero. *Circ Res* 1976;39: 536–541.
104. Friedman WF: The intrinsic physiologic properties of the developing heart. *Prog Cardiovasc Dis* 1972;15:87–111.
105. Blackstone EH, Kirklin JW, Bradley EL, DuShane JW, Appelbaum A: Optimal age and results in repair of large ventricular septal defects. *J Thorac Cardiovasc Surg* 1976;72:661–679.
106. Cartmill TB, DuShane JW, McGoon DC, Kirklin JW: Results of repair of ventricular septal defect. *J Thorac Cardiovasc Surg* 1966;52:486–501.
107. Hoffman JIE, Rudolph AM: The natural history of isolated ventricular septal defect. *Adv Pediatr* 1970;17:57–79.
108. Beckman RH, Rocchini AP, Rosenthal A: Hemodynamic effects of nitroprusside in infants with a large ventricular septal defect. *Circulation* 1981;64:553–558.
109. Beckman RH, Rocchini AP, Rosenthal A: Hemodynamic effects of hydralazine in infants with a large ventricular septal defect. *Circulation* 1982;65:523–528.
110. Lister G, Hellenbrand WE, Kleinman CS, Talner NS: Physiologic effects of increasing hemoglobin concentration in left-to-right shunting in infants with ventricular septal defects. *N Engl J Med* 1982;306:502–506.
111. Vogel JHK, McNamara DG, Blount SG Jr: Role of hypoxia in determining pulmonary vascular resistance in infants with ventricular septal defects. *Am J Cardiol* 1967;20:346–349.
112. Heath D, Helmholz HF Jr, Burchell HB, DuShane JW, Kirklin JW, Edwards JE: Relation between structural changes in the small pulmonary arteries and the immediate reversibility of pulmonary hypertension following closure of ventricular and atrial septal defects. *Circulation* 1958; 18:1167–1174.
113. Dammann JF Jr, McEachen JA, Thompson WM Jr, Smith R, Muller WH Jr: The regression of pulmonary vascular disease after the creation of pulmonic stenosis. *J Thorac Cardiovasc Surg* 1961;42:722–734.
114. Hallidie-Smith KA, Hollman A, Cleland WP, Bentall HH, Goodwin JF: Effects of surgical closure of ventricular septal defects upon pulmonary vascular disease. *Br Heart J* 1969;31:246–260.
115. Hallidie-Smith KA, Wilson RSE, Hart A, Zeidifard E: Functional status of patients with large ventricular septal defect and pulmonary vascular disease 6 to 16 years after surgical closure of their defect in childhood. *Br Heart J* 1977;39:1093–1101.
116. Clarkson PM, Frye RL, DuShane JW, Burchell HB, Wood EH, Weidman WH: Prognosis for patients with ventricular septal defect and severe pulmonary vascular obstructive disease. *Circulation* 1968;38:129–135.
117. Rosenthal A, Nathan DG, Marty AT, Button LN, Miettinen OS, Nadas AS: Acute hemodynamic effects of red cell volume reduction in polycythemia of cyanotic congenital heart disease. *Circulation* 1970;42:297–307.

CHAPTER 4

DIAGNOSIS AND MANAGEMENT OF PRIMARY PULMONARY HYPERTENSION

E. Kenneth Weir

INTRODUCTION

"Yet Nature desiring that the blood should be strained through the lungs, was forc'd to add the right ventricle, by whose pulse the blood should be forc'd through the very lungs . . . " (De Motu Cordis, William Harvey).[1] The basic problem in primary pulmonary hypertension is that there is increased resistance to blood being strained through the lungs and this may ultimately lead to right ventricular failure. The term "primary pulmonary hypertension" may be used to describe a clinical condition characterized by pulmonary hypertension in the absence of any demonstrable cause, sometimes referred to as "unexplained pulmonary hypertension."[2] However, such a definition requires amplification. What constitutes pulmonary hypertension and how rigorously are other conditions to be excluded? Although the physical examination and noninvasive studies may indicate pulmonary hypertension, cardiac catheterization is necessary for definitive diagnosis and accurate measurement of pulmonary arterial pressure. The normal mean pulmonary arterial pressure for a young adult at rest is 13 ± 4 (SD) mm Hg. (See Chapter 1, Table 1). For the purposes of the current NIH primary pulmonary hypertension registry, patients are accepted as having pulmonary hypertension if the mean pulmonary arterial pressure is greater than 25 mm Hg at rest or greater than 30 mm Hg on exercise. A resting pulmonary arterial pressure of 25 mm Hg or greater is also used as a criterion by the Japanese primary pulmonary hypertension research committee.[3] These figures are clearly outside the normal range but are low enough to include patients who may be identified early in the course of their disease. Many diseases can give rise to pulmonary hypertension and the means by which they can be recognized will be discussed in the section on differential diagnosis. Other conditions, such as portal hypertension and Raynaud's disease, occur more frequently in patients with primary pulmonary hypertension than in the general population, but the significance of the association is unclear. These conditions will be considered in the discussion of possible etiologic factors in primary pulmonary hypertension.

Unfortunately, even when the diagnosis of primary pulmonary hypertension has been made by cardiac catheterization and the clinical exclusion of other conditions, the selected patients do not form a homogeneous group. In one study of 47 open lung biopsies taken from patients with a clinical diagnosis of primary pulmonary hypertension, 15 showed plexogenic pulmonary arteriopathy, 15 had the changes of chronic thromboembolism and in 2 there was pulmonary veno-occlusive disease.[4] These 32 patients demonstrate three distinct histologic appearances as discussed in Chapter 11, but using the criteria adopted by a World Health Organization conference in 1973,[5] all would be grouped pathologically under the term "primary pulmonary hypertension." In addition to these three pathologic subgroups, the lung biopsy study also revealed 15 patients with other reasons for the development of pulmonary hypertension: 10 had lung fibrosis, 2 showed changes suggestive of pulmonary venous hypertension, 2 had changes compatible with chronic hypoxia, and one was diagnosed as primary pulmonary hemosiderosis. As lung biopsy has been performed very infrequently in patients with primary pulmonary hypertension, it is easy to understand that all the published information based on the clinical diagnosis of the disease will include data from a variety of conditions.

Our knowledge of primary pulmonary hypertension has also been limited by several other facts: (i) the disease is uncommon and even a major center may only admit 5 to 10 new patients each year; (ii) measurement of pulmonary arterial pressure for diagnosis, studies of natural history, or assessment of therapy, requires right-heart catheterization; (iii) symptoms only occur when moderate or severe pulmonary hypertension has already developed and because of this, patients present relatively late in the course of the disease; and (iv) there is no animal model of primary pulmonary hypertension.

This chapter will review the information available on primary pulmonary hypertension in the sense of unexplained pulmonary hypertension.[2] Consequently, it should be remembered that the selection of patients reported in various papers as suffering from primary pulmonary hypertension may vary widely, depending on the diagnostic facilities at hand, the availability of lung tissue for histology, and the knowledge and application of the investigator.

EPIDEMIOLOGY

Primary pulmonary hypertension was seldom reported before the development of cardiac catheterization. Autopsy findings suggestive of primary pulmonary hypertension were described in 1891[6] and 1907.[7] A total of 16 cases was covered in a review of the pathology of "primary pulmonary arteriosclerosis" compiled by Brenner in 1935.[8] Only 2 cases were described in a series of 10,000 autopsies in 1954 (0.02%).[9]

Paul Wood gave a brief account of the condition in 1950,[10] but the first detailed clinical description, together with cardiac catherization data, were published in 1951.[11] Subsequent clinical studies have yielded higher percentages than the earlier autopsy data, although from more selected populations. Paul Wood found 17 instances of primary pulmonary hypertension out of a consecutive series of 10,000 patients seen in his cardiovascular clinic (0.17%: 14 female and 3 male).[12] In Denmark 14 cases were identified out of 6,000 patients examined in a cardiological laboratory between 1947 and 1960 (0.23%: 8 female, 6 male).[13] Primary pulmonary hypertension was diagnosed 17 times in 1,550 right heart catherizations performed in Norway between 1960 and 1966 (1.1%: 10 female, 7 male).[14]

Wagenvoort and Wagenvoort in 1970 discussed the histologic changes in the pulmonary vasculature of 110 patients with "vasoconstrictive primary pulmonary hypertension" and found 467 additional adult cases in the literature.[15] Assuming that the incidence of the disease did not rise, this rapid increase in the recognition of primary pulmonary hypertension was due mainly to the introduction of right heart catheterization[16] and better techniques of differential diagnosis.

Primary pulmonary hypertension can occur at any age but symptoms appear most commonly in young adults (15–35 years). In childhood the sex incidence is approximately equal. One report, which described 39 patients up to the age of 15 years with autopsy-proven primary pulmonary hypertension, included 21 boys and 18 girls.[15] Most authors state that after childhood the incidence is greater in women, with a ratio (F:M) of about 2.5:1.[13-15,17] However, a large Japanese survey (137 cases), noted a greater number of males in the third decade of life.[18] At present no differences have been documented in the geographical or racial incidence of the disease.

PROGNOSIS

After the onset of symptoms, the length of survival of patients with primary pulmonary hypertension is very variable, but the average time tends to be short. The age at the time of death in 110 patients studied by Wagenvoort and Wagenvoort was an average of 23 years.[15] In their experience the disease seemed to progress more rapidly in the young. Four children were only known to be symptomatic during 4 to 6 weeks before death.

Unfortunately, patients usually present when the disease is relatively far advanced both hemodynamically and histologically. Consequently, there is little information on the duration of the presymptomatic phase. In one instance, a girl who became symptomatic at age 10, was shown retrospectively on chest x-ray to have had pulmonary hypertension at age 3.[19] Even then she must have had significantly elevated pulmonary arterial pressures. Pregnancy is poorly tolerated in women with primary pulmonary hypertension, and death from right heart failure during pregnancy, or occurring at the time of delivery, is common.[13] Occasional patients live for many years after the symptoms first appear: four have been reported between 20 and 29 years,[15] one patient 27 years, and another 38 years.[20] Spontaneous regression of the disease has also been documented.[21,22]

In one study the size of the hilar vessels on chest x-ray was found to correlate with the length of survival.[23] This is somewhat surprising as the absolute level of pulmonary arterial pressure recorded has not been helpful in the assessment of prognosis. By the time the patient develops symptoms, the pulmonary arterial pressure is usually already high[18] and does not correlate with the length of survival.[24] Possibly the size of the pulmonary arteries reflects not only the pressure but also the duration of the condition. The cardiac output tends to fall with increasing time after the onset of symptoms[17] and the pulmonary vascular bed becomes less responsive to vasodilator agents. Thus, the finding at catheterization of low cardiac output and unresponsive pulmonary vasculature suggest more advanced disease. In one study the cardiac index was known in 55 patients,[24] and those who died were noted to have had lower cardiac outputs (2.6 ± 0.7 SE. L/min/M^2) than those who survived (3.3 ± 1.1). The same authors found that a systemic arterial oxygen tension below 70 mm Hg was associated with an extremely bad prognosis. The presence of right heart failure is a bad prognostic sign. In one report, all 6 patients with right heart failure died, at an average of 1 year post-catheterization.[13]

ETIOLOGY

No single etiologic factor has been recognized in primary pulmonary hypertension. It may be that several different etiologic stimuli can in the long-term give rise to a common final pathway which is classified clinically and pathologically as primary pulmonary hypertension. The World Health Organization (WHO) pathologic classification of primary pulmonary hypertension mentioned in the introduction[5] includes thromboembolism and pulmonary venous thrombosis, as well as plexogenic pulmonary arteriopathy. Consequently, it is reasonable to ask whether all primary pulmonary hypertension might not be the result of thrombosis-in-situ, or embolism, or a combination of both.

Thromboembolism

Several authors have suggested that numerous, small, clinically silent emboli might cause most, if not all, cases of primary pulmonary hypertension.[25,26] However, subsequent pathologic studies have shown that thromboembolic pulmonary hypertension can be differentiated histologically from plexogenic primary pulmonary hypertension, using tissue obtained by lung biopsy or at autopsy.[4,15] As discussed in detail in Chapter 11, in primary pulmonary hypertension the characteristic histologic features are marked medial hypertrophy, laminar "onion skin" intimal fibrosis, and plexiform lesions. In thromboembolic pulmonary hypertension the medial hypertrophy tends to be mild, and the intimal fibrosis is patchy. It might be thought that micro-thromboemboli could give rise to a different histologic picture than larger emboli but, in cases with both large and small emboli, the lesions in the small vessels still do not resemble those seen in primary hypertension.[15] The presence of the small peripheral vessels can be appreciated on post-mortem arteriography as a background haze in normal or embolized lungs, but not in primary pulmonary hypertension.[27] Dilatation and plexiform lesions do not occur in thromboembolic pulmonary hypertension,[15] but thromboembolism may occur in patients with primary pulmonary hypertension, giving rise to a confusing histologic picture. Despite these cases, it is clear that primary pulmonary hypertension cannot be explained on the basis of recurrent pulmonary embolism alone.

A recent study in 13 patients with longstanding primary pulmonary hypertension showed that 7 had markedly reduced fibrinolytic activity following occlusion of a peripheral systemic vein, in comparison to normal controls.[28] This might indicate a defect in fibrinolysis or endothelial cell function which could predispose to the development of thrombosis-in-situ. Alternatively, the reduced fibrinolytic activity might not be etiologically important, but could be a marker of a more generalized abnormality in endothelial cell function.

Vasoconstriction

In the WHO classification, the term plexogenic arteriopathy refers to a morphologic pattern of lesions in the lung vessels that may eventually produce plexiform lesions. Consequently, Edwards and Edwards[29] and Wagenvoort and Wagenvoort[15] consider that medial hypertrophy alone is the first structural change in this form of primary pulmonary hypertension. Certainly, hypertrophy of the media of the pulmonary arterioles, and/or distal extension of the medial layer into arterioles of approximately 50 diameter, is present in most cases of primary pulmonary hypertension with demonstrated plexiform lesions. In many children with primary pulmonary hypertension and in the occasional adult, who is identified very early in the course of the disease and submitted to lung biopsy, it may be the only histologic change.[29] These morphologic observations suggest that vasoconstriction is the initial mechanism of pulmonary hypertension in many patients with primary pulmonary hypertension. The fact that a number of vasodilators can reduce pulmonary arterial pressure and resistance in some patients (as discussed under Treatment), further strengthens the supposition that vasoconstriction is involved. This point has been illustrated by Paul Wood in terms of the vasodilation produced by acetylcholine.[30]

The correlations of Raynaud's disease and migraine with variant angina[31,32] have raised the possibility of a more generalized vasospastic condition in some patients. The frequent association of Raynaud's disease with primary pulmonary hypertension[33-35] provides additional circumstantial evidence in favor of vasoconstriction as an etiologic factor. In fact, primary pulmonary hypertension has been referred to as "pulmonary Raynaud's disease." The vasoconstriction concept suggests an early stage characterized by medial hypertrophy and an increase in pulmonary vascular resistance reversible by vasodilators. Later in the course of the disease the predominant lesion is intimal fibrosis and the elevated vascular resistance is relatively fixed. This progression of histologic features has not been observed over time in a single patient with primary pulmonary hypertension, but the physiologic equivalent has been reported: on one occasion acetylcholine produced a marked decrease in pulmonary arterial pressure, but 3 years later had no effect.[36] It is interesting to note that the ability to reduce pulmonary hypertension by the use of vasodilators does not exclude thromboembolism as an etiologic factor. Some decrease in pulmonary arterial pressure and resistance was obtained with 1 or more vasodilators in each of 5 patients who had clear evidence of pulmonary embolism.[37]

Anderson et al. have proposed an alternative to the explanation that medial hypertrophy occurs first, and the intimal change follows later.[27] They suggest that intimal proliferation may occur intially and that the medial hypertrophy could arise, either because of the mechanical obstruction downstream, or because of a vasoconstrictor effect of the intimal cells. Several items of circumstantial evidence support the contention that endothelial cell function is altered, although they do not necessarily indicate that this is the first step in the pathogenesis of primary pulmonary hypertension. For instance, a reduced ability of the pulmonary vascular endothelium to extract endogenous norepinephrine has been demonstrated in patients with several forms of pulmonary hypertension and probably represents diminished function occurring as a result of the pulmonary hypertension.[38] It is not known whether the norepinephrine that is not extracted may itself exacerbate the pulmonary hypertension. The relationship of the pulmonary vascular endothelium to the reactivity of the adjacent smooth muscle has only recently been recognized. The relaxation of rabbit pulmonary artery rings by acetylcholine is dependent upon the integrity of the endothelium.[39] The same holds true for the relaxation caused by bradykinin in dogs.[40] As mentioned earlier,[28] reduced fibrinolytic activity has been described in the systemic venous endothelium of patients with primary pulmonary hypertension, which might suggest a more widespread endothelial abnormality, not merely occurring as a result of increased pulmonary arterial pressure. If endothelial cell function is indeed impaired, this could reduce the formation of the endogenous pulmonary vasodilator, prostacyclin.

Information obtained from the study of lung histology sometimes suggests an initial change in the pulmonary vascular endothelium. Electron micrographs in one patient with primary pulmonary hypertension showed a marked increase in the thickness of the endothelial cells of the capillaries and small non-muscular arteries, together with numerous pinocytotic vesicles which suggested an increase in cellular activity.[41] Light microscopy in this case revealed medial hypertrophy but intimal fibrosis is occasionally observed in the absence of medial hypertrophy.[42] These clues indicate that abnormalities of endothelial function should be considered in the search for the pathogenesis of primary pulmonary hypertension. However, regardless of whether medial hypertrophy or intimal change comes first, these ideas propose mechanisms, not etiologic stimuli. The cause, or causes, of the vasoconstriction of endothelial cell malfunction remain unknown.

Auto-immune Disease

The greater incidence of primary pulmonary hypertension in young women and its occurrence in patients with known collagen disease raise the possibility that there is an underlying immune process. Primary pulmonary hypertension has been reported in association with systemic lupus erythematosus,[43,44] Raynaud's disease,[17,45] Raynaud's disease as part of the CREST syndrome,[46] scleroderma,[47] rheumatoid arthritis,[48] dermatomyositis,[49] polymyositis,[50] and mixed connective tissue disease.[51] Sera from 31 of 52 patients with scleroderma and 11 of 19 patients with Raynaud's disease were found to contain cytotoxic activity specific for endothelial cells, compared to only 1 of 24 patients with other active connective tissue diseases.[52] The authors of this report speculated that initial endothelial cell damage may lead to platelet activation and associated smooth muscle proliferation. The cells involved in the intimal thickening of scleroderma have ultrastructural features of smooth muscle,[53] and platelets are known to release a factor which causes smooth muscle proliferation in vitro[54,55] The possible role of platelets is discussed in more detail at the end of this section.

The severity of pulmonary hypertension in scleroderma is not related to the degree of interstitial fibrosis.[46,47] This disparity and the effectiveness of vasodilators in some patients led Sackner et al. to propose that vasospasm might in part be responsible for the pulmonary hypertension which can occur in scleroderma.[56] More recently, pulmonary vasoconstriction has been documented in a patient with scleroderma who was exposed to cold.[57] Another interesting report concludes that patients with isolated Raynaud's disease develop pulmonary vasospasm when their hands are immersed in cold water, thus suggesting a more generalized form of vasoconstriction in this condition.[58] This suggestion parallels the possibility, mentioned earlier, that there is an association between Raynaud's disease, variant angina, and migraine headaches.[31,32] Recently, 7 out of 8 patients with the CREST syndrome (calcinosis, Raynaud's disease, esophageal dysmotility, sclerodactyly, and telangiectasia) were documented to have pulmonary hypertension.[59] The strongest association of primary pulmonary hypertension seems to be with that part of the autoimmune spectrum represented by Raynaud's disease and scleroderma. It is possible that primary pulmonary hypertension shares some etiologic factor or factors with them, and thus information concerning endothelial damage or vasoconstriction in Raynaud's disease or scleroderma that may provide insight into the pathophysiology of primary pulmonary hypertension. The fact that Raynaud's phenomenon is commonly induced by combination chemotherapy with vinblastine and bleomycin for malignant disease[60,61] suggests a potential model for the study of vasospastic disease.

Familial Factors

The first description of a single family in which more than 1 member had unexplained pulmonary hypertension was published by Clarke et al. in 1927.[62] By 1980, the experience of Wagenvoort and Wagenvoort, combined with cases in the literature, recorded 58 patients in 28 families.[15] In one instance, primary pulmonary hypertension was documented to occur in twins.[63] In many cases an autosomal dominant mode of inheritance has been demonstrated, although it has incomplete penetrance and may skip several generations and consequently appear to be sporadic. Alternatively, it may persist in a family for several generations.[64] The association between primary pulmonary hypertension and autoimmune disease is strengthened by the observation that the family of a patient with primary pulmonary hypertension may include others with Raynaud's disease, but no overt pulmonary hypertension.[65] This could imply that the genetic substrate is such that another stimulus can cause pulmonary hypertension, or that the Raynaud's disease and the pulmonary hypertension are manifestations of the same disease. One family has been reported to have abnormal fibrinolysis, and the suggestion was made that the mechanism of the pulmonary hypertension might involve impaired lysis of recurrent microemboli.[66] However, in another family, which included 3 cases of primary pulmonary hypertension, no deficiencies of the fibrinolytic system could be found.[67] An experimental model of the genetic propensity to develop pulmonary hypertension has been described in cattle,[68,69] which may be helpful in defining the genetic component that contributes to the individual reactivity of pulmonary vessels.

Persistent fetal circulation in the neonate, which is described in detail in Chapter 2, is a form of unexplained pulmonary hypertension. However, survivors of persistent fetal circulation have not been reported to have long-term pulmonary hypertension. In addition, children and adults presenting with unexplained pulmonary hypertension seldom give a history of problems in the neonatal period. Studies of the elastic pattern of the main pulmonary artery indicate that most primary pulmonary hypertension is acquired, rather than congenital. In the congenital form, the elastic fibers retain the closely packed, parallel appearance present in the fetus. In the adult form the fibers are shorter and more irregular.[70,71] It is also significant that in the persistent fetal circulation there is considerable extension of smooth muscle into the small, normally non-muscular arteries, while this feature is less prominent in primary pulmonary hypertension. In the latter condition there is a marked loss of small arteries on angiography,[72] which is not seen in persistent fetal circulation.

Factors Related to Pregnancy and the Menstrual cycle

Primary pulmonary hypertension is often first noticed during pregnancy. However, it may well be that the condition was present earlier and was exacerbated by the hemodynamic changes of pregnancy, or came to light at an antenatal examination. Normally, pulmonary arterial pressure in women is lower than usual during pregnancy,[73] and the pulmonary vascular reactivity in dogs is known to be reduced during pregnancy.[74]

The care of the pregnant patient with primary pulmonary hypertension will be considered in the section on management. The menstrual cycle involves changes in systemic vascular reactivity. The pattern of vasoconstriction during menstruation, followed by vasodilatation, occurs not only in the spiral arteries supplying the endometrium but has also been described in the vascular bed of the conjunctiva.[75] Whether similar changes occur in pulmonary vascular reactivity has not been studied. The reason for the increased incidence of primary pulmonary hypertension in women of child-bearing age is unknown. While it is obviously not the sole etiologic factor, the high incidence in this group should be remembered as a possible clue to the underlying mechanism.

Shepard et al. suggested that amniotic fluid embolism might be an etiologic factor in primary pulmonary hypertension.[76] However, histologic examination in one of the patients who had been pregnant "showed no features that could be interpreted as residue of amniotic embolism." Amniotic fluid embolism is usually apparent clinically,[77,78] and survivors have not been recognized to have a high incidence of chronic pulmonary hypertension. As discussed earlier, it is clear that the ratio of women to men developing primary pulmonary hypertension increases markedly at puberty, but there is no evidence that this is related to amniotic embolism or any other form of pulmonary embolism.

Drugs and Diet

Most patients with primary pulmonary hypertension do not give an atypical history of drug ingestion or abnormal diet. However, between 1967 and 1970 in central Europe, a sudden increase in the incidence of primary pulmonary hypertension occurred approximately a year after the introduction of aminorex, an appetite suppressant.[79] The "epidemic" subsided shortly after the drug was withdrawn. The details of the pulmonary hypertension related to aminorex are discussed in Chapter 9. About 2% of the population taking aminorex were shown to develop pulmonary hypertension. These may have been people who were genetically susceptible or they may have coincidentally taken other common drugs, such as acetaminophen, which can alter hepatic metabolism. At least 1 report states that following the discontinuation of aminorex these patients seem to have a somewhat better prognosis than patients with primary pulmonary hypertension who have no documented intake of anorectic agents.[79] It may be that if the etiologic stimuli could be recognized in primary pulmonary hypertension and removed, the prognosis in this condition would also improve.

Besides the appetite suppressant agents, the oral contraceptives form another group of drugs whose relationship to primary pulmonary hypertension is uncertain. It has been suggested that in some cases oral contraceptives may be involved in the etiology.[80] Another report on 3 patients with congenital septal defects of the heart indicated that the use of oral contraceptives may have accelerated the course of the pulmonary vascular disease.[81] The incidence of venous thrombosis, whether apparent[82,83] or subclinical,[84] is about 3 times more common in women taking oral contraceptives than in those who do not. For the reasons discussed earlier, it is not thought that pulmonary embolism is the underlying etiologic stimulus in primary pulmonary hypertension. However, the increased tendency to thromboembolism in women taking oral contraceptives highlights another factor. It has been mentioned that fibrinolytic activity is sometimes found to be reduced in patients with primary pulmonary hypertension. After cessation of oral contraceptives, patients who have recovered from thromboembolism show a greater than expected number with decreased plasminogen activators in vein biopsy specimens and reduced fibrinolytic responses to venous occlusion.[85,86] In connection with the previous subsection, it is worth noting that fibrinolytic activity is also reduced during pregnancy.[87] In view of these associations, the potential significance of decreased fibrinolytic activity in the etiology of primary pulmonary hypertension needs to be assessed further.

Cirrhosis and Portal Hypertension

Patients with cirrhosis occasionally develop pulmonary hypertension which is histologically indistinguishable from the primary form.[88,89] This combination of conditions is very rare: 0.26% of patients with cirrhosis and 0.016% of all autopsies.[90] When both cirrhosis and pulmonary hypertension are present in 1 patient, they may be part of a more generalized autoimmune disease.[91] Although it has been suggested that pulmonary embolism from portal venous thromboses might be responsible,[92] the histology usually resembles the diffuse involvement seen in primary pulmonary hypertension rather than the patchy changes of thromboembolism. In addition, it is unusual for thrombosis to be apparent in the portal venous system of these patients at autopsy. Other etiologic possibilities include the hypothesis that endogenous or exogenous vasoconstrictor substances from the splanchnic circulation bypass the liver and are not detoxified prior to reaching the pulmonary vasculature.

The experimental creation of a portocaval shunt results in several metabolic changes which might be relevant, including a decrease in hepatic monoamine oxidase activity[93] and a reduction in oxidative metabolism in the brain.[94] However, it is not known whether these changes also occur in lung tissue, and attempts to provoke pulmonary vascular alterations by the surgical production of portal hypertension in rats have failed.[95] Bile duct ligation in the rat leads to ultrastructural changes in both alveolar cells and pulmonary capillary endothelium.[96] It is interesting to note that the relationship between hepatic function and pulmonary vascular reactivity is somewhat contradictory. Some patients with cirrhosis may have a diminished or absent pulmonary pressor response to hypoxia,[97] in contrast to the occasional patient who develops a condition akin to primary pulmonary hypertension. Patients who die in hepatic failure have been shown to have diffuse dilatation of the pulmonary vascular bed.[98]

Other Etiologic Clues

Platelet survival in vivo was found to be decreased in 7 of 13 patients with primary pulmonary hypertension. This change might be secondary to the pulmonary hypertension itself, but recent work suggesting an etiologic role for platelets in other forms of pulmonary hypertension,[99-101] raises the possibility that the platelets might be involved in the etiology of primary pulmonary hypertension. As mentioned earlier, platelets can release a factor which stimulates smooth muscle proliferation in vitro.[54,55] Proliferation of smooth muscle after endothelial injury in the intact rabbit is markedly inhibited when thrombocytopenia is induced first,[102] thus suggesting that platelets also play a part in vivo.

Thromboxane A_2 is known to cause both platelet aggregation and pulmonary vasoconstriction. In an 8-year-old girl with primary pulmonary hypertension the circulating level of the breakdown product, thromboxane B_2, was 850 pg/ml (normal 65 pg/ml).[103] It is not known whether this increase was primary or secondary. However, 1 patient has been reported to show a reduction in pulmonary arterial pressure following administration of indomethacin, an inhibitor of prostaglandin-like substances, including thromboxane A_2.[104] Further research is needed to determine whether platelets or prostaglandin-like substances, including leukotrienes, are involved in the etiology of primary pulmonary hypertension. Granulocyte aggregation and sequestration in the lung is known to cause endothelial damage[105] and this pathophysiologic mechanism should also be considered. It may be relevant to note that the bronchial arteries, which share some of the environmental conditions of the pulmonary arteries, are histologically normal in primary pulmonary hypertension. This consideration might place more emphasis on the role of components of the blood returning to the lungs from the body.

CLINICAL MANIFESTATIONS

Symptoms

Patients who have primary pulmonary hypertension almost invariably suffer from breathlessness on exertion. In addition to being the most common symptom, it is usually the first. However, by the time breathlessness appears, the disease is already far advanced and the pulmonary arterial pressure is markedly elevated. The breathlessness cannot be explained on the basis of hypoxemia in most cases. Pulmonary ventilation studies may be normal, but frequently patients show a reduction in vital capacity[106] and sometimes a decrease in lung compliance.[107] It has been suggested that the breathlessness may be related to an inability to increase cardiac output during exertion.[108] In some patients the cardiac output does increase during exercise and, because the pulmonary vascular resistance is relatively fixed, the pulmonary arterial pressure rises rapidly. This acute, more severe pulmonary hypertension may contribute to the dyspnea in these instances. As the disease progresses, breathlessness also occurs at rest and fatigue becomes a frequent complaint. Somewhat surprisingly, orthopnea is a relatively common late symptom, though paroxysmal dyspnea is seldom described.

Other symptoms which are often noted include: chest pain, palpitations, ankle swelling and syncope, or a feeling of faintness. Again, the fixed pulmonary vascular resistance and associated low cardiac output probably provide the explanation for much of the fatigue and syncope occurring with exertion. In some cases a vagally induced bradycardia may be responsible. It has also been suggested that the arteries supplying the sinus and atrioventricular nodes are involved in the pathologic vascular process and that this observation might explain some of the syncopal episodes.[109] With this possible exception, the coronary arteries are usually normal and the angina may be the result of relative underperfusion of hypertrophied right ventricular muscle. A contributory factor may be the stretching of the large pulmonary arteries.[110] If the chest pain is pleuritic, other causes of pulmonary hypertension, such as embolism or collagen disease, should be considered.

Other symptoms are less common and tend to occur late in the course of the disease. These include hemoptysis, which may be fatal[111]; hoarseness, caused by the pressure of the main pulmonary artery on the recurrent laryngeal nerve[111]; abdominal pain associated with hepatic distension; and cyanosis. The cyanosis can be the result of a right-to-left shunt across a patent foramen ovale. Significant intrapulmonary shunting is uncommon. In addition to the central cyanosis, peripheral cyanosis occurs because of the low cardiac output. A persistent dry cough is sometimes a distressing symptom.

Signs

Prior to the onset of right heart failure, the clinical signs are those of pulmonary hypertension and a diminished cardiac output. The degree of breathlessness at rest varies from patient to patient. It is unusual for cyanosis to be prominent at the initial presentation. The pulse is rapid and its volume is small. The hands and feet are cold. Because of the diminished compliance of the right ventricle, the a wave of the jugular venous pulse is easily seen (Figure 1). A left parasternal lift is usually detectable as a result of right ventricular hypertrophy, but as this is a pressure overload situation, it is less impressive than that caused by volume changes, such as the left atrial expansion which occurs in severe mitral regurgitation. Quite often the systolic impulse of the pulmonary artery can be felt in the second left intercostal space and the closure of the pulmonary valve is also palpable. On auscultation, a pulmonary systolic ejection click is sometimes heard, followed by a relatively soft systolic ejection murmur. The pulmonary component of the second heart sound is as loud, or louder than, the aortic component[112] and the splitting of the 2 components may be normal or close. When severe pulmonary hypertension is present, an early diastolic murmur of pulmonary insufficiency is occasionally audible. A right ventricular fourth heart sound is frequently heard at the left sternal border.

With the onset of right ventricular failure the presence of cyanosis may be more apparent. Clubbing is rarely seen. Leg edema, elevation of the jugular venous pressure, and hepatomegaly are evident. If tricuspid insufficiency occurs, the liver will be felt to be pulsatile and the v wave becomes equal to, or more prominent than, the a wave in the jugular venous pulse. The pansystolic murmur of tricuspid regurgita-

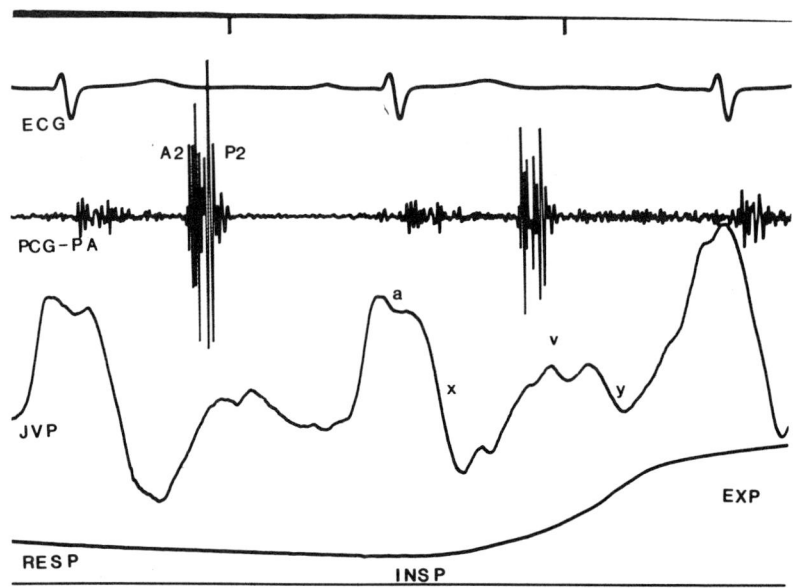

Figure 1. Phonocardiogram and jugular venous pulse (JVP) tracing of a patient with moderately severe primary pulmonary hypertension (PA pressure 84/28). P_2 is as loud as A_2 on the phonocardiogram (PCG) recorded in the pulmonary area (PA). There is a prominent "a" wave in the JVP. The respiratory trace shows inspiration and expiration.

tion is heard over the fourth left intercostal space and is loudest on inspiration. If the liver is not pulsatile and the murmur fails to change with respiration, the possibility of a ventricular septal defect should be considered. The tricuspid regurgitation is usually secondary to dilatation of the right ventricle, but spontaneous rupture of one of the papillary muscles has also been described in primary pulmonary hypertension.[113] The splitting of the second heart sound may become wider and fixed in patients with right heart failure. On the basis of the physical examination alone, it is usually impossible to differentiate between primary pulmonary hypertension and other causes of pulmonary hypertension, including Eisenmenger's syndrome.

LABORATORY INVESTIGATIONS

Because the history and the physical examination may be inconclusive, additional investigations are necessary to establish the diagnosis of pulmonary hypertension and to reduce the number of possible etiologies. However, none of these tests has specificity for primary pulmonary hypertension, with the exception of the lung biopsy. If arterial oxygen desaturation is present, the hematocrit may be increased and in some patients the erythrocyte sedimentation rate and plasma levels of γ-globulin are elevated.

The electrocardiogram reflects right ventricular hypertrophy and right atrial abnormality (See Figure 2, Chapter 1). The P waves tend to be tall and peaked (> 3 mm). The mean QRS axis is shifted to the right (> 90°). Tall dominant R waves are present in the anterior chest leads. ST depression and T wave inversion may occur in the same leads.

The chest x-ray can be helpful by suggesting the presence of pulmonary hypertension, but none of the measurements of pulmonary arterial size give an accurate indication of the severity of pulmonary hypertension in individual patients.[3] The routine PA and lateral projections show right ventricular enlargement, prominence of the main pulmonary artery segment, and dilatation of the right and left pulmonary arteries (Figures 2a and b). The peripheral lung fields may appear normal or oligemic. An increase in the cardiothoracic ratio correlates with a rise in right atrial pressure and consequently with right ventricular failure.[3]

Pulmonary function tests may be normal, although, as discussed earlier, the vital capacity and lung compliance are diminished in some patients.[106,107] The tests are helpful in assessing the potential contribution of chronic obstructive or restrictive lung diseases in the etiology of the pulmonary hypertension. The arterial blood gases are normal initially, but a reduction in oxygen tension occurs in the later stages of the disease. If hypoxemia and a respiratory alkalosis are present early in the course of the disease, pulmonary embolism should be considered.

The role of echocardiography in the diagnosis of pulmonary hypertension is similar to that of the chest x-ray; namely, it may sometimes suggest the presence of pulmonary hypertension but does little to quantitate it. It plays a more important part in excluding other conditions, such as mitral stenosis and left ventricular dysfunction. On the M-mode echocardiogram, pulmonary hypertension has been associated with mid-systolic notching (Figure 3), a diminution of the "a" dip (Figure 4), and prolongation of the right ventricular pre-ejection period.[114–116] However, more recent observations have failed to correlate pulmonary arterial pressure with "a" wave amplitude.[117] Mid-systolic notching lacks sensitivity[117] and can also occur in the absence of pulmonary hypertension.[118] Paradoxical movement of the inter-

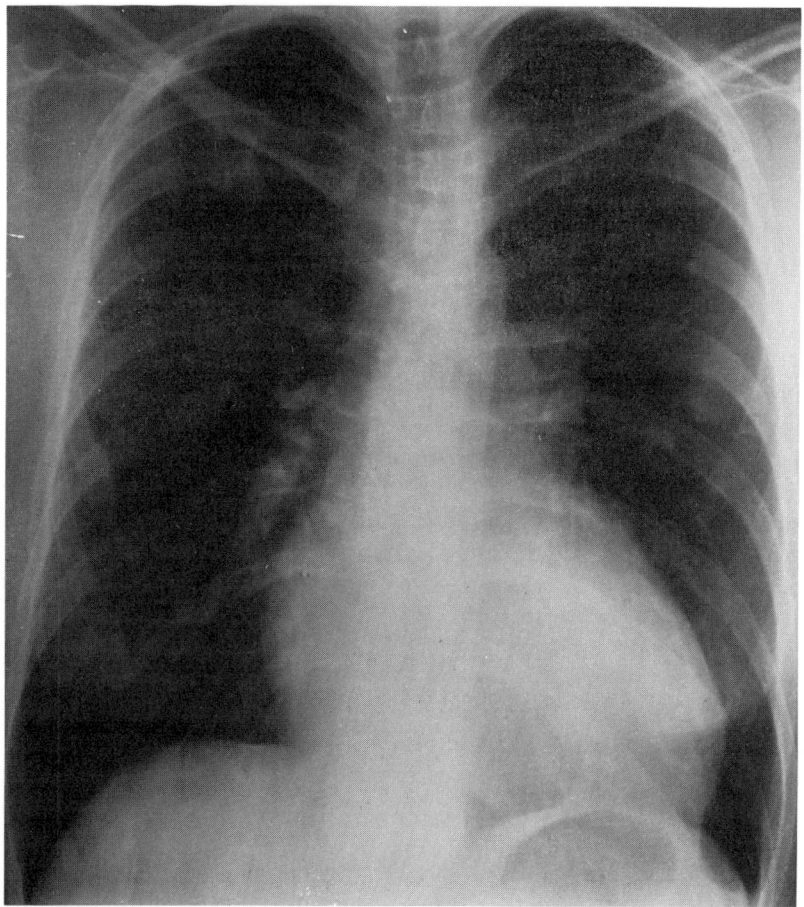

Figure 2a. Chest x-ray (PA) of patient with moderately severe primary pulmonary hypertension. Prominent main pulmonary artery. (Courtesy of Dr. J.W. Erdahl.)

ventricular septum can be demonstrated by M-mode or two-dimensional echocardiography in patients with primary pulmonary hypertension and also in other forms of right ventricular pressure overload.[119] Technical difficulties frequently make it impossible to obtain adequate studies of the pulmonary valve and thus limit the usefulness of M-mode echocardiography.[117] Two-dimensional echocardiography usually demonstrates some dilatation of the right ventricle when pulmonary hypertension is present (Figure 5). It can also be used to detect the presence of a right-to-left shunt at atrial or ventricular level when microbubbles cross the septum following the intravenous injection of indocyanine green dye or saline.

Diagnosis and Management of Primary Pulmonary Hypertension

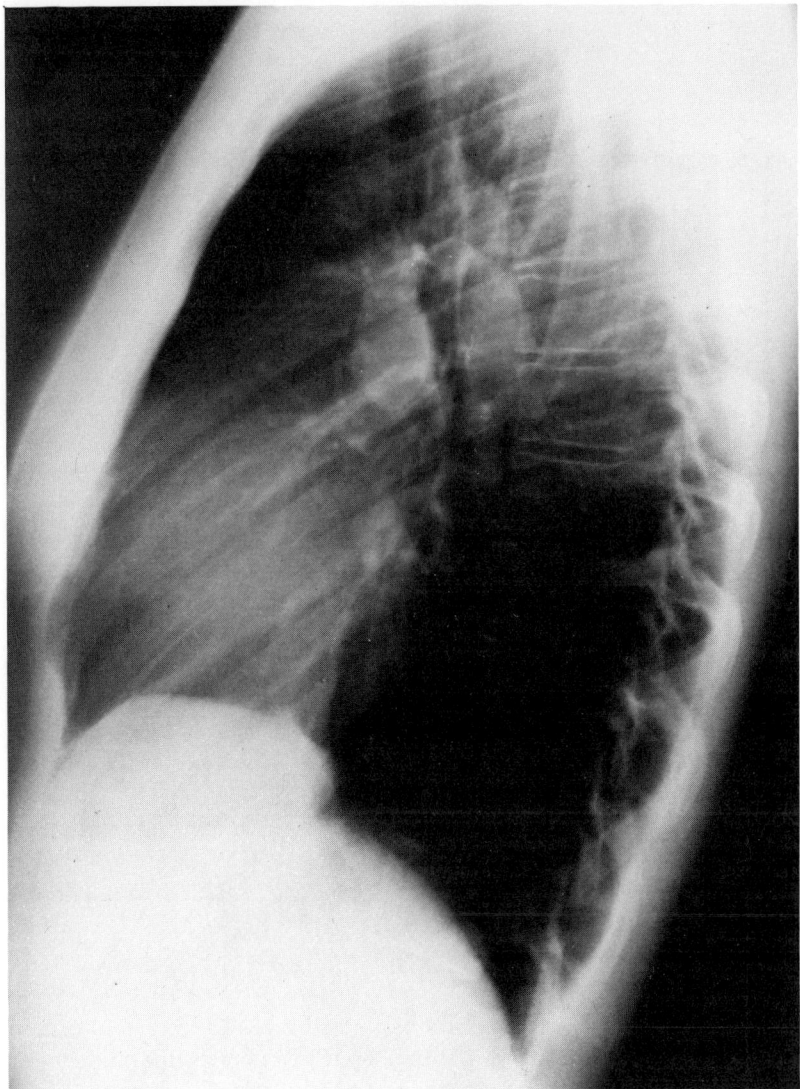

Figure 2b. Chest x-ray (Lateral) showing filling in of the retrosternal air-space, compatible with right ventricular enlargement. (Courtesy of Dr. J.W. Erdahl.)

Perfusion/ventilation lung scans are often used in an attempt to exclude major discrete perfusion defects, caused by thromboemboli, in patients already diagnosed as having pulmonary hypertension. The perfusion scan can be very helpful if it shows such large diagnostic segmental or lobar defects. In primary pulmonary hypertension the

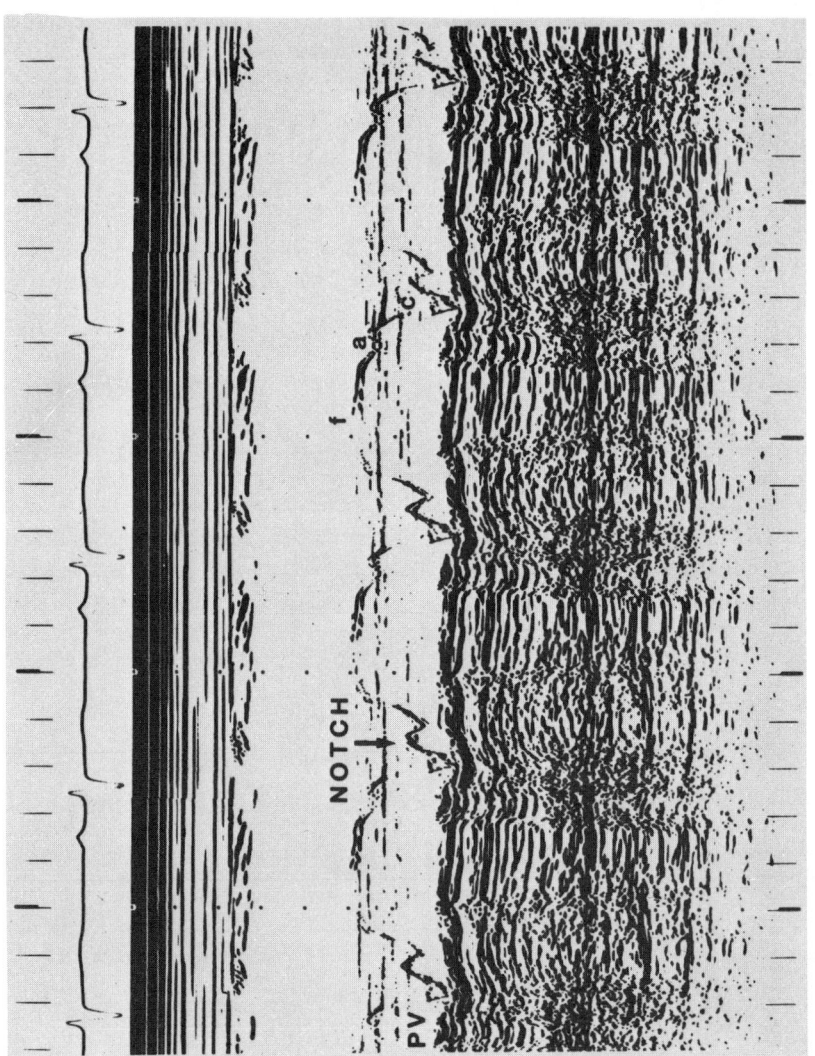

Figure 3. Echocardiogram from patient with severe primary pulmonary hypertension showing systolic notching of the posterior pulmonary valve cusp (PV), but continued presence of the "a" wave dip.

Diagnosis and Management of Primary Pulmonary Hypertension 135

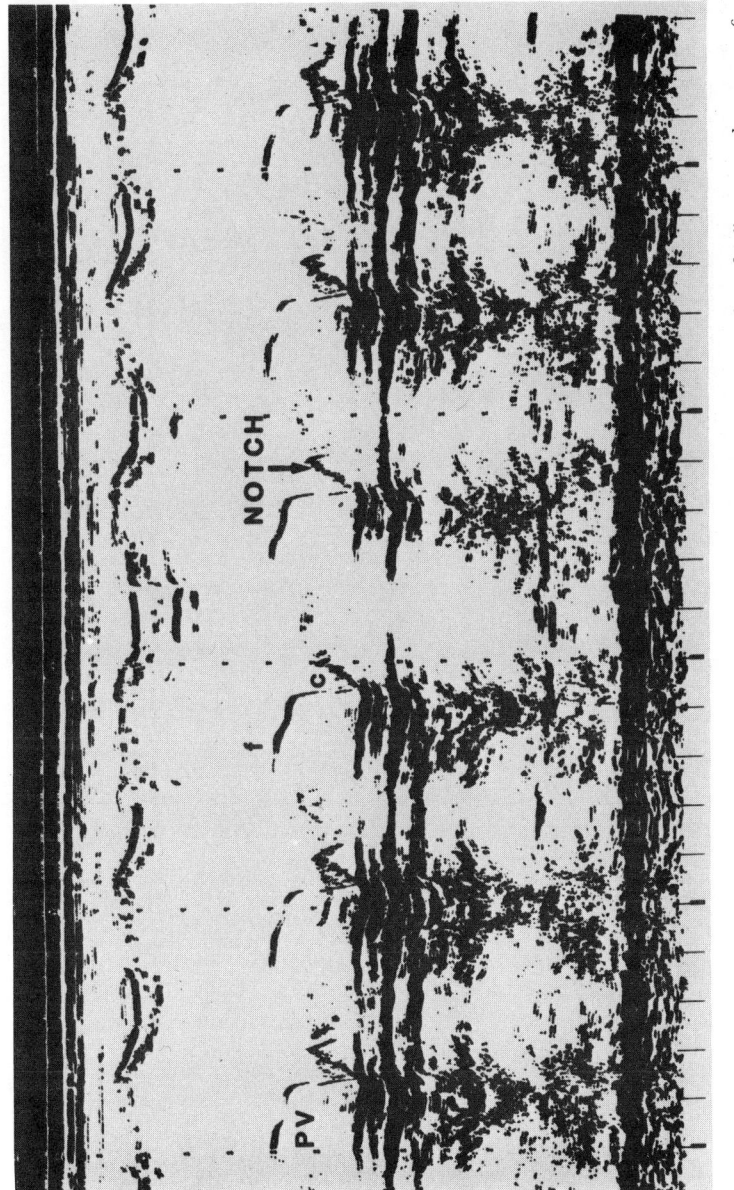

Figure 4. Echocardiogram from patient with severe primary pulmonary hypertension to show loss of "a" wave and presence of systolic notching on posterior pulmonary valve cusp (PV).

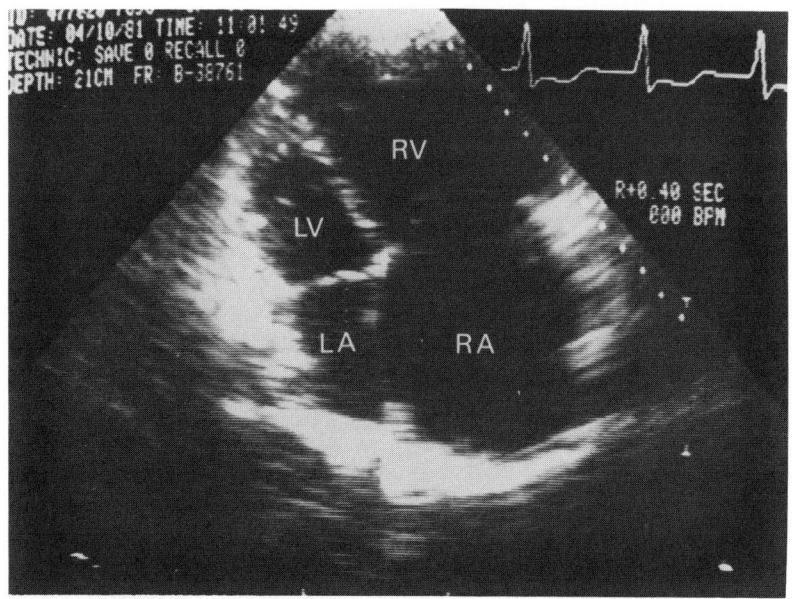

Figure 5. Two-dimensional echocardiogram illustrating marked dilatation of the right atrium (RA) and ventricle (RV) in a patient with severe primary pulmonary hypertension.

ventilation and perfusion lung scans may both be normal, or the perfusion scan may have a diffuse spotty appearance, without large filling defects.[120,121] Unfortunately, there is also an intermediate group with multiple, small, poorly-defined defects on the perfusion scan, which does not clearly include or exclude embolism,[120] similar to the pattern seen in Figure 6. It should be noted that in the presence of pulmonary hypertension the injection of macroaggregated albumin for perfusion scans has been reported to have caused several deaths.[122]

It has recently been demonstrated that ventilation/perfusion lung scans could be used to detect pulmonary hypertension.[123] In patients with pulmonary hypertension, the distribution of blood flow from the apex to the base of the lung in the erect position is more uniform than in normal subjects. Consequently, the change in the ratio of upper to lower zone perfusion, which occurs on moving from the supine to the erect position, is much smaller in patients with pulmonary hypertension. This change can be measured from the lung scan and corrected for lung volume. The gated pool scan, in the 45° left anterior oblique view, can demonstrate right ventricular enlargement and hypokinesis, if present.[124] It is also a very useful method of excluding left ventricular dysfunction as a cause of pulmonary hypertension.

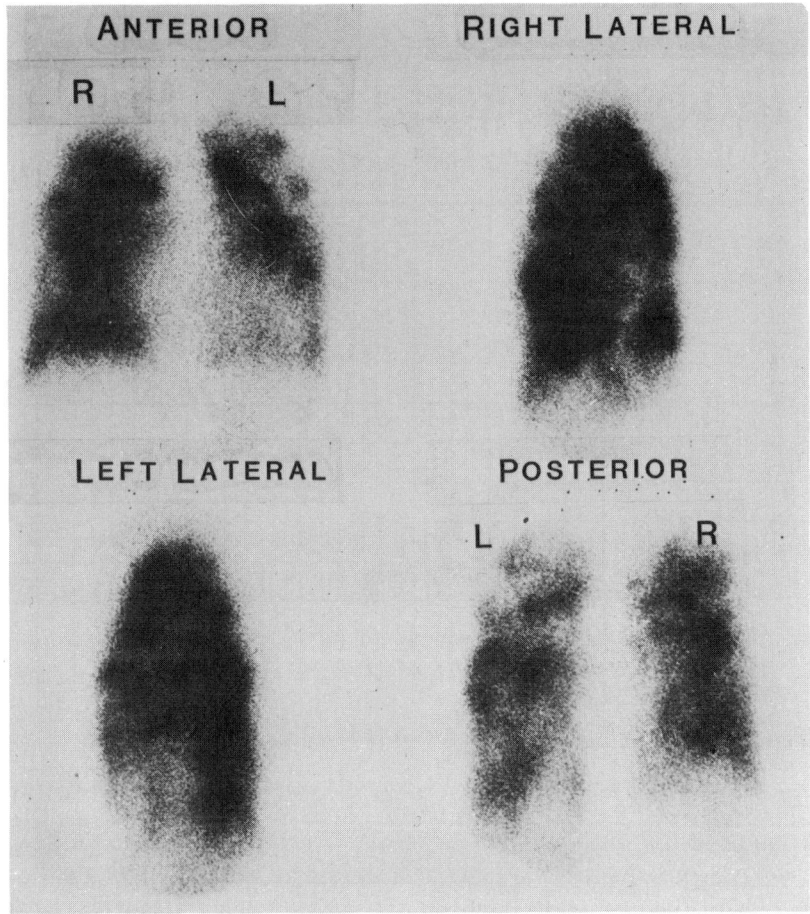

Figure 6. Technetium 99m MAA perfusion lung scan demonstrating multiple non-specific perfusion defects in a 20-year-old patient with severe pulmonary hypertension (PA 120/60 mm Hg), found at autopsy to have the rare form of primary pulmonary hypertension caused by pulmonary venous thrombosis, but no pulmonary thromboembolism. The non-specific perfusion pattern is the same as that seen in some patients with primary plexogenic pulmonary hypertension, but is indistinguishable from the scan produced by multiple small emboli.

Right heart catheterization is essential for the accurate measurement of pulmonary arterial pressure and resistance (Figure 7). However, as discussed in Chapter 1, the risk of catheterization in patients with severe pulmonary hypertension is relatively high, and it should only be performed in centers with experience in treating such patients. It is important to realize that pulmonary arterial pressure can fluctuate

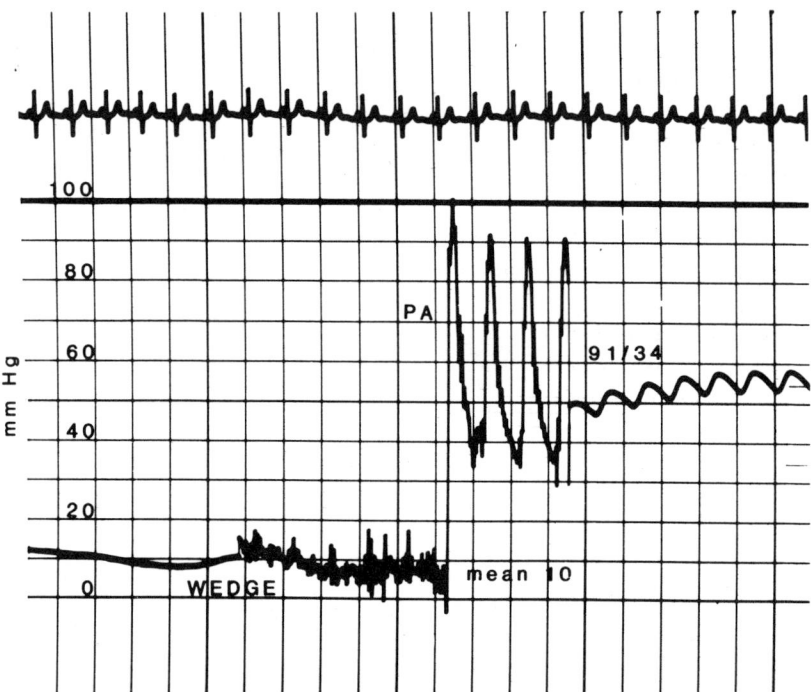

Figure 7. Markedly elevated pulmonary arterial pressure (PA) and normal pulmonary arteral wedge pressure (WEDGE), in a patient with severe primary pulmonary hypertension.

spontaneously, independent of changes in aortic pressure or heart rate.[125] Consequently, baseline data should be obtained over a period of at least 20 minutes. In relatively mild cases the measurements can be made both at rest and during supine bicycle exercise (as discussed in the section on treatment). Documentation of a normal pulmonary arterial wedge pressure (< 12 mm Hg) is an important step in excluding left-sided heart disease. The finding of a mean pulmonary artery pressure above 25 mm Hg confirms the diagnosis of pulmonary hypertension but leaves the question of etiology unanswered. Occasionally, pulmonary arterial pulsus alternans can be documented.[126]

Indicator dilution studies are the most reliable method for the exclusion of congenital intra-cardiac shunts, such as an atrial or ventricular septal defect. Pulmonary angiography has been used in an attempt to demonstrate the presence or absence of thromboembolic disease. This procedure is useful if filling defects or obstruction of major vessels by emboli can be seen. However, even large emboli can undergo lysis within 2 weeks and thrombosis-in-situ can be mistaken for embolism. Consequently, the angiogram is frequently inconclusive.[127] Wedge pulmonary arteriography can demonstrate emboli in arteries only 1 to 2 mm in diameter,[128] but the clinical value of the technique in the differential diagnosis of primary pulmonary hypertension has not been assessed. The postmortem injection of lungs with barium sulfate, followed by microradiography demonstrates the loss of small peripheral arteries which occurs in primary pulmonary hypertension.[72] The same loss of small arteries has been appreciated as a loss of background haze in clinical wedge angiograms obtained in patients with pulmonary hypertension secondary to congenital heart defects.[129]

The increased risk of pulmonary angiography in patients with primary pulmonary hypertension is well recognized.[15,130] Pulmonary arterial pressure is reported to increase by 10 to 15 mm Hg after pulmonary angiography.[131] Because of the risk and the lack of specificity, some centers do not perform pulmonary angiography and empirically treat with anticoagulants. If angiography is performed, the injection should be selective (preferable into one lobe at a time) and should be recorded on bi-plane film.

Open lung biopsy has been used for the definitive diagnosis of primary pulmonary hypertension during life for over 20 years[132] and recently has been used more frequently.[133] It permits histologic distinction between primary and thromboembolic pulmonary hypertension, as discussed in Chapter 11. It also allows the exclusion of pulmonary venous thrombosis. The latter is of questionable advantage, as pulmonary venous thrombosis is rare and has a poor prognosis, which is not improved by current treatment. Occasionally lung biopsy may reveal a previously unsuspected interstitial lung disease or autoimmune process, but the benefit for the individual patient undergoing the procedure is likely to be relatively low, unless there are symptoms or laboratory findings which suggest the possibility of collagen-vascular disease. In terms of our understanding of the natural history and treatment of the disease in general, lung biopsy could be very important. For instance, a vasodilator cannot be expected to be effective if there is widespread intimal fibrosis. Consequently, biopsy information is necessary for the definition of subgroups within the category of primary pulmonary hypertension, for the accurate comparison of different modes of treatment and for the exclusion of other diseases. There is likely to be a continuing debate of the merits, or otherwise, of lung biopsy. The author is not aware of any report of a death attributable to open lung biopsy in a patient with primary pulmonary hypertension.

DIFFERENTIAL DIAGNOSIS

Many diseases may give rise to pulmonary hypertension. Often the diagnosis of an underlying condition can be made from the history, physical examination, and a few routine laboratory tests. Occasionally more sophisticated studies are required as indicated in Table 1. Some conditions are relatively uncommon but may still merit consideration if the history is appropriate, such as: schistosomiasis[134]; choriocarcinoma[135]; sickle cell disease[136]; tumor emboli[137]; and the intravenous injection of pulverized pills, which can cause a granulomatous pulmonary vasculitis.[138] At the time that cardiac catheterization is performed to confirm the diagnosis of pulmonary hypertension and to obtain baseline hemodynamic data, many potential causes can be excluded. However, as discussed in the introduction, the remaining "primary pulmonary hypertension" patients do not represent a homogeneous population. The only way to ensure an accurate diagnosis is to subject the patient to open lung biopsy. This may be appropriate depending on the condition of the patient and the assessment of whether any likely change in diagnosis will result in a significant change in management.

While some diseases clearly provide a pathologic basis for pulmonary hypertension, in other instances, such as cirrhosis, scleroderma, and Raynaud's disease, it seems more appropriate to consider that the patient may have primary pulmonary hypertension associated, genetically or otherwise, with the other condition.

PATHOLOGY

The histologic changes which occur in the pulmonary vasculature of patients with plexogenic primary pulmonary hypertension are described in detail in Chapter 11. The early lesions include thickening of the media of the small arteries and intimal proliferation. The medial thickening is the result of hypertrophy of the smooth muscle cells, rather than hyperplasia.[41] "Onion-skin" intimal fibrosis, dilatation lesions, fibrinoid necrosis with or without arteritis, plexiform lesions, and pulmonary hemosiderosis are observed in more severe cases[15,27,29,133] as the disease progresses. Medial thickening is prominent in infants

TABLE 1
Causes of Pulmonary Hypertension

Potential Cause of Pulmonary Hypertension	Possible Diagnostic Studies
a) Pulmonary embolic disease:	ventilation/perfusion scans and/or selective, lobar pulmonary angiography (preferably biplane).
b) Pulmonary venous thrombosis or obstruction:	chest x-ray, angiography, lung biopsy.
c) Congenital intra-cardiac shunts causing increased pulmonary blood flow:	indicator dilution studies.
d) Increased left atrial pressure; secondary to mitral or aortic valve disease, left ventricular dysfunction or systemic hypertension	pulmonary artery wedge pressure or left atrial pressure (via patent foramen ovale) (> 15 mm Hg).
e) Pulmonary airways disease (e.g., chronic bronchitis and emphysema):	respiratory function tests (FVC/FEV_1).
f) Hypoxic pulmonary hypertension associated with (i) impaired ventilation; either central (CNS) or peripheral (chest wall problems or upper airway obstruction). (ii) residence at high altitude:	sleep apnea studies and respiratory tests.
g) Interstitial lung disease, pneumoconioses and fibrosis (e.g. silicosis, rheumatoid disease and sarcoidosis):	chest x-ray, spirometry and carbon monoxide diffusion, rheumatoid factor, lymph node biopsy.
h) Collagen disease (e.g., SLE, polyarteritis nodosa, scleroderma):	LE cells, FANA, skin, muscle, or other tissue biopsy, esophageal motility studies.
i) Parasitic disease (schistosomiasis or filariasis):	rectal biopsy, complement fixation, skin tests, blood smears.
j) Cirrhosis or portal vein thrombosis:	liver function tests.
k) Peripheral pulmonary artery stenosis (including Takayasus disease and fibrosing mediastinitis):	selective pulmonary angiography, or pressure gradient at catheterization.
l) Sickle cell disease:	erythrocyte morphology, hemaglobin electrophoresis.
m) Choriocarcinoma and hydatidiform mole:	serum or urinary β-subunit of chorionic gonadotrophin
n) Intravenous injection of pulverized pills:	lung biopsy.

and young children, while intimal proliferation and fibrosis usually become more marked in older children and adults.[15] The 1973 World Health Organization report[5] required the histologic demonstration of plexiform lesions in order to substantiate the diagnosis of plexogenic pulmonary hypertension. However, as medial thickening appears to be the initial change, it has been suggested that this early form should be included in the general category of plexogenic pulmonary arteriopathy.[29] It is important to remember that plexogenic lesions are not specific for primary pulmonary hypertension and are also seen when pulmonary hypertension is associated with congenital left-to-right shunts, cirrhosis, aminorex, or schistosomiasis.

MANAGEMENT

Changes in Life-style

While interest has recently focused on the use of vasodilators in patients with primary pulmonary hypertension, there are a number of general considerations which are also important. Patients with primary pulmonary hypertension have been noted to deteriorate during pregnancy and consequently, conception should be avoided.[13,21] Although oral contraceptives have not been demonstrated to cause primary pulmonary hypertension, an association between the two has been suggested,[80] and some other means of contraception is indicated. The little published information available suggests that continuing a pregnancy to term in the presence of primary pulmonary hypertension carries a considerable risk of maternal death.[13,139] Obviously, the extent of the risk will vary somewhat according to the severity of the pulmonary hypertension, but any patient who is symptomatic is likely to be intolerant of hypoxia, acidosis, or a demand for increased cardiac output. The possible advantages which may follow the termination of pregnancy are illustrated by two anecdotal cases. One patient (27 years) was found to be completely unresponsive to hydralazine when catheterized during the first trimester of pregnancy (Table 2). The pregnancy was terminated at the time and 9 months later, the same hydralazine regimen produced a significant reduction in pulmonary arterial pressure and resistance.[140] Another patient (23 years) was referred with severe primary pulmonary hypertension at the end of the first trimester of pregnancy.[141] Her initial pulmonary arterial

TABLE 2
Altered Response to Hydralazine after Termination of Pregnancy[140]

		Ppa	PVR
1st trimester of pregnacy	Control	61	7.9
	Hydralazine	61	8.3
9 months after termination	Control	61	9.5
	Hydralazine	52	7.9

Hydralazine was admnistered 50 mg orally q 6 hours for 48 hours. Ppa: mean pulmonary arterial pressure, mm Hg. PVR: pulmonary vascular resistance, mm Hg/L/min.

pressure was 166/75 (mean 104) mm Hg and total pulmonary resistance was 25.4 mm Hg/L/min. There was no response to oxygen, isoproterenol, or hydralazine. After 3 doses of diltiazem her pulmonary arterial pressure the next day was 128/38 (mean 77) mm Hg. The pregnancy was terminated using an intravenous infusion of oxytocin. Six days later her pulmonary arterial systolic pressure was less than 130 mm Hg despite discontinuation of the diltiazem. These two cases suggest that a modest improvement may follow termination of pregnancy and that the dangers of later pregnancy can be avoided. If the decision to terminate a pregnancy is made, prostaglandin $F_2\alpha$ should not be used by any route, as it is known to cause an increase in pulmonary arterial pressure even in normal women undergoing abortion.[73] At the time of termination, cardiac output, systemic arterial blood gases, pulmonary and systemic arterial pressures should be monitored carefully. Loss of blood or acidosis should be corrected quickly.

Primary pulmonary hypertension may be more common at high altitude.[142] It is not known whether there is any relationship between the mechanism of hypoxic pulmonary vasoconstriction and the pathophysiology of primary pulmonary hypertension, but any vasoconstrictor stimulus is likely to be deleterious and patients should be advised to move to low altitude if possible. One 16-year-old girl in Leadville (10,200 feet) was found to have pulmonary hypertension (pulmonary arterial pressure 67/27 mm Hg), possibly on the basis of chronic hypoxic pulmonary vasoconstriction. After living at sea level for 11 months her pressure was 33/8 mm Hg.[143] While it is unlikely that she suffered from primary pulmonary hypertension, the case illustrates the potential benefit of moving to a lower altitude. Smoking has not been shown to be an etiologic factor in primary pulmonary hypertension, but as nicotine inhibits the vascular production of prostacyclin, while leaving the platelet synthesis of thromboxane intact,[144] it is likely in theory to exaccerbate pulmonary hypertension.

Potential Iatrogenic Problems

In one paper published in 1955 the intravenous administration of barbiturates was reported to cause hypotension and death in 2 patients with primary pulmonary hypertension.[145] Subsequent papers have not specifically incriminated barbiturates but have indicated an increased risk of anesthesia, surgical procedures, and cardiac catheterization.[15,146] Data from animal experiments suggest that it may be advisable to avoid the use of histamine H_2 blockers, such as cimetidine, and prostaglandin synthetase inhibitors, such as indomethacin, because they can increase the severity of hypoxic pulmonary vasoconstriction.[147,148] At present these remain theoretical considerations.

Anticoagulation and Antiplatelet Agents

In the clinical situation it can be very difficult to make the differential diagnosis between primary pulmonary hypertension and pulmonary hypertension produced by multiple occult thromboemboli. Even with pulmonary angiography it is not always possible to distinguish one condition from the other. Of 156 cases submitted to Wagenvoort and Wagenvoort as primary pulmonary hypertension, 31 showed a histologic pattern suggesting thromboembolism.[15] Goodwin et al. have also stressed the difficulty of making the differential diagnosis.[149] Because it may be impossible to exclude thromboembolism, it is relatively easy to justify the use of anticoagulants, although they are not routinely used by many centers. Another reason for their administration is the possibility that the etiology of primary pulmonary hypertension might involve microthromboemboli. Goodwin et al. recommend using oral anticoagulants in both thromboembolic and primary pulmonary hypertension. However, they and others[14,149-151] have been unable to document any improvement in patients with primary pulmonary hypertension on this treatment. One retrospective study has suggested a beneficial effect of anticoagulants on survival.[152]

A case can also be made for the administration of antiplatelet agents. Abnormalities of platelet function have been recorded in primary pulmonary hypertension[153] and could be important in the pathogenesis, as discussed in the section on etiology. In addition, animal laboratory experiments have shown that dipyridamole can cause pulmonary vasodilatation, an effect which is independent of its action on platelets.[154]

VASODILATORS: GENERAL CONSIDERATIONS

Vasodilators have been tried in the management of primary pulmonary hypertension since 1951[11] and recently there has been a surge of interest in this mode of treatment.[155-158] Up to this time a number of factors have made a prospective controlled trial impossible: (i) as mentioned in the introduction, the clinical diagnosis of primary pulmonary hypertension often includes patients with other conditions; (ii) any one medical center admits comparatively few patients with primary pulmonary hypertension (perhaps 5 to 10 patients/year in a major medical center with a known interest in the condition); (iii) cardiac catheterization is necessary to establish both the baseline pulmonary hemodynamics and the response to treatment; (iv) even when the hemodynamic data have been obtained, histologic staging of the severity of the disease, to allow more accurate comparison between patients, can only be made after open lung biopsy; (v) the natural history is quite variable. Because of these factors the difficulty of comparing different vasodilator regimes will be apparent. Despite this, useful information can be obtained on the relative efficacy of 2 agents if they are given sequentially in a random, double-blind manner, for several months each, so that each patient is their own control.

There are several additional major problems to be considered in the use of vasodilators. One such problem is the fact that no vasodilator is specific for pulmonary vascular smooth muscle. Consequently, if the vasodilator induces systemic vasodilatation in the face of a relatively fixed pulmonary vascular resistance (e.g., with widespread intimal fibrosis), systemic hypotension will follow. Alternatively, the systemic vasodilatation quite often results in an increase in cardiac output and, although the calculated pulmonary vascular resistance may fall, the pulmonary arterial pressure actually rises, thus increasing right ventricular work. This sequence is potentially fatal,[159] and it is imperative that vasodilator therapy be initiated only when sequential cardiac output and pulmonary arterial pressure measurements can be obtained.

The ideal acute response to the vasodilator is both a reduction in pulmonary arterial pressure and an increase in cardiac output to within the normal range. However, it is more common to observe an increase in cardiac output and a fall in the calculated pulmonary vascular resistance but little or no reduction in pulmonary arterial pressure. It has been suggested that such a response may not be beneficial,[160] but in 9 patients with pulmonary hypertension (including 2 with primary pulmonary hypertension), who showed this pattern when treated with hydralazine, the mean right ventricular end-diastolic pressure fell from 18 + 6 to 12 + 5 (S.D.) mm Hg[161] (See Figure 10 of Chapter 7). The reduction in end-diastolic pressure was correlated with the reduction in pulmonary vascular resistance and suggests an improvement in the right ventricular failure. Patients who have an increase in cardiac output, but no change in pulmonary artery pressure, often report a lessening of fatigue. While patients with a low cardiac output have a poor prognosis,[24] it is not known whether a drug-induced increase in cardiac output will improve longevity. It is not even known whether the long-term reduction in pulmonary arterial pressure and resistance achieved by vasodilator drugs in a few patients will prolong life. Although an improvement would seem likely, it may be relevant to recall that in patients with cor pulmonale treated with home oxygen, the group of patients who showed a large fall in pulmonary arterial pressure tended to have a higher mortality than patients with small decreases in pressure.[162]

Some centers advocate testing the effect of vasodilators during supine bicycle exercise as well as at rest, in an attempt to demonstrate that a vasodilator, which may have little effect on resting hemodynamics, can reduce the increase in pulmonary arterial pressure occurring on exercise. While this occurs occasionally, patients with symptomatic primary pulmonary hypertension can seldom exercise for long and the procedure increases the discomfort and risk involved. If exercise is used, the upright bicycle should be avoided in the acute test because of systemic hypotension.

Many investigators at present try several pulmonary vasodilator drugs during one cardiac catheterization study. The response of the individual patient is unpredictable and a person who develops pulmonary vasodilatation with one drug may not respond to another. Many do not respond to any vasodilator therapy. While additional data can be obtained by studying the patient on 2 consecutive days, observation in an intensive care unit is necessary if the Swan-Ganz catheter is to be left in place overnight and there is small but real danger of ventricular ectopy or pulmonary infarction from a wedged catheter. The potential dangers of catheterization are discussed in Chapter 1.

An acute response to a particular drug given orally or intravenously does not guarantee a long-term response. However, one recent study found that patients who responded acutely to prostacyclin and nifedipine had an improved exercise capacity after 3 months of treatment with calcium blockers, while those who did not respond acutely did not improve on chronic treatment.[163] Consequently, the acute screening process seems to be a logical approach to the problem. Some patients claim symptomatic improvement despite a lack of objective improvement in their hemodynamic status. For this reason it is important that the catherization should be repeated 2 or 3 months after the initiation of oral therapy, in order to evaluate progress. Although this may appear to be an overly invasive form of management, the disease often progresses rapidly and an aggressive attempt to reverse its course can be justified. Only a minority of patients with systemic hypertension require multiple drug regimes. Although the management of primary pulmonary hypertension is currently at the stage where the efficacy of each drug has to be demonstrated, it is likely that the majority of patients will benefit from the simultaneous use of several interventions. The NIH registry of patients with primary pulmonary hypertension may indicate which of the agents discussed below are most useful.

Historically, acetylcholine and tolazoline hydrochloride (Priscoline) have been given to determine whether there might be a reversible component of vascular spasm contributing to pulmonary hypertension. Paul Wood observed a decrease in pulmonary arterial pressure and resistance in 5 out of 6 patients with primary pulmonary hypertension given acetylcholine into the pulmonary artery.[164] However, prolonged intravenous infusion of acetylcholine is not a practical proposition for the management of primary pulmonary hypertension. Pulmonary vasodilatation has also been seen in patients with primary pulmonary hypertension after the intravenous administration of tolazoline.[11] Unfortunately, a fatality has been reported following the injection of tolazoline,[165] and its oral use for primary pulmonary hypertension has not been found effective.[150,166] Thus, although tolazoline may be useful in the acute management of persistent fetal circulation,[167] it is seldom used now in the management of primary pulmonary hypertension.

VASODILATORS: DRUGS UNDER STUDY

The vasodilators currently being used can be divided into four categories: α-adrenergic blockers, β-adrenergic agonists, calcium channel blockers, and agents acting directly on vascular smooth muscle. The β-adrenergic agonists are seldom used at present and most interest is focused on the calcium blockers and direct-acting agents. The rationale for the use of these particular agents can be more easily appreciated with a knowledge of the physiologic control mechanisms of the pulmonary vasculature.[168-170] As in other areas of therapy, initial enthusiasm is often tempered somewhat on reappraisal (Table

3). In addition to those agents listed in the table, contrasting results have also been reported for prostacyclin[183,184] and captopril.[125,185] It will be apparent from Table 3 that vasodilators have been used extensively in primary pulmonary hypertension during the last few years. The marked variation in the reported responses to vasodilator administration probably reflects the lack of homogeneity within the clinical diagnosis of primary pulmonary hypertension and the different histologic stages discussed earlier. In this review of vasodilators the doses quoted are those which have been used during investigational studies, performed in several different countries.

β-adrenergic Stimulators

The sublingual administration of isoproterenol (20 mg) was reported in 1963 to decrease pulmonary vascular resistance, though not pulmonary arterial pressure, in 14 patients, including 3 with primary

TABLE 3
Varying Experience with Certain Vasodilators in Primary Pulmonary Hypertension

Hemodynamic Improvement in Some	*Adverse Effects*
1978—Isoproterenol as a potential pulmonary vasodilator in primary pulmonary hypertension.[171]	1978—Unfavorable hemodynamic and clinical effects of isoproterenol in primary pulmonary hypertension.[172]
1978—Diazoxide in treatment of primary pulmonary hypertension.[173]	1981—Hazards of diazoxide in pulmonary hypertension.[174]
1979—Primary pulmonary hypertension treated with oral phentolamine.[175]	1981—Adverse hemodynamic effects of phentolamine in primary pulmonary hypertension.[176]
1980—Oral hydralazine therapy for primary pulmonary hypertenson.[177]	1982—Deleterious effects of hydralazine in patients with pulmonary hypertension.[178]
1982—The role of hydralazine therapy for pulmonary arterial hypertension of unknown cause.[179]	1982—Adverse effect of hydralazine in patients with primary pulmonary hypertension.[180]
1981—Primary pulmonary hypertension: effects of nifedipine.[181]	1982—Failure of nifedipine treatment in primary pulmonary hypertension.[182]

pulmonary hypertension.[186] Several subsequent studies using both sublingual and intravenous isoproterenol generally supported these hemodynamic results of acute administration,[171,187,188] although some patients showed a rise in pulmonary arterial pressure as cardiac output increased.[160] Both pulmonary vascular resistance and pressure decreased in a few cases. Prolonged (30–36 months) hemodynamic improvement has been recorded in 3 patients on chronic sublingual isoproterenol (15 mg, from 6 to 20 times/day).[171,188] Unfortunately, the isoproterenol sometimes has to be decreased or stopped because of palpitations, tremulousness, a feeling of apprehension, and even angina.[172] It has been suggested that isoproterenol therapy may only produce symptomatic improvement, without prolonging life.[151,189] As discussed earlier, this comment can be made about any of the vasodilators currently in use. Terbutaline, a relatively selective β_2 agonist, has been tried unsuccessfully (both subcutaneously and orally), in 1 patient who responded to sublingual isoproterenol.[104] It seems likely that β-stimulators will soon be replaced by other pulmonary vasodilators which are better tolerated and have a longer duration of action.

α-adrenergic Blockers

Tolazoline hydrochloride, which was discussed above, causes competitive α blockade, in addition to several other actions. Phentolamine is a more potent α-blocker and its other effects are less prominent. In 1 patient phentolamine (5 mg) given intravenously caused a moderate reduction in resting pulmonary arterial pressure and resistance, and a considerable fall in these variables measured during exercise.[175] This patient continued to show hemodynamic benefit after 7 months on oral phentolamine (50 mg every 3 hours while awake; total daily dose, 250 mg). Another patient had a small reduction in pulmonary vascular resistance during exercise following 50 mg intravenous phentolamine (0.3 mg/min), but developed orthostatic hypotension on oral therapy.[190] A subsequent study reported 2 patients who responded well to intravenous phentolamine (5 mg iv), and also had a reduction in pulmonary arterial pressure and resistance during rest and exercise when given another α-blocker, prazosin (2–5 mg orally).[191] However, after 3 months oral prazosin therapy (15 mg/day), the pulmonary arterial pressure was the same in one and higher in the other. One patient given phentolamine (5 mg iv) developed a marked fall in systemic vascular resistance, a small increase in cardiac output, and an alarming rise in pulmonary arterial pressure.[176] The authors discuss the possibility that she had fixed anatomic vascular changes. This type of response strengthens the argument that only vasodilators which are rapidly reversible should be used to determine whether a vasoconstrictive element is present. Phenoxybenzamine is a longer acting α-blocker than phentolamine. In conjunction with oxygen administration at night, oral administration has been associated with improvement in pulmonary arterial pressure and resistance over a 7-month period in 1 patient.[192] Alpha-blockade will remain an important option in the treatment of primary pulmonary hypertension, but the current data do not indicate which specific blocker will be best.

Calcium Blockers

There are an increasing number of calcium channel blockers in clinical use or under study. However, only 3 have been tried in the management of primary pulmonary hypertension at this time. The pharmacology of these 3 calcium antagonists has been compared.[193] Verapamil has been tried acutely in 9 patients with primary pulmonary hypertension.[194] A total of 0.15 mg/kg was infused into the pulmonary artery at a rate of 1 mg/min. A significant reduction in mean pulmonary arterial pressure ($>$ 5 mm Hg) was achieved in only 3 patients with pulmonary vascular resistance increasing in 6 because of an alarming tendency for cardiac output to fall. Diltiazem (0.25 mg/kg iv) caused a modest fall in pulmonary arterial pressure, both during exercise and at rest, in 4 women with primary pulmonary hypertension.[195] In another report, diltiazem, given either intravenously (10 mg) or orally (30 mg), was found to reduce pulmonary arterial pressure and resistance acutely in 1 patient.[196] Eleven months after starting diltiazem (30 mg, 3 times daily) she was asymptomatic. Similar acute hemodynamic effects have been demonstrated with nifedipine (20 mg sublingually) in 4 patients.[181,197] After several months on oral nifedipine therapy, catheterization was repeated in 3 and all showed continued improvement. In 1 acute study, which included several subjects with primary pulmonary hypertension, sublingual nifedipine produced a greater mean fall in pulmonary arterial pressure and resistance than hydralazine, with less decrease in systemic arterial pressure.[198] Some patients, however, have not shown acute[182] or chronic[199] improvement with nifedipine. It is likely that calcium antagonists will be used in the future treatment of primary pulmonary hypertension, but there is insufficient clinical evidence at present to indicate which will be most effective. Because of its negative inotropic effect, verapamil is probably contraindicated. Experimental data indicate that nifedipine is a more effective acute pulmonary vasodilator in a dog model of pulmonary hypertension than diltiazem or verapamil.[200] Nifedipine may also be advantageous in some patients as it appears to inhibit experimentally-induced bronchoconstriction.[201]

Direct-acting Vasodilators

Diazoxide

Diazoxide was first suggested for the treatment of primary pulmonary hypertension in 1969.[202] The pharmacology and systemic actions of the drug have been well summarized.[203] In 1978 diazoxide was reported to cause an acute reduction in pulmonary arterial pressure and resistance when given intravenously in increasing doses (90, 180, and 300 mg), to 3 patients with primary pulmonary hypertension.[173] One had symptomatic improvement on oral diazoxide (400 mg/day) but died 2 years after the start of treatment. The other patient who had long-term oral diazoxide (up to 600 mg/day), was asymptomatic after 33 months follow-up and continued to show a lower pulmonary arterial pressure and resistance. Similar symptomatic and hemodynamic improvement has been noted when diazoxide was used in 2 other cases; 300 mg/day for 6 months[204] and 600 mg/day for 15 months.[205] In the latter instance pulmonary hypertension recurred when the diazoxide was stopped.

The injection of diazoxide into the pulmonary artery of patients with severe primary pulmonary hypertension can precipitate dramatic systemic hypotension[174] and should be avoided. The potential danger associated with the use of all vasodilators in primary pulmonary hypertension has been documented in 1 such case.[159] As increasing doses of diazoxide were given into the pulmonary artery of this patient, the heart rate, cardiac output, and pulmonary arterial pressure increased. After injection of 300 mg, seizures, ventricular tachycardia, systemic hypotension, and death ensued. In the face of a relatively unresponsive pulmonary vasculature, administration of vasodilators will cause systemic hypotension and an increase in pulmonary arterial pressure. Other known side effects of diazoxide administration have been described in 9 patients with primary pulmonary hypertension: peripheral edema, diabetes, postural hypotension, hirsutism, nausea, and vomiting.[206] Acute injection of diazoxide into the pulmonary artery of these patients was noted to reduce pulmonary vascular resistance but had little effect on pulmonary arterial pressure. One out of 5 of these patients who were recatheterized after long-term oral therapy, showed a fall in pulmonary arterial pressure, while 4 had a reduction in pulmonary vascular resistance. In summary, diazoxide can induce varying degrees of hemodynamic remission and occasionally improve symptoms, but has frequent serious side effects, especially in those patients who have severe pulmonary hypertension (pulmonary arterial systolic pressure > 100 mm Hg).

Hydralazine

Hydralazine has been widely used since it was reported that oral hydralazine (50–75 mg every 6 hours) reduced pulmonary vascular resistance in 4 patients during rest and exercise, both in the short and long-term.[177] The change in pulmonary arterial pressure was small. Since that time, two groups of investigators have described a total of 8 patients with primary pulmonary hypertension in whom hydralazine did not reduce pulmonary arterial pressure but did cause significant systemic hypotension.[178,180] A third group has shown that patients who subsequently benefited from long-term oral hydralazine could be identified by initial hemodynamic monitoring of the effect of infusing hydralazine (0.33 mg/kg over 3 minutes) into the pulmonary artery.[179] They did not comment on symptomatic systemic hypotension. The patients who did respond had lower mean pulmonary arterial pressures (36 ± 3 (SEM) mm Hg) than those who did not respond (80 ± 6 mm Hg). This finding, that less severe pulmonary hypertension was more susceptible to the effects of hydralazine, is usually also true of other vasodilators, although exceptions occur.[146] It should be remembered that hydralazine, like diazoxide and verapamil, is bound to albumin and may interact with other albumin-bound drugs, such as oral anticoagulants.

Prostacyclin

The pulmonary vasodilator action of hydralazine is thought to arise in part through its ability to stimulate prostacyclin production.[207] Direct prostacyclin infusion has been reported in two groups of adults[183,184] a child,[103] and a neonate.[208] Although prostacyclin is not selective for the pulmonary vasculature, it can decrease pulmonary arterial pressure as well as resistance. In addition, it has the advantage that the dose can be titrated according to the hemodynamic effect and the action can be rapidly stopped by discontinuing the infusion (Figure 8).

Dipyridamole/Minoxidil

An analogue with a much longer biologic half-life will have to be found if prostacyclin is to be useful in long-term treatment. Dipyridamole stimulates endogenous prostacyclin production,[209] and it is known to be able to prevent acute hypoxic pulmonary hypertension in the dog.[154] Because dipyridamole could oppose both pulmonary vasoconstriction and platelet aggregation, a trial in primary pulmonary hypertension may be reasonable. A clinical trial of the vasodilator,

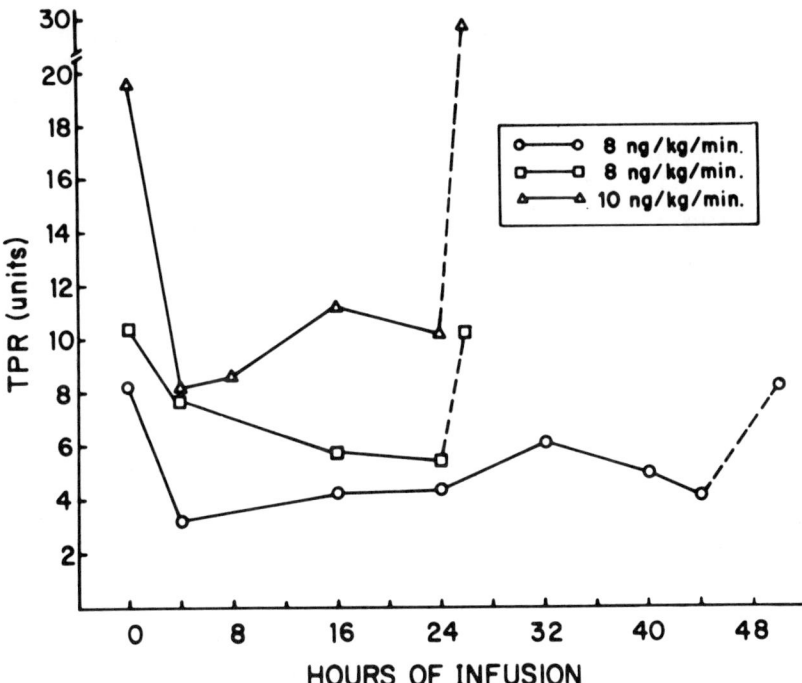

Figure 8. Effects of a continuous infusion of prostacyclin on total pulmonary resistance (TPR) in 3 patients with primary pulmonary hypertension. Interrupted lines represent discontinuation of the infusion and subsequent control measurements. (Reprinted by permission of the American Heart Association, Inc. from Rubin LJ, Groves BM, Reeves JT, Frosolono M, Handel F, Cato AE: Prostacyclin-induced acute pulmonary vasodilation in primary pulmonary hypertension. Circulation 1982;66:334.

minoxidil, has also been suggested.[206] This drug is known to cause pulmonary vasodilatation in experimental models of pulmonary hypertension[210] and tended to reduce slightly elevated pulmonary arterial pressure and resistance in patients treated for systemic hypertension.[211]

Nitroprusside

Like prostacyclin, sodium nitroprusside is also used widely as a screening agent to determine whether there is an element of reversible vasospasm in patients with an elevated pulmonary vascular resistance.[212] The intravenous infusion can be started at 10 μg/min and increased by 10 μg/min every 4 minutes, unless there is a significant fall in systemic systolic pressure (e.g., below 95 mm Hg), or an increase in pulmonary systolic pressure (> 5 mm Hg above control). Because sodium nitroprusside has both arterial and venous dilating actions, a logical oral combination to mimic its effect would be hydralazine and isosorbide dinitrate. However, sublingual isosorbide dinitrate has not been shown to have an acute hemodynamic effect in primary pulmonary hypertension.[213]

Captopril

Captopril is not, strictly speaking, a direct acting pulmonary vasodilator as it has several mechanisms of action. By inhibiting the angiotensin converting enzyme it decreases circulating levels of the pulmonary vasoconstrictor angiotensin II, while increasing levels of the vasodilator, bradykinin. Possibly through the effect of bradykinin, captopril also causes an increase in the plasma levels of prostaglandin E_2.[214] In 1 patient with severe primary pulmonary hypertension (pulmonary arterial pressure 100/36 mm Hg) the administration of captopril over 3 months was associated with a remarkable clinical recovery.[185] However, in a series of 4 patients given captopril over 48 hours, no improvement in hemodynamics was noted during rest or exercise,[125] and the same was true of 4 other patients treated for 12 weeks.[215]

Oxygen

Although oxygen is not considered a drug, it does cause pulmonary vasodilatation. Oxygen administration is known to be effective in the treatment of pulmonary hypertension secondary to chronic parenchymal lung disease.[216] It may have contributed to the long-term improvement of 1 patient with primary pulmonary hypertension,[192] but it usually has little effect on hemodynamics.[146,171,187]

OTHER INTERVENTIONS

Inhibition of the Synthesis of Prostaglandin-like Substances

Markedly increased levels of circulating thromboxane B_2 have been measured in 1 patient.[103] If thromboxane, a vasoconstrictor, was responsible for the pulmonary hypertension, then inhibition of the synthesis of all prostaglandin-like substances might be helpful. In a different patient, indomethacin (50 mg orally every 8 hours) was associated with a modest reduction in pulmonary arterial pressure after 24 hours.[104] However, administration of indomethacin to 7 patients in a recent study did not alter pulmonary arterial pressure but tended to increase pulmonary vascular resistance.[146] Equally, a single 50 mg rectal dose of indomethacin (1 patient)[192] and the intravenous administration of 1 g sodium salicylate (2 patients)[171] have both been found to be ineffective. Experimentally, the inhibition of prostaglandin synthesis tends to augment pulmonary hypertension,[148] and consequently this form of treatment should only be tried if an increased level of constrictor prostaglandin-like-substances has been documented.

Steroids and Azothiaprine

Steroids and azothiaprine, each given separately for at least 3 months failed to decrease pulmonary arterial pressure in 3 patients.[171]

Isovolumic Hemodilution

Isovolumic hemodilution should be considered if the hematocrit is above 50%.[217] A gradual reduction in mean hematocrit (60 ± 2 to 50 ± 1%) by repeated venesections was associated with a fall of both pulmonary arterial pressure and resistance in 8 of 9 patients with cor pulmonale, secondary to chronic airways disease.[218]

Intravenous Fibrinolytic Therapy

Intravenous fibrinolytic therapy in 3 patients did not cause a demonstrable improvement in pulmonary pressure when administered over 1 to 3 days. One patient developed a cerebral hemorrhage.[219]

Surgical Approaches to Treatment

Pulmonary artery banding, combined with an anastomosis between the subclavian artery and the pulmonary artery, has been reported to improve 3 patients symptomatically, although the operation also decreased the systemic arterial oxygen tension.[14] Left stellate ganglion blockade was ineffective in 1 patient and the procedure led to bilateral pneumothoraces and death.[220] Stripping of the sympathetic nerves to the pulmonary vasculature is also said to be disappointing.[130]

Heart–lung Transplantation

Many young patients with primary pulmonary hypertension are unresponsive to vasodilators or other forms of medical treatment. When they are incapacitated by breathlessness and right heart failure, heart–lung transplantation may provide functional improvement and the hope of increased longevity. This operation was first performed successfully at the Stanford Medical Center in March 1981. In 3 previous attempts at other centers the patients had died within a month of operation. At present, a total of 6 patients have been reported by the Stanford group, including 3 with primary pulmonary hypertension.[221,222] It seems likely that the use of cyclosporin A and endomyocardial biopsy will make long-term management of rejection feasible. If so, the demand for this operation will greatly exceed supply and will pose major logistic and philosophical problems.

SUMMARY OF TREATMENT

While a few patients obtain symptomatic and/or hemodynamic improvement from one or other of the drugs discussed above, at present there is no long-term treatment which has been shown to improve longevity. Consequently, in choosing which agents to try, it is important to avoid those with serious side effects. Many patients will eventually be treated with several drugs simultaneously, but these should be added one by one under careful hemodynamic monitoring in an intensive care environment, by physicians with experience in the management of pulmonary hypertension. For those end-stage patients who are unresponsive to medical treatment, heart–lung transplantation may offer the only chance of improving the poor prognosis.

Acknowledgment: I am most grateful to Miss Mary Bougetz and Mrs. Margaret Chelmo for their assistance in the preparation of this chapter. Supported by VA research funds and NHBLI Grant HL 23211.

REFERENCES

1. Harvey W: De Motu Cordis. Geoffrey Keynes English Translation. p. 4. London: Nonesuch Press, 1928.
2. Fishman AP: Editorial: Unexplained pulmonary hypertension. *Circulation* 1982;65:651.
3. Kanemoto N, Furuya H. Etoh T, Sasamoto H, Matsuyama S: Chest roentgenograms in primary pulmonary hypertension. *Chest* 1979; 76:45.
4. Wagenvoort CA: The use of lung biopsies in the diagnosis of primary pulmonary hypertension. *Bull Eur Physiopathol Respir* 1982;18:87P.
5. World Health Organization. *Primary Pulmonary Hypertension.* Report on a WHO meeting, edited by Hatano S, Strasser T., Geneva, 1975.
6. Romberg E: Ueber sklerose der lungenarterien. *Deutsch Arch Klin Med* 1891;48:197.
7. Monckeberg JG: Uber die genuine arteriosklerose der lungenarterie. *Deutsch Med Wschr* 1907;33:1243.
8. Brenner O: Pathology of the vessels of the pulmonary circulation. IV. *Arch Intern Med* 1935;56:976.
9. Goodale F, Thomas WA: Primary pulmonary arterial disease, observations with special reference to medial thickening of small arteries and arterioles. *Arch Path* 1954;58:568.
10. Wood P: Congenital heart disease. *Br Med J* 1950; ii:693.
11. Dresdale DT, Schultz M, Michtom RJ: Primary pulmonary hypertension. 1. Clinical and hemodynamic study. *Am J Med* 1951;11:686.
12. Wood P: Pulmonary hypertension. In: Wood P, ed. *Diseases of the Heart and Circulation.* 3rd ed. London: Eyre and Spottiswoode, 1968:976.
13. Nielsen NC, Fabricius J: Primary pulmonary hypertension, with special reference to prognosis. *Acta Med Scand* 1961:170:731.
14. Storstein O, Efskind L, Muller C, Rokseth R, Sander S: Primary pulmonary hypertension with emphasis on its etiology and treatment. *Acta Med Scand* 1966;79:197.
15. Wagenvoort CA, Wagenvoort N: Primary pulmonary hypertension. A pathologic study of the lung vessels in 156 clinically diagnosed cases. *Circulation* 1970;42:1163.
16. Forssman W: Die sondierung des rechten herzens. *Klin Wschr* 1929; 8:2085.

17. Walcott G, Burchell HB, Brown AL: Primary pulmonary hypertension. Am J Med 1970;49:70.
18. Watanabe S, Ogata T: Clinical and experimental study upon primary pulmonary hypertension. Jpn Heart J 1976;40:603.
19. Ahlquist J, Burstein J: A case of idiopathic pulmonary hypertension. Acta Med Scand 1958;160:1.
20. Suarez LD, Sciandro EE, Llera JJ, Perosio AM: Long-term follow-up in primary pulmonary hypertension. Br Heart J 1979;41:702.
21. Bourdillon PDV, Oakley CM: Regression of primary pulmonary hypertension. Br Heart J 1976; 38:264.
22. Fujii A, Rabinovitch M. Matthews EC: A case of spontaneous resolution of idiopathic pulmonary hypertension. Br Heart J 1981;46:574.
23. Anderson G, Reid L, Simon G: The radiographic appearances in primary and in thromboembolic pulmonary hypertension. Clin Radiol 1973;24:113.
24. Kanemoto N, Sasamoto H: Pulmonary hemodynamics in primary pulmonary hypertension. Jpn Heart J 1979;20:395.
25. Blount SG: Primary pulmonary hypertension. Mod Con Cardiovasc Dis 1967;36:67.
26. Rosenberg SA: A study of the etiologic basis of primary pulmonary hypertension. Am Heart J 1964; 68:484.
27. Anderson EG, Simon G, Reid L: Primary and thrombo-embolic pulmonary hypertension: A quantitative pathological study. J Path 1973; 110:273.
28. Fuchs J, Mlczoch J, Niessner H: Abnormal fibrinolysis in primary pulmonary hypertension. Eur Heart J 1981;2:A168.
29. Edwards WD, Edwards JE: Clinical primary pulmonary hypertension. Three pathologic types. Circulation 1977;56:884.
30. Wood P: Pulmonary hypertension. Mod Con Cardiovasc Dis 1959;28:513.
31. Miller D, Waters DD, Warnica W, Szlachcic J, Kreeft J, Theroux P: Is variant angina the coronary manifestation of a generalized vasospastic disorder. N Engl J Med 1981;304:763.
32. Coffman JD, Cohen RA: Vasospasm-Ubiquitous? N Engl J Med 1981: 304:780.
33. Smith W, Kroop I: Raynaud's disease in primary pulmonary hypertension. JAMA 1957;165:1245.
34. Celoria G, Friedell G, Sommers S: Raynaud's disease and primary pulmonary hypertension. Circulation 1960;22:1055.
35. Rawson A, Woske HA: Study of etiologic factors in so-called primary pulmonary hypertension. Arch Int Med 1960;105:233.
36. Samet P, Bernstein WH: Loss of reactivity of the pulmonary vascular bed in primary pulmonary hypertension. Am Heart J 1963;66:197.
37. Dantzker DR, Bower JS: Partial reversibility of chronic pulmonary hypertension caused by pulmonary thromboembolic disease. Am Rev Respir Dis 1981;124:129.
38. Sole MJ, Drobac M, Schwartz L, Hussain MN, Vaughan-Neil EF: The extraction of circulating catecholamines by the lungs in normal man and in patients with pulmonary hypertension. Circulation 1979;60:160.
39. Furchgott RF, Zawadzki JV: The obligatory role of endothelial cells in relaxation of arterial smooth muscle by acetylcholine. Nature 1980; 288:373.

40. Cherry PD, Furchgott RF, Zawadzki JV, Jothianandan D: Role of endothelial cells in relaxation in isolated arteries by bradykinin. *Proc Natl Acad Sci* 1982;79:2106.
41. Meyrick B, Clarke SW, Symons C, Woodgate DJ, Reid L: Primary pulmonary hypertension. A case report including electronmicroscopic study. *Br J Dis Chest* 1974;68:11.
42. Brill IC, Krygier JJ: Primary pulmonary vascular sclerosis. *Arch Int Med* 1941;68:560.
43. Cummings P: Primary pulmonary hypertension and SLE. *N Engl J Med* 1973; 288:1078.
44. Nair SS, Askari AD, Popelka CG, Kleinerman JF: Pulmonary hypertension and systemic lupus erythematosus. *Arch Int Med* 1980:140:109.
45. Kanemoto N, Gonda N, Katsu M, Fukuda J: Two cases of pulmonary hypertension with Raynaud's Phenomenon. *Jpn Heart J* 1975;16:354.
46. Salerni R, Rodnan GP, Leon FL, Shaver JA: Pulmonary hypertension in the CREST syndrome variant of progressive systemic sclerosis (scleroderma). *Ann Int Med* 1977;86:394.
47. Young RH, Mark G: Pulmonary vascular changes in scleroderma. *Am J Med* 1978; 64:998.
48. Gardner DL, Onthie JJ, Macleod J, Allan WS: Pulmonary hypertension in rheumatoid arthritis. Report of a case with intimal sclerosis of the pulmonary and digital arteries. *Scot Med J* 1957; 2:183.
49. Caldwell IW, Aitchison JD: Pulmonary hypertension in dermatomyositis. *Br Heart J* 1956;18:273.
50. Bunch TW, Tancredi RG, Lie JT: Pulmonary hypertension in polymyositis. *Chest* 1981;79:105.
51. Jones MB, Osterholm RK, Wilson RB, Martin FH, Commers JR, Bachmayer JD: Fatal pulmonary hypertension and resolving immunecomplex glomerulonephritis in mixed connective tissue disease. *Am J Med* 1978;65:855.
52. Kahaleh MB, Leroy EC: Specific endothelial cell injury produced by scleroderma serum in vitro. *J Exp Med* 1979;149:1326.
53. Sinclair RA, Antonovych TT, Mostofi FK: Renal proliferative arteriopathies and associated glomerular changes. A light and electron microscopic study. *Hum Pathol* 1976;7:565.
54. Ross R, Glomset J, Kariya B, Harker L: Platelet-dependent serum factor that stimulates the proliferation of arterial smooth muscle cells in vitro. *Proc Natl Acad Sci USA* 1974;71:1207.
55. Witte LD, Kaplan LK, Nossel HL, Lages BA, Weiss HJ, Goodman DS: Studies of the release from human platelets of the growth factor for cultured human arterial smooth muscle cells. *Circ Res* 1978;42:402.
56. Sackner MA, Akgun N, Kimbel P, Lewis DH: The pathophysiology of scleroderma involving the heart and respiratory system. *Ann Intern Med* 1964;60:611.
57. Naslund MJ, Pearson TA, Ritter JM: A documented episode of pulmonary vasoconstriction in systemic sclerosis. *Johns Hopkins Med J* 1981; 148:78.
58. Fahey PJ, Utell MJ, Condemi JJ, Green RM, Hyde RW: Raynaud's phenomenon of the pulmonary vasculature. *Chest* 1980;78:515.
59. Howard TP, Solomon DA, Germain B, Golman AL: Clinically silent pulmonary hypertension in the CREST syndrome. *Chest* 1980;78:522.

60. Vogelzang MJ, Bosl GJ, Johnson K, Kennedy BJ: Raynaud's phenomenon: A common toxicity after combination chemotherapy for testicular cancer. *Ann Int Med* 1981;95:288.
61. Scheulen ME, Schmidt CG: Raynaud-syndrom nach kombinierter zytostatischer behandlung von patienten mit malignen hodentumoren. *Dtsch Med Wschr* 1982;107:1640.
62. Clarke RC, Coombes CF, Hadfield G: On certain abnormalities, congenital and acquired, of the pulmonary artery. *Q J Med* 1927;21:51.
63. Czarnecki SW, Rosenbaum HM, Wachtel HL: The occurrence of primary pulmonary hypertension in twins with a review of etiological considerations. *Am Heart J* 1968;75:240.
64. Newman JH, Loyd JE, Prima RK: Genetic aspects of familial primary pulmonary hypertension. *Am Rev Resp Dis* 1982;125:132.
65. Rawson AJ, Woske HM: A study of etiologic factors in so-called primary pulmonary hypertension. *Arch Int Med* 1960;105:233.
66. Inglesby TV, Singer JW, Gordon DA: Abnormal fibrinolysis in familial pulmonary hypertension. *Am J Med* 1973;55:5.
67. Tubbs RR, Levin RD, Shirey EK, Hoffman GC: Fibrinolysis in familial pulmonary hypertension. *Am J Clin Path* 1979;71:384.
68. Weir EK, Tucker A, Reeves JT, Will DH, Grover RF: The genetic factor influencing pulmonary hypertension in cattle at high altitude. *Cardiovasc Res* 1974;8:745.
69. Cruz JC, Reeves JT, Russel BE, Alexander AF, Will DH: Embryo transplanted calves: The pulmonary hypertensive trait is genetically transmitted. *Proc Soc Exper Biol Med* 1980;164:142.
70. Heath D, Edwards JE: Configuration of elastic tissue of pulmonary trunk in idiopathic pulmonary hypertension. *Circulation* 1960;21:59.
71. Roberts WC: The histologic structure of the pulmonary trunk in patients with "primary" pulmonary hypertension. *Am Heart J* 1963;65:230.
72. Reeves JT, Noonan JA: Microarteriographic studies of primary pulmonary hypertension. *Arch Pathol* 1973:95:50.
73. Weir EK, Greer BE, Smith SC, Silvers GW, Droegemueller W, Reeves JT, Grover RF: Bronchoconstriction and pulmonary hypertension during abortion induced by 15-methyl-prostaglandin $F_2\alpha$. *Am J Med* 1976;60:556.
74. Moore LG, Reeves JT: Pregnancy blunts pulmonary vascular reactivity in dogs. *Am J Physiol* 1980;239:H297.
75. Landersman R, Douglas RG, Dreishpoon G, Holze E: The vascular bed of the bulbar conjunctiva in normal menstrual cycle. *Am J Obstet Gynecol* 1953;66:988.
76. Shepard JT, Edwards JE, Burchell HB, Swan HJC, Wood EH: Clinical, physiological and pathological considerations in patients with idiopathic pulmonary hypertension. *Br Heart J* 1957;19:70.
77. Moser KM: Pulmonary vascular obstruction due to embolism and thrombosis. In: Moser KM ed. *Pulmonary Vascular Diseases*. New York: Marcel Dekker, 1979:374.
78. Roche WD, Norris HJ: Detection and significance of maternal pulmonary amniotic fluid embolism. *Obstet Gynecol* 1974;43:729.
79. Gurtner HP: Pulmonary hypertension, plexogenic pulmonary arteriopathy and the appetite depressant drug aminorex: Post or propter? *Bull Eur Physiopath Resp* 1979;15:897.

80. Kleiger RE, Boxer M, Ingham RE, Harrison DC: Pulmonary hypertension in patients using oral contraceptives. *Chest* 1976;69:143.
81. Oakley C, Somerville J: Oral contraceptives and progressive pulmonary vascular disease. *Lancet* 1968;1:890.
82. Royal College of General Practitioners oral contraception study. *J R Coll Gen Pract* 1978;28:393.
83. Vessey MP: Steroid contraception, venous thromboembolism and stroke; data from countries other than the United States. In: Sciarra JJ, Zatuchni GI, Spiedel JJ, eds. *Risks, Benefits and Controversies in Fertility Control*. Hagerstown, Md.: Harper & Row, 1978:113.
84. Alkjaersig N, Fletcher A, Burstein R: Association between oral contraceptive use and thromboembolism: A new approach to its investigation based on plasma fibrinogen chromatography. *Am J Obstet Gynecol* 1975; 122:199.
85. Astedt B, Isacson S, Nilsson IM, Pandolfi M: Thrombosis and oral contraceptives: Possible predisposition. *Br Med J* 1973;4: 631.
86. Dreyer NA, Pizzo SV: Blood coagulation and idiopathic thromboembolism among fertile women. *Contraception* 1980;22:123.
87. Howie PW: Thromboembolism. *Clin Obstet Gynecol* 1977;4:397.
88. Segel N, Kay JM, Bayley TJ, Paton A: Pulmonary hypertension with hepatic cirrhosis. *Br Heart J* 1968;30:575.
89. Senior RM, Britton RL, Turino GM, Wood JA, Langer GA, Fishman AP: Pulmonary hypertension associated with cirrhosis of the liver and with porta-caval shunts. *Circulation* 1968;37:88.
90. Ruttner JR, Bartschi JP, Niedermann, R, Schneider J: Plexogenic pulmonary arteriopathy and liver cirrhosis. *Thorax* 1980; 35:133.
91. Morrison EB, Gaffney FA, Eigenbrodt EH, Reynolds RC, Buya LM: Severe pulmonary hypertension associated with macronodular (postnecrotic) cirrhosis and autoimmune phenomena. *Am J Med* 1980;69:513.
92. Naeye RL: "Primary" pulmonary hypertension with coexisting portal hypertension. *Circulation* 1960;22:376.
93. Faraj BA, Camp VM, Ansley J, Ali FM, Malveaux EJ: Impaired monoamine oxidase activity in dogs with portacaval shunt. *Biochem Pharmacol* 1980;29:2831.
94. Nieto C, Arias J, Alsasua A, Garcia de Jalon PD: Changes in brain oxidative metabolism in rats with portocaval shunt. *Experientia* 1980; 36:1403.
95. Kibria G, Smith P, Heath D, Sagar S: Observations on the rare association between portal and pulmonary hypertension. *Thorax* 1980;35:945.
96. Popovic NA, Mullane JF: Effects of biliary obstruction on pulmonary ultrastructure in the rat. *Am J Pathol* 1972;68:97.
97. Daoud FS, Reeves JT, Schaefer JW: Failure of hypoxic pulmonary vasoconstriction in patients with liver cirrhosis. *J Clin Invest* 1972;51:1076.
98. Williams A, Trewby P, Williams R, Reid L: Structural alterations to the pulmonary circulation in fulminant hepatic failure. *Thorax* 1979;34:447.
99. Van Benthuysen KM, Dauber IM, Hyers TA, Steele PP, Weil JV: The role of platelets in hypertensive pulmonary vascular disease. *Fed Proc* 1982;40:3210.
100. Keith IM, Will JA, Weir EK: Pharmacologic attenuation of hypoxia-induced arterial hypertrophy in rat lungs. *Fed Proc* 1982;41:1686.

101. Nenci GG, Berrettini M, Todisco T, Costantini V, Grasselli S: Platelet activation in hypoxic pulmonary hypertension. *Bull Eur Physiopath Resp* 1982;18:115P.
102. Friedman RJ, Stemerman MB, Wenz B, Moore S, Gauldie J, Gent R, Tiell ML, Spaet TH: The effect of thrombocytopenia on experimental arteriosclerotic lesion formation in rabbits. *J Clin Invest* 1977;60:1191.
103. Watkins WD, Peterson MB, Crone RK, Shannon DC, Levine L. Prostacyclin and prostaglandin E_1 for severe idiopathic pulmonary artery hypertension. *Lancet* 1980;1:1083.
104. Person B, Proctor RJ: Primary pulmonary hypertension. Response to indomethacin, terbutaline and isoproterenol. *Chest* 1979;76:601.
105. Jacob HS: Complement-induced vascular leukostasis. Its role in tissue injury. *Arch Path Lab Med* 1980;104:617.
106. Horn M, Ries A, Neveu C, Moser K: Restrictive ventilatory pattern in precapillary pulmonary hypertension. *Am Rev Resp Dis* 1983;128:163-165.
107. Scharf SM, Feldman NT, Graboys TB, Wellman JJ: Restrictive ventilatory defect in a patient with primary pulmonary hypertension. *Am Rev Resp Dis* 1978;118:609.
108. Gatewood RP, Yu PN: Primary pulmonary hypertension. In: Goodwin JF, Yu PN eds. *Progress in Cardiology*. Philadelphia: Lea and Febiger, 1979:325.
109. James TN: On the cause of syncope and sudden death in primary pulmonary hypertension. *Ann Intern Med* 1962;56:252.
110. Viar WN, Harrison TR: Chest pain in association with pulmonary hypertension: Its similarity to the pain of coronary disease. *Circulation* 1952;5:1.
111. Yuceoglu YZ, Dresdale DT, Valensi QJ, Narvas RM, Gottleib NT: Primary pulmonary hypertension with hoarseness and massive (fatal) hemoptysis. *Vasc Dis* 1967;4:290.
112. Stein PD, Sabbah HN, Anbe DT, Khaja F: Hemodynamic and anatomic determinants of relative differences in amplitude of the aortic and pulmonary components of the second heart sound. *Am J Cardiol* 1978;42:539.
113. Kunhali K, Gherian G, Bakthaviziam A, Abraham MT, Krishnaswami S: Rupture of a papillary muscle of the tricuspid valve in primary pulmonary hypertension. *Am Heart J* 1980;99:225.
114. Weyman AE, Dillon JC, Feigenbaum H, Chang S: Echocardiographic patterns of pulmonic valve motion with pulmonary hypertension. *Circulation* 1974;50:905.
115. Shah PM: Echocardiography of the aortic and pulmonary valves. *Prog Cardiovasc Disc* 1978;20:451.
116. Lew W, Karliner JS: Assessment of pulmonary valve echogram in normal subjects and in patients with pulmonary arterial hypertension. *Br Heart J* 1979;42:147.
117. Acquatella H, Schiller NB, Sharpe DN, Catterjee K: Lack of correlation between echocardiographic pulmonary valve morphology and simultaneous pulmonary arterial pressure. *Am J Cardiol* 1979;43:946.
118. Bauman W, Wann LS, Childress R, Weymann AE, Feigenbaum H, Dillon J: Mid systolic notching of the pulmonary valve in the absence of pulmonary hypertension. *Am J Cardiol* 1979;43:1049.

119. Tanaka H, Tei C, Nakao S, Tahara M, Sakurai S, Kashima T, Kanehisa T: Diastolic bulging of the interventricular septum toward the left ventricle. *Circulation* 1980;62:558.
120. Wilson AG, Harris CN, Lavender JP, Oakley CM: Perfusion lung scanning in obliterative pulmonary hypertension. *Br Heart J* 1973;35:917.
121. Brune J, Emonot A, Wiesendanger T, Munsch C, Galy P: Comparative study of alterations of respiratory function tests in chronic pulmonary thromboembolism and primary pulmonary hypertension. *Thorax* 1979; 34:697.
122. Child JD, Wolfe JD, Tashkin D, Nakano F: Fatal lung scan in a case of pulmonary hypertension due to obliterative pulmonary vascular disease. *Chest* 1975;67:308.
123. Horn M, Hooper W, Brach B, Ashburn W, Moser K: Postural changes in pulmonary blood flow in pulmonary hypertension: A noninvasive technique using ventilation-perfusion scans. *Circulation* 1982; 66:621.
124. Bianco JA, Shafer RB: Abnormal images of right heart disorders. *Clin Nuc Med* 1979;4:368.
125. Rich S, Martinex J, Lam W, Rosen KM: Captopril as treatment for patients with pulmonary hypertension. *Br Heart J* 1982; 48:272.
126. Meyer BL, Bogart DB, Carley JE, Wong BYS, Dunn MI: Pulmonary arterial pulsus alternans secondary to primary pulmonary hypertension. *Chest* 1976;70:374.
127. Dalen JE, Banas JS, Brooks HL, Evans GL, Paraskos JA, Dexter L: Resolution rate of acute pulmonary embolism in man. *N Engl J Med* 1969;280:1194.
128. Stein PD: Wedge arterography for the identification of pulmonary emboli in small vessels. *Am Heart J* 1971;82:618.
129. Rabinovitch M, Keane JF, Fellows KE, Castaneda AR, Reid L: Quantitative analysis of the pulmonary wedge angiogram in congenital heart defects. *Circulation* 1981;63:152.
130. Chapman DW, Abbott JP, Latson J: Primary pulmonary hypertension. Review of the literature and results of cardiac catheterization in ten patients. *Circulation* 1957;15:35.
131. Messer JA: Primary pulmonary hypertension: A fatality during pulmonary angiography (in discussion). *Chest* 1973;64:628.
132. Charms BL: Primary pulmonary hypertension. Effect of unilateral pulmonary artery occlusion and infusion of acetylcholine. *Am J Cardiol* 1961;8:94.
133. Wagenvoort CA: Lung biopsy specimens in the evaluation of pulmonary vascular disease. *Chest* 1980;77:614.
134. Sadigursky M, Andrade ZA: Pulmonary changes in schistosomal cor pulmonale. *Am J Trop Med Hyg* 1982;31:779.
135. Walden PAM: Primary pulmonary hypertension. *Br Med J* 1981; 282:652.
136. Collins FS, Orringer EP: Pulmonary hypertension and cor pulmonale in the sickle hemoglobinopathies. *Am J Med* 1982; 73:814.
137. Fanta CH, Compton CC: Microscopic tumour emboli to the lungs: A hidden cause of dyspnoea and pulmonary hypertension. *Thorax* 1979; 43:794.
138. Houk RJ, Bailey GL, Daroca PH, Brazda F, Johnson FB, Klein RC: Pentazocine Abuse: Report of a case with pulmonary arterial cellulose granulomas and pulmonary hypertension. *Chest* 1980;77:277.

139. Jewett JF, Ober WB: Primary pulmonary hypertension as a cause of maternal death. *Am J Obstet Gynec* 1956;71:1335.
140. Personal communication from L.J. Rubin, M.D.
141. Personal communication from B.M. Groves, M.D. and J.T. Reeves, M.D.
142. Khoury GH, Hawes CR: Primary pulmonary hypertension in children living at high altitude. *J Pediat* 1963;62:177.
143. Grover RF, Vogel JHK, Voigt GC, Blount SG: Reversal of high altitude pulmonary hypertension. *Am J Cardiol* 1966;18:928.
144. Wennmalm A: Interaction of nicotine and prostaglandins in the cardiovascular system. *Prostaglandins* 1982;23:139.
145. Inkley SR, Gillespie L, Funkhouser RK: Two cases of primary pulmonary hypertension with sudden death associated with the administration of barbiturates. *Ann Int Med* 1955;43:396.
146. Hermiller JB, Bambach D, Thompson MJ, Huss P, Fontana ME, Magorien RD, Unverferth DV, Leier CV: Vasodilators and prostaglandin inhibitors in primary pulmonary hypertension. *Ann Int Med* 1982;97:480.
147. Tucker A, Weir EK, Reeves JT, Grover RF: Failure of histamine antagonists to prevent hypoxic pulmonary vasoconstriction in dogs. *J Appl Physiol* 1976;40:496.
148. Weir EK, McMurtry IF, Tucker A, Reeves JT, Grover RF: Prostaglandin synthetase inhibitors do not decrease hypoxic pulmonary vasoconstriction. *J Appl Physiol* 1976;41:714.
149. Goodwin JF, Harrison CV, Wilcken DEL: Obliterative pulmonary hypertension and thromboembolism. *Br Med J* 1963;1:777.
150. Sleeper JC, Orgain ES, McIntosh HD: Primary pulmonary hypertension. *Circulation* 1962;26:1358.
151. Hultgren HN, Shettigar VR: Isoproterenol in primary hypertension. *Am J Cardiol* 1980;45:529.
152. Fuster V, Giuliani ER, Brandenbury RO, Weidman WH, Edwards WD: The natural history of idiopathic pulmonary hypertension. *Am J Cardiol* 1981;47:422.
153. Stuard ID, Heusinkveld RS, Moss AJ: Microangiopathic hemolytic anemia and thrombocytopenia in primary pulmonary hypertension. *N Engl J Med* 1972;287:869.
154. Mlczoch J, Weir EK, Grover RF: Inhibition of hypoxic pulmonary vasoconstriction by dipyridamole is not platelet mediated. *Can J Physiol Pharmacol* 1976;55:448.
155. Reeves JT: Hope in primary pulmonary hypertension? *N Engl J Med* 1980;302:112.
156. Klinke WP: Treatment for primary pulmonary hypertension. *Am Heart J* 1980;100:587.
157. Rubin LJ: Primary pulmonary hypertension: New approaches to therapy. *Am Heart J* 1980;100:757.
158. Elkayam V: Vasodilator therapy in primary pulmonary hypertension. *Chest* 1981;79:253.
159. Rubino JM, Schroeder JS: Diazoxide in the treatment of primary pulmonary hypertension (letter). *Br Heart J* 1979; 42:362.
160. Rich S, Martinez J, Lam W, Levy PS, Rosen KM: Reassessment of the effects of vasodilator drugs in primary pulmonary hypertension: Guidelines for determining a pulmonary vasodilator response. *Am Heart J* 1983;105:119.

161. Rubin LJ, Handel F, Peter RH: The effects of oral hydralazine on right ventricular end-diastolic pressure in patients with right ventricular failure. *Circulation* 1982;65:1369.
162. Nocturnal Oxygen Trial Group: Continuous or nocturnal oxygen therapy in hypoxemic chronic obstructive lung disease. *Ann Intern Med* 1980;93:391.
163. Rozkovec A, Minty K, Stradling J, Shephard G, MacDermot J, Oakley CM, Dollery CT, Hughes JMB: Value of acute vasodilator studies in management of primary pulmonary hypertension. *Circulation* 1982:66:196.
164. Wood P: The vasoconstrictive factor in pulmonary hypertension. *Br Heart J* 1958;20:557.
165. Wade EG, Rowlands DJ: Diazoxide in treatment of primary pulmonary hypertension (reply to letter). *Br Heart J* 1979;42:362.
166. Rao BNS, Moller JH, Edwards JE: Primary pulmonary hypertension in a child. Response to pharmacologic agents. *Circulation* 1969;40:583.
167. Korones SB, Fabien GA. Successful treatment of "persistent fetal circulation" with tolazoline. *Pediatr Res* 1975;9:367.
168. Downing SE, Lee JC: Nervous control of the pulmonary circulation. *Ann Rev Physiol* 1980;42:199.
169. Fishman AP: Vasomotor regulation of the pulmonary circulation. *Ann Rev Physiol* 1980;42:211.
170. Bergofsky EH: Humoral control of the pulmonary circulation. *Ann Rev Physiol* 1980;42:221.
171. Daoud FS, Reeves JT, Kelly DB: Isoproterenol as a potential pulmonary vasodilator in primary pulmonary hypertension. *Am J Cardiol* 1978; 42:817.
172. Elkayam V, Frishman WH, Yoran C, Strom J, Sonnenblick EH, Cohen M: Unfavorable hemodynamic and clinical effects of isoproterenol therapy in primary pulmonary hypertension. *Cardiovasc Med* 1978;3:1177.
173. Wang SWS, Pohl JEF, Rowlands DJ, Wade EG: Diazoxide in treatment of primary pulmonary hypertension. *Br Heart J* 1978;40:572.
174. Buch J, Wennevold A: Hazards of diazoxide in pulmonary hypertension. *Br Heart J* 1981;46:401.
175. Ruskin JN, Hutter AM: Primary pulmonary hypertension treated with oral phentolamine. *Ann Int Med* 1979;90:772.
176. Cohen ML, Kronzon I: Adverse hemodynamic effects of phentolamine in primary pulmonary hypertension. *Ann Int Med* 1981;95:591.
177. Rubin LJ, Peter RH: Oral hydralazine for primary pulmonary hypertension. *N Engl J Med* 1980;302:69.
178. Packer M, Greenberg B, Massie B, Dash H: Deleterious effects of hydralazine in patients with pulmonary hypertension. *N Engl J Med* 1982;306:1326.
179. Lupi-Herrera E, Sandoval J, Seoane M, Bialostozky D: The role of hydralazine therapy for pulmonary arterial hypertension of unknown cause. *Circulation* 1982;65:645.
180. Kronzon I, Cohen M, Winer HE: Adverse effect of hydralazine in patients with primary pulmonary hypertension. *JAMA* 1982;247:3112.
181. Camerini F, Alberti E, Klugmann S, Salvi A: Primary pulmonary hypertension: Effects of nifedipine. *Br Heart J* 1980;44:352.

182. Berkenboom G, Sobolski J, Stoupel E: Failure of nifedipine treatment in primary pulmonary hypertension. Br Heart J 1982;47:511.
183. Rubin LJ, Groves BM, Reeves JT, Frosolono M, Handel F, Cato AE: Prostacyclin-induced acute pulmonary vasodilation in primary pulmonary hypertension. Circulation 1982;66:334.
184. Guadagni DN, Ikram H, Maslowski AH: Haemodynamic effect of prostacyclin (PGI_2) in pulmonary hypertension. Br Heart J 1981;45:385.
185. Kokubu T, Kazatani Y, Hamada M, Matsuzaki K, Ito T, Nishimura K, Ochi T, Daimon F, Joh T: Is captopril effective in primary pulmonary hypertension? Jpn Circ J 1982;46:1095.
186. Lee TD, Roveti GC, Ross RS: The hemodynamic effects of isoproterenol on pulmonary hypertension in man. Am Heart J 1963;65:361.
187. Shettingar VR, Hultgren HN, Specter M, Martin R, Davies DH: Primary pulmonary hypertension. Favorable effect of isoproterenol. N Engl J Med 1976; 295:1414.
188. Lupi-Herrera E, Bialostozky D, Sobrino A: The role of isoproterenol in pulmonary artery hypertension of unknown etiology (primary). Chest 1981;79:292.
189. Pantano JA: Isoproterenol in primary pulmonary hypertension. N Engl J Med 1980;302:919.
190. Cha SD, Kirschbaum M, Maranhao V, Paine E, Gooch AS. Phentolamine for primary pulmonary hypertension. Ann Int Med 1979;91:927.
191. Levine TB, Rose T, Kane M, Weir EK, Cohn JN: Treatment of primary pulmonary hypertension by alpha adrenergic blockade. Circulation 1980; 62,III:75.
192. Nagaska Y, Akutsu H, Lee YS, Fujimoto S: Longterm favorable effect of oxygen administration on a patient with primary pulmonary hypertension. Chest 1978;74:299.
193. Henry PD: Comparative pharmacology of calcium antagonists: Nifedipine, Verapamil and Diltiazem. Am J Cardiol 1980;46:1047.
194. Landmark K, Refsum AM, Simonsen S, Starstein O: Verapamil and pulmonary hypertension. Acta Med Scand 1978;204:299.
195. Crevey BJ, Dantzker DR, Bower JS, Popat KD, Walker SK: Hemodynamic and gas exchange effects of intravenous diltiazem in patients with pulmonary hypertension. Am J Cardiol 1982;49:578.
196. Kambara H, Fujimoto K, Wakabayashi A, Kawai C. Primary pulmonary hypertension: Beneficial therapy with diltiazem. Am Heart J 1981; 101:230.
197. McLeod AA, Wise JR, Daly K, Jewitt D: Nifedipine in treatment of primary pulmonary hypertension. Br Heart J 1981;34:619.
198. Fisher J, Borer JS, Moses JW, Goldberg HL, Niarchos A, Whitman H, Parikh D, Mermelstein P: Pulmonary hypertension: Comparative effects of nifedipine versus hydralazine. Circulation 1982;66,II:194.
199. Dalal JJ, Griffiths BE, Henderson AH: Primary pulmonary hypertension: Effects of nifedipine. Br Heart J 1981;46:230.
200. Young TE, Lundquist LJ, Chesler E, Weir EK: Comparative effects of nifedipine, verapamil and diltiazem on experimental pulmonary hypertension. Am J Cardiol 1983;51:195.

201. Fanta CH, Venugopalan CS, Lacouture PG, Drazen JM: Inhibition of bronchoconstriction in the guinea pig by a calcium blocker, nifedipine. *Am Rev Respir Dis* 1982;125:61.
202. Just H, Stein V: Untersuchungen uber die Wirkung von Diazoxid, einer neuen blutdrucksenkenden Substanz, auf den groBen und den kleinen Kreislauf beim Hypertoniker. *Z Kreislaufforsch* 1969;58:925.
203. Koch-Weser: Diazoxide. *N Engl J Med* 1976;294:1271.
204. Klinke WP, Gilbert JAL: Diazoxide in primary pulmonary hypertension. *N Engl J Med* 1980;302:91.
205. Hall DR, Petch MC: Remission of primary pulmonary hypertension during treatment with diazoxide. *Br Med J* 1981;282:1118.
206. Honey M, Cotter L, Davies N, Denison D: Clinical and hemodynamic effects of diazoxide in primary pulmonary hypertension. *Thorax* 1980;35:269.
207. Rubin LJ, Lazar JD: Influence of prostaglandin synthesis inhibitors on pulmonary vasodilatory effects of hydralazine in dogs with hypoxic pulmonary vasoconstriction. *J Clin Invest* 1981;67:193.
208. Lock JE, Olley PM, Coceani F, Swyer PR, Rowe RD: Use of prostacylin in persistant fetal circulation. *Lancet* 1979;1:1343.
209. Blass KE, Block HV, Forster W, Ponicke K: Dipyridamole: A potent stimulator of prostacyclin biosynthesis. *Br J Pharmacol* 1980;68:71.
210. Weir EK, Chidsey CA, Weil JV, Grover RF: Minoxidil reduces pulmonary vascular resistance in dogs and cattle. *J Lab Clin Med* 1976;88:885.
211. Alpert MA, Bauer JH, Parker BM, Brooks CS, Freeman JA: Pulmonary hemodynamics in systemic hypertension. Long-term effect of minoxidil. *Chest* 1979;76:379.
212. Fuleihan DS, Mookherjee S, Potts JL, Obein AI, Warner RA, Eich RH: Sodium nitroprusside: A new role as a pulmonary vasodilator. *Am J Cardiol* 1979;43:405.
213. McKay C, Norman A, Chatterjee K, Ader R, Ports T, Brundage B, Parmley W: Comparative hemodynamics of sublingual isosorbide dinitrate and intravenous isoproterenol in precapillary pulmonary hypertension. *Clin Res* 1980;28:10A.
214. Swartz SL, Williams GH, Hollenberg NK, Levine L, Dluhy RG, Moore TJ: Captopril-induced changes in prostaglandin production. *J Clin Invest* 1980;65:1257.
215. Leier CV, Bambach D, Nelson S, Hermiller JB, Huss P, Magorien RD, Unverferth DV: Captopril in primary pulmonary hypertension. *Circulation* 1983;67:155.
216. Stark RD, Finnegan P, Bishop JM. Daily requirements of oxygen to reverse pulmonary hypertension in patients with chronic bronchitis. *Br Med J* 1972;3:724.
217. LeVeen HH, Ip M, Ahmed N, Mascardo T, Guinto RB, Falk G, D'Ovidio N: Lowering blood viscosity to overcome vascular resistance. *Surg Gyn Obstet* 1980;150:139.
218. Weisse AB, Moschos CB, Frank MJ, Levinson GE, Cannilla JE, Regan TJ: Hemodynamic effects of staged hematocrit reduction in patients with stable cor pulmonale and severely elevated hematocrit levels. *Am J Med* 1975;58:92.

219. Fischer M, Mosslacher H, Slany J: Thrombolytische therapie bie primar vaskularen pulmonaler hypertension. *Med Wett* 1971;8:299.
220. Gorlin R, Clare FB, Zuska JJ. Evidence for pulmonary vasoconstriction in man. *Br Heart J* 1958;20:346.
221. Reitz BA, Wallwork JL, Hunt SA, Pennock JL, Billingham ME, Oyer PE, Stinson EB, Shumway NE. Heart-lung transplantation: Successful therapy for patients with pulmonary vascular disease. *N Engl J Med* 1982;306:557.
222. Reitz BA. Heart-lung transplantation: A review. *Heart Transplantation* 1982;1:291.

CHAPTER 5

THROMBOEMBOLIC PULMONARY HYPERTENSION

Joseph V. Messer

"How is it possible to expect mankind to take advice when they will not so much as heed warnings?"

J. Swift, 1667–1745

With few exceptions, severe pulmonary hypertension when first diagnosed is irreversible and leads inexorably to progressive incapacitation and death. Notable exceptions include some cases of congenital or acquired disease of the heart and great vessels and many cases in which pulmonary hypertension occurs as a result of venous thromboembolism. Although schistosomiasis is the commonest cause of chronic pulmonary hypertension, affecting 200,000,000 of the world's population, venous thromboembolism occupies a central position in the etiology of pulmonary hypertension since it is the commonest cause of acute pulmonary hypertension, is highly responsive to proper therapy, and is frequently mismanaged. Diagnosis and prevention, rather than treatment, represent the continuing challenges of this major health problem. In hospitalized patients, pulmonary emboli are the most common cause of acute pulmonary disease,[1] and are among the most misdiagnosed conditions encountered in hospital practice. In a 1972 postmortem study, the frequency of missed diagnoses was 67%, while positive diagnoses were incorrect in 63% of the patients.[2] Numerous angiographic studies suggest that the clinical diagnosis of pulmonary embolism is correct in only about one-third of patients.[3] Data from three carefully performed studies demonstrated negative pulmonary angiograms in 80% of patients in whom pulmonary embolism was diagnosed by clinical findings, blood gases, and perfusion lung scans.[4-6] The extent of this diagnostic paradox is illustrated in Figure 1.

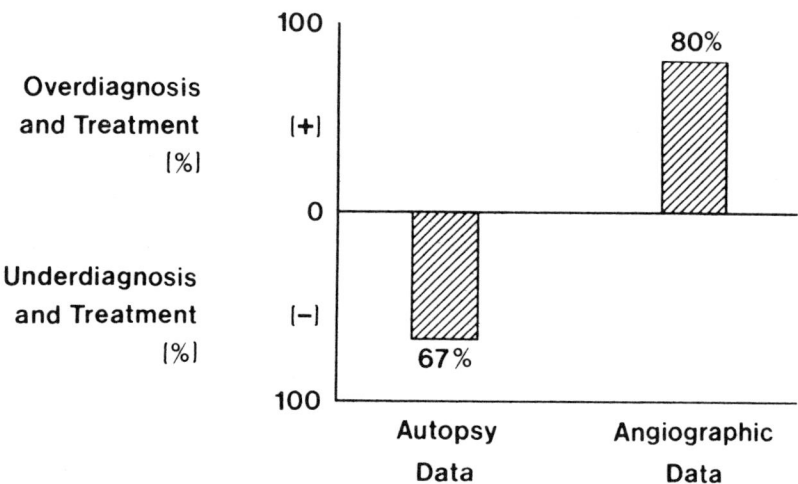

Figure 1. Graphic representation of the accuracy of widely employed diagnostic criteria for pulmonary embolism when judged by autopsy[1] and angiographic studies.[4-6] (Reproduced with permission from Reference 83.)

The ability to prevent thromboembolic pulmonary hypertension depends almost entirely on the prophylaxis, or early detection and treatment, of deep venous thrombosis of the lower extremities. Although more than a century has passed since Virchow postulated the triad of vascular injury, venous stasis, and hypercoagulability as conditions predisposing to venous thrombosis,[7] no uniformly successful methods exist to control these preconditions in patients at high risk. When the classical signs of lower extremity deep venous thrombosis are present, the diagnosis can be made with ease and therapy is usually highly effective. Unfortunately, the physical examination of the legs is normal in nearly one-half of patients with deep venous thrombosis, although reasonably reliable invasive and non-invasive methods are available for its diagnosis.

The implications of these data are obvious. Apparently, the diagnostic tools employed by many clinicians are inadequate and require improvement based on recent advances in our understanding of the pathophysiology of venous thromboembolism. Therapeutically, the results of misdiagnosis are particularly hazardous. In most patients the primary goal of treatment is the prevention of *recurrent* thromboembolism, which occurs in nearly 50% of untreated patients and is fatal in approximately half of these recurrences.[8] Furthermore, most patients with chronic pulmonary hypertension secondary to thromboembolism have been misdiagnosed and therefore untreated for *symptomatic* episodes of pulmonary embolism.[9] Thus, failure to treat is an avoidable and potentially fatal error.

Conversely, treatment for venous thromboembolism is costly, inconvenient, and associated with significant morbidity and mortality. Well conducted studies have reported mortality rates as high as 2.4% in short term, fully heparinized patients and 2%/patient year during long-term oral anticoagulation.[10-12] While these risks may be unavoidable in patients with documented deep venous thrombosis or pulmonary embolism, they cannot be tolerated in the case of falsely positive diagnosis.

Several studies during the past decade provide a basis for avoiding the cruel paradox of venous thromboembolism: underdiagnosis and inadequate treatment according to autopsy data, and overdiagnosis and inappropriate treatment according to pulmonary angiographic validations. Since therapy for venous thromboembolism is highly effective and significantly hazardous, diagnostic accuracy is of utmost importance. Although some issues remain unanswered or controversial, knowledge is now available to improve the management of venous thromboembolism, a major cause of pulmonary hypertension.

THE INCIDENCE AND PREVALENCE OF THROMBOEMBOLIC PULMONARY HYPERTENSION

The true incidence of acute thromboembolic pulmonary hypertension and the prevalence of chronic pulmonary hypertension secondary to recurrent thromboembolism are unknown. This is not unexpected considering the serious inaccuracy of clinical diagnosis in acute pulmonary embolism and the difficulty encountered in properly separating the rare condition of chronic thromboembolic pulmonary hypertension from the equally rare conditions generally referred to as primary pulmonary hypertension and pulmonary venoocclusive disease.

Acute Thromboembolic Pulmonary Hypertension

It is reasonable to assume that a majority of symptomatic patients with acute pulmonary embolism have transient or more persistent pulmonary hypertension. Thus, some appreciation of the incidence of acute thromboembolic pulmonary hypertension can be obtained from estimates of the incidence of acute pulmonary embolism and physiologic studies in selected patients. The majority of such estimates are derived from autopsy series or from approximations based on clinical correlation studies.

Autopsy Studies

Because only limited incidence and prevalence data are available from living patient populations, autopsy data frequently are used to obtain prevalence estimates for pulmonary embolism. Although markedly differing results have been reported by various authors, 3 studies deserve special consideration. Smith et al. in 1962 utilized postmortem pulmonary arteriography to demonstrate a 26% prevalence of pulmonary emboli in one year's autopsies at the Peter Bent Brigham Hospital.[13] The finding of emboli varied from 15% in nonselected autopsies to 60% in cases with the clinical diagnosis of pulmonary embolism. During this period, 14% of autopsy cases died from pulmonary embolism, the single most common cause of death observed. Frieman et al.[14] utilized meticulous dissection to demonstrate pulmonary emboli in 64% of 61 consecutive adult autopsies, a prevalence in close agreement with that of 52% reported by Morrell and Dunnill[15] from a painstaking postmortem investigation of 263 right lungs. The prevalence of emboli in the left lungs was only 12% when studied routinely.

Thus, the patient population, the pathologist, and the procedures employed appear to influence the reported prevalence of pulmonary emboli from autopsy studies. Overall, the 40–50% autopsy prevalence of pulmonary emboli suggested by Rosenow[16] seems reasonable, with emboli contributing directly to 15% of adult deaths in acute general hospitals. Acute thromboembolic pulmonary hypertension undoubtedly plays a role in nearly all of these deaths.

Although autopsy studies may encourage unwarranted and potentially erroneous extrapolations to incidence data for acute and chronically recurring pulmonary embolism, they have been invaluable in emphasizing the need for improved diagnostic methods and in elucidating the pathophysiology of thromboembolic pulmonary hypertension. In a reasonable extrapolation based on autopsy studies, biostatistical reports and data on treatment effects in acute pulmonary embolism, Dalen and Alpert have estimated the annual incidence of *symptomatic* pulmonary embolism in the United States.[17] Their analysis, summarized in Table 1, emphasizes the importance of accurate diagnosis and appropriate therapy in determining ultimate outcome, and provides some insight into the incidence and consequences of acute thromboembolic pulmonary hypertension. Over 200,000 patients die of symptomatic pulmonary embolism each year, and it is probable that such patients experience significant pulmonary hypertension whether due to massive embolism or from submassive emboli superimposed on preexisting cardiopulmonary disease.

Clinical Studies

The National Cooperative Trials of Thrombolytic Therapy provided definitive data concerning the incidence of acute thromboembolic pulmonary hypertension in patients with documented, quantified pulmonary embolism.[18,19] In earlier studies, McIntyre and Sasahara[20] had observed that pulmonary hypertension, defined as a mean pulmonary artery pressure greater than 20 mm Hg, occurred in 70% of pulmonary emboli patients without preexisting cardiopulmonary disease.

Utilizing the same definition of thromboembolic pulmonary hypertension, Phase 1 of the Urokinase Pulmonary Embolism Trial demonstrated acute pulmonary hypertension in approximately 60% of patients with documented pulmonary embolism.[18] In Phase 2 of the Trial, 99% of the patients had right ventricular systolic pressures greater than 25 mm Hg when initially measured.[19] From these studies, an 80% estimated incidence of pulmonary hypertension in acute pulmonary embolism is not unreasonable. Applying these data to the

TABLE 1
Annual Incidence of Pulmonary Embolism in the United States*

	Survival	Deaths	Total (%)
Within 1 Hour	—	67,000	67,000[11]
Beyond 1 Hour			
Diagnosed and Treated	150,000	13,000	163,000[26]
Not Diagnosed or Treated	280,000	120,000	400,000[63]
	430,000	200,000	630,000[100]

*From data in reference 17.
(Reproduced with permission from Reference 83.)

Dalen-Alpert estimate of 430,000 *survivors* of symptomatic pulmonary embolism predicts an additional 340,000 cases of acute thromboembolic pulmonary hypertension in the United States each year.

Thus, acute thromboembolic pulmonary hypertension probably occurs in a total of over 540,000 patients annually, contributing to the morbidity of acute thromboembolism which is the third most frequent cause of death in the United States, more common than cerebrovascular accidents and half as frequent as acute myocardial infarction. Because of the significant effects of prophylaxis and acute treatment, a large proportion of these fatalities are probably avoidable.

The Incidence of Acute Venous Thromboembolism in Various Patient Populations

Although overall incidence data define the importance of venous thromboembolism and pulmonary hypertension as a major health problem, management of individual patients is enhanced by knowledge concerning the incidence of the disease in specific patient populations. Such knowledge influences the clinician's index of suspicion, and often determines the aggressiveness of surveillance, prophylaxis, and early detection. In addition, since the prevalence of disease in a given patient population strongly influences the predictive accuracy of diagnostic tests,[21] an appreciation of expected incidence is essential to proper interpretation of diagnostic results.

Only limited incidence data are available for specific subgroups of the patient population. McNeil has reported a pulmonary embolism incidence of 10% in hospitalized patients over 40 years of age presenting with multiple complaints suggesting pulmonary embolism, and 20% in patients below 40 years of age with the single symptom of pleuritic chest pain.[22]

Angiographically diagnosed pulmonary embolism is present in 17–40% of patients with a suggestive clinical history, arterial hypoxemia, and a positive perfusion lung scan.[4-6] In a more recent prospective study of 139 consecutive patients with clinically suspected pulmonary embolism and abnormal perfusion lung scans, 62% of patients undergoing adequate pulmonary angiography had pulmonary emboli.[23] Despite widespread belief that oral contraceptives are an important risk factor for pulmonary embolism, Moser[24] estimates that the annual incidence of embolism in women on "the pill" is, at maximum, only 8 in 100,000. Estimated incidences of pulmonary embolism and, therefore, indications of the incidence of acute thromboembolic pulmonary hypertension in various patient subgroups are presented in Table 2. These data suggest that the occurrence of pulmonary embolism varies widely in the most predisposed subgroups of the patient population, with reported incidences ranging from 1–50%. The vast majority of predisposed populations, however, have an incidence of less than 25%, considerably lower than that observed in most groups studied to determine the accuracy of diagnostic tests in thromboembolic disease.

Additional studies of the incidence of acute pulmonary embolism and thromboembolic pulmonary hypertension are urgently needed. It appears that their incidence is increasing as oral contraceptive use increases, more extensive surgery is performed, the older population increases in size, and especially, as saphenous veins are increasingly harvested for coronary artery bypass surgery.

TABLE 2
Incidence of Pulmonary Embolism in Various Patient Groups

Patient Population	Incidence of Pulmonary Embolism (%)	References
Sudden death, ages 15–45	.0003	25
Abdominal-thoracic surgery	1–4	26
Hip surgery	2–12	26
Heart failure, clinical diagnosis	8–15	26
Post myocardial infarction	9	26
Post mitral valve surgery	10	26
Fractures, pelvis, and lower extremities	10	27
Over 40 years, multiple symptoms of pulmonary embolism	10	22
Under 40 years, pleuritic chest pain	20	22
General hospital, positive history, hypoxemia, perfusion scan	17–40	4–6
Heart failure at autopsy	48	28

Chronic Thromboembolic Pulmonary Hypertension

If the estimates made of the incidence of *acute* thromboembolic pulmonary hypertension are subject to criticism, suggestions concerning the prevalence of chronic pulmonary hypertension caused by recurrent thromboemboli are even more tenuous. This unfortunate circumstance reflects the fact that this condition is commonly undiagnosed during life and requires specialized examination for its postmortem detection.

It is generally agreed that pulmonary hypertension secondary to repeated emboli emerges from two clinical backgrounds. In most patients, the embolic episodes are symptomatic, but go undiagnosed and untreated.[9] In very rare cases, recurring thromboemoli are clinically silent. The resulting chronic pulmonary hypertension and cor pulmonale are judged to be idiopathic, and are usually clinically indistinguishable from primary pulmonary hypertension or pulmonary venoocclusive disease. In nearly all cases, definitive diagnosis requires histologic examination at biopsy or autopsy. (See Chapter 11.)

Symptomatic Pulmonary Emboli

The potential for pulmonary emboli to produce anatomic abnormalities leading to chronic pulmonary hypertension is well documented in pathologic studies. Totally occluded vessels, organized emboli with incomplete recanalization, fibrous bands, and webs are common at autopsy.

It is generally agreed that a single episode of massive pulmonary embolism does not lead to chronic pulmonary hypertension and cor pulmonale.[17,29,30] Recurrent embolism is the essential etiologic factor in this usually fatal complication of thromboembolic disease and, unfortunately, occurs commonly. In the Urokinase Pulmonary Embolism Trial population, 15% of the patients had had 2 or more prior episodes of pulmonary embolism, and 20% had recurrent embolism in the first 2 weeks following treatment.[18] Autopsy studies suggest an even higher frequency of recurrence in patients dying with pulmonary embolus. Smith[13] found emboli of varying ages in 42 of 54 patients, and Morrell and Dunnill[15] found evidence of recurrent emboli in a significant proportion of their cases.

If recurrent embolism is central to the development of chronic thromboembolic pulmonary hypertension, are data available concerning the size of predisposed patient populations from which the prevalence of chronic thromboembolic pulmonary hypertension can be estimated? Certainly the most likely population to develop this complication is that in which symptomatic pulmonary emboli are undiagnosed and untreated, estimated by Dalen and Alpert to number 400,000 patients annually. Fifty percent of these patients may be expected to have recurrent thromboembolism.[8] The studies of Riedel et al.[29] suggest that even when treated after diagnosis, 17% of patients with prior recurrent pulmonary embolism die from severe pulmonary hypertension an average of 2 years after the initial examination, while the remainder do not develop severe pulmonary hypertension even after several years. Without treatment, a significantly higher percentage of such patients with recurrent pulmonary embolism might be expected to develop chronic changes, and constitute the major patient population contributing to the prevalence of chronic thromboembolic pulmonary hypertension and cor pulmonale in the United States.[31]

What is known concerning the development of chronic pulmonary hypertension in patients diagnosed and treated for acute pulmonary embolism? The Urokinase Pulmonary Embolism Trial demonstrated the importance of adequate anticoagulation in preventing recurrent thromboembolism. The rate of recurrence was significantly lower, 16 versus 35 percent, in patients with adequate levels of anticoagulation.[18] Dalen observed only 1 death from chronic cor pulmonale in 60 patients followed 1 to 7 years after major pulmonary embolism had been diagnosed and adequately treated.[17] It appears that chronic thromboembolic pulmonary hypertension is extremely unlikely when pulmonary embolism is recognized and recurrence is prevented by appropriate therapy.

Clinically Silent Pulmonary Emboli

It is well appreciated that pulmonary emboli may occur without clinically recognizable consequences, resulting in the widespread obliteration of both central and peripheral pulmonary arteries, chronic pulmonary hypertension, and cor pulmonale. Reliable data are not available concerning the prevalence of this chronic, progressive disease since nearly all estimates rely on autopsy studies.

Silent or occult thromboembolism is the most malignant form of thromboembolic pulmonary hypertension. Rarely diagnosed before irreversible changes have occurred, silent pulmonary embolism frequently is associated with severe pulmonary hypertension when objective studies are first obtained, and usually progresses to death in 2 or 3 years after initial detection.[29] The patient population with silent thromboembolic pulmonary hypertension probably is a continuum of the larger population with symptomatic, but undiagnosed, pulmonary embolism, patient classification being more a function of the physician's diagnostic acumen than of the underlying pathophysiologic process. In Riedel's series[29] of occult pulmonary embolism, clinically apparent pulmonary embolus occurred in 7 of 13 patients *after* the diagnosis of silent pulmonary embolism was established, and 5 of the 12 patients in Owen's autopsy series[32] of "unrecognized" thromboembolic cor pulmonale had had single or recurrent episodes of hemoptysis.

When defined as pulmonary hypertension or cor pulmonale caused by previously unrecognized pulmonary emboli, this form of chronic thromboembolic pulmonary hypertension is very rare.[33] The diagnosis usually is first entertained in the context of idiopathic or primary pulmonary hypertension, itself an extremely rare condition reported by Paul Wood in only 0.17% of his patients over a 10-year period.[34] Owen et al.[32] found only 12 cases of unrecognized thromboembolic chronic cor pulmonale among 8,000 autopsies over a period of 20 years, but cautioned that this figure is misleadingly low since patients with other complicating cardiorespiratory diseases were excluded from analysis.

Autopsy studies in patients with idiopathic or primary pulmonary hypertension are the usual source of prevalence data for chronic silent thromboembolic pulmonary hypertension. The Wagenvoorts demonstrated recurrent, apparently silent pulmonary emboli in 20% of 156 autopsied cases previously diagnosed as primary pulmonary hypertension.[35] In a recent report by Steele et al.[36] only 120 patients with idiopathic pulmonary hypertension were diagnosed at the Mayo Clinic over a 20-year period. Follow-up studies revealed thromboembolism in 58% of the cases available for autopsy analysis. In a careful clinical study of 21 patients diagnosed as having chronic obliterative pulmonary hypertension over a 5-year period at Hammersmith Hospital, Wilson et al.[37] concluded that 38% had chronic thromboembolic disease. It seems unlikely, however, that these were truly unrecognized embolic cases since the majority had histories suggestive of thromboembolic disease.

Although an extremely rare condition accounting for perhaps one-third to one-half of chronic idiopathic pulmonary hypertension, silent recurring thromboembolism is sufficiently amenable to therapy to warrant Dexter's often repeated dictum[38] that primary (or idiopathic) pulmonary hypertension should not be diagnosed during life and that all such patients should be treated as though they had recurrent pulmonary emboli (Figure 2).

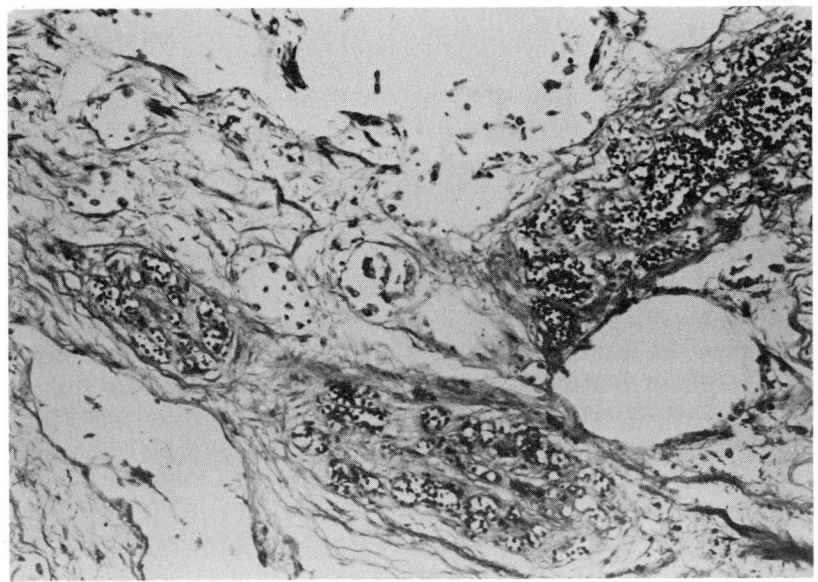

Figure 2, a and b. *Organizing and recanalized unsuspected thromboemboli in small pulmonary vessels observed in a young male at autopsy with right heart failure and sudden death. (Courtesy of J. Coon, M.D., Ph.D., Department of Pathology, Rush-Presbyterian-St. Luke's Medical Center.)*

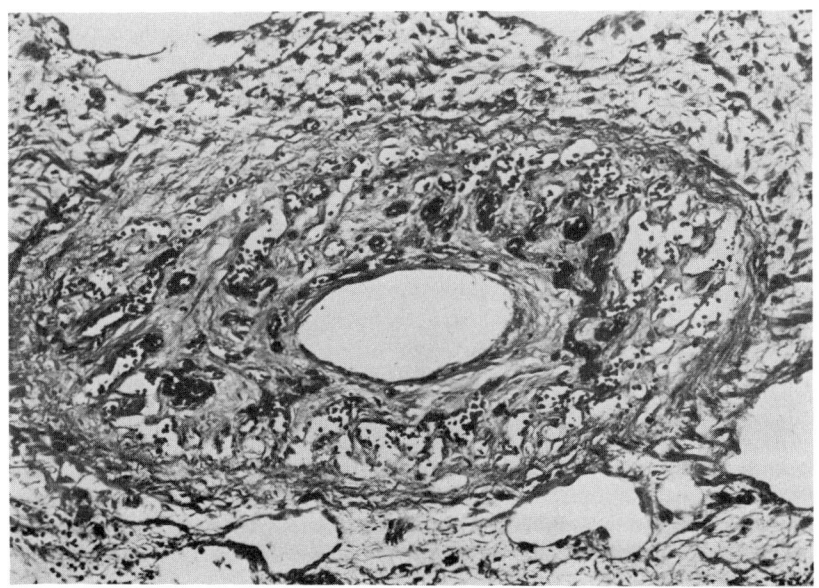

Figure 2 b.

Deep Venous Thrombosis and Pulmonary Embolism

Since deep venous thrombosis is the precursor of thromboembolic pulmonary hypertension in most patients, its incidence and relation to pulmonary embolization warrant consideration. In a recent editorial emphasizing the importance of early detection and prophylaxis, Moser suggests that 20 million episodes of deep venous thrombosis may occur each year in the United States, giving rise to pulmonary embolism in somewhat less than 10% of the cases.[39]

Although these estimates probably overstate the case, several clinical studies demonstrate the serious magnitude of deep venous thrombosis in selected populations. In a prospective study, Rossi et al.[40] reported the development of deep venous thrombosis in 72% of patients hospitalized with acute spinal cord injury. Seventy-one percent of patients over the age of 70 admitted with acute myocardial infarction developed deep venous thrombosis in a prospective study by Emerson et al.[41] There was a 12% incidence of deep venous thrombosis in patients less than 50 years old and an overall incidence of 34% in the entire myocardial infarction population studied. These figures are somewhat higher than those reported in prospective studies of patients following surgery. Kakkar et al.[42] reported extensive deep venous thrombosis in 20% and the International Multicentre Trial observed the development of deep venous thrombosis in only 7% of the untreated control group following general surgery.[43]

Reports of the incidence of pulmonary embolism complicating deep venous thrombosis also vary widely, with the effects of treatment having a major influence on incidence and ultimate outcome. According to Gallus,[44] before anticoagulants 26–27% of patients with clinical evidence of postpartum or postoperative venous thrombosis developed signs and symptoms of embolism which was fatal in 11–23%. More recently, Moreno-Cabral et al.[45] reported lung scan evidence of silent pulmonary embolism in 50% of patients with deep venous thrombosis confirmed by venography. In Kakkar's study,[42] approximately 40% of patients with untreated silent postoperative popliteal or femoral vein thrombosis had significant pulmonary emboli. Emphasizing the greater risk of embolization when deep venous thrombosis occurs proximally, Bell and Simon[46] estimate overall embolic rates of 15–20% in deep venous thrombosis, while Rosenow, et al.[16] report that approximately 50% of iliofemoral deep venous thrombi will embolize to the lungs (Figure 3).

Given the frequent occurrence of deep venous thrombosis and the high incidence of embolization, it is not unexpected that a significant

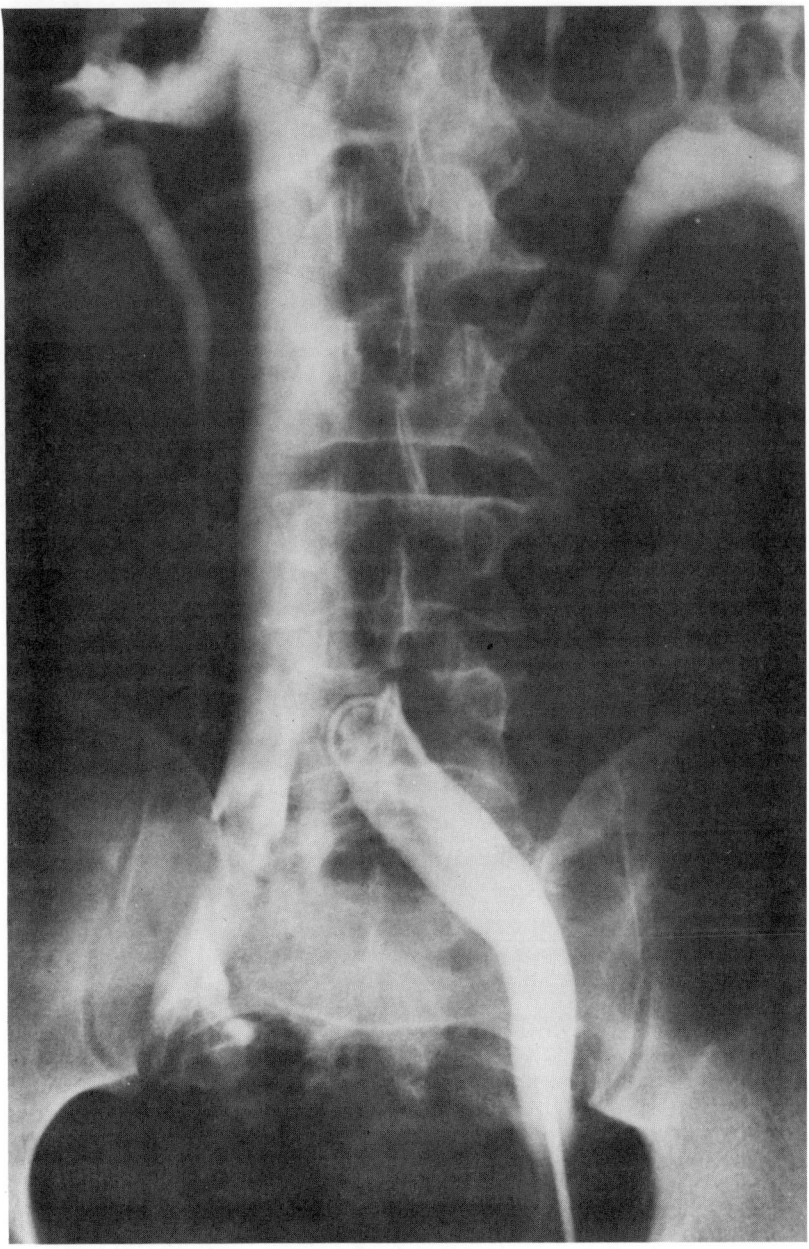

Figure 3. Right ileofemoral clot in patient with clinically apparent deep venous thrombosis of right leg. (Courtesy of M.D. Bogdonoff, M.D., Department of Diagnostic Radiology, Rush-Presbyterian-St. Luke's Medical Center.)

percentage of patients with angiographically proven pulmonary embolism have deep venous thrombosis. Hull et al.[23] found deep venous thrombosis in 71% of patients with pulmonary embolism and in an additional third of patients with abnormal perfusion lung scans but negative pulmonary angiograms. In a similar angiographic study, Bynum and Wilson[47] found that 54% of patients with pulmonary embolism had deep venous thrombosis distributed about evenly between calf and thigh veins. Thromboembolism recurred most frequently in chronic medical conditions or illnesses of unknown cause, 20% and 40% respectively, and in only 12% of surgical, traumatic, and obstetrical illness.

The implications of these data are clear. The major opportunity to reduce the morbidity and mortality of thromboembolic pulmonary hypertension resides in the prevention or early detection and effective treatment of deep venous thrombosis.

THE ETIOLOGY AND PATHOPHYSIOLOGY OF THROMBOEMBOLIC PULMONARY HYPERTENSION

The Origin and Destination of Thromboemboli

Pathogenesis

Virchow postulated that venous stasis, hypercoagulability, and venous wall injury were all important pathogenetic factors in venous thrombosis. Venous stasis appears to be the most important member of the classic triad,[48] but probably is not a sufficient single precipitating factor. The importance of hypercoagulability has been debated, but undoubtedly plays some role in the increased predisposition to deep venous thrombosis of women in whom oral contraceptives increase circulating estrogen levels and in certain malignancies such as pancreatic carcinoma. The interaction of venous endothelial damage and the hypercoagulable state has been emphasized by Green,[49] who has suggested that hypercoagulability can be detected in routine testing by assays for Antithrombin III levels β-thromboglobulin (β-TG) to platelet factor 4 (PF4) ratios, and the platelet aggregate ratio. He suggests these studies in patients without an obvious cause for their venous thrombosis.

Venous intimal injury may result from mechanical trauma, prolonged hypoxia, and immune complex deposition. Exposure of the subendothelial collagen tissue stimulates platelet adhesion and aggregation initiating a chain of reactions that enhance clotting.[49] Clearly, venous intimal injury plays an important initiating and prepetuating role in venous thrombosis following trauma and extensive surgical procedures.

Anatomical Sources of Thromboemboli

Disagreement persists concerning the relative importance of calf versus femoral and iliac venous thrombi as sources of pulmonary emboli. It is generally agreed that calf vein thrombi propagate proximally before posing the threat of serious thromboembolism, and that the vast majority of significant pulmonary emboli arise from the iliac, femoral, or popliteal veins.[46] Important exceptions include septic and bland thrombi arising from the pelvic veins, especially following obstetrical or prostatic surgery, septic emboli from superficial phlebitis or tricuspid endocarditis in drug users, thrombi associated with intracardiac catheters, and very rarely, right atrial thrombi.

Propagation and Embolization

Venous thrombi usually adhere to the vein wall at the point of origin, commonly above valve leaflets. Through accretion of successive layers of fibrin, enmeshed red cells, and platelets, thrombi propagate centrally in the direction of flow until the free floating segment breaks loose and is propelled by the venous current to the right heart. The age of the dislodged thrombotic fragment is important to its ultimate fate within the pulmonary tree. Fresh thrombi are more susceptible to fragmentation in transit through the contracting right ventricle and often produce multiple smaller emboli. Older organized thrombi are more likely to pass intact into the pulmonary circulation, lodging at bifurcations to produce partial obstruction of major pulmonary vessels.

Anatomical Locations and Massivity of Pulmonary Emboli

The relative frequencies of thromboembolism to various portions of the pulmonary vasculature are usually ascribed to corresponding differences in blood flow, an explanation for which Harris and Heath find little supporting evidence.[50] A detailed analysis of 1,272 embolized vessels from angiographic data collected in the Urokinase Pulmonary Embolism Trial[51] is presented in Table 3, and clearly indicates a preponderence of emboli in the right lung and in the lower lobes. Segmental level arteries are involved most frequently with lobar arteries being the next most common site of embolization. Intermediate and main branches contained fewer than 10% of the emboli and the main trunk pulmonary artery contained less than 1% of the emboli. These observations from living patients agree closely with the autopsy findings of Smith et al.[13] whose observations are included in Table 3. The only important difference in Smith's study was the considerably more frequent involvement of the main pulmonary trunk, a not unexpected finding in autopsy patients in whom death was attributed primarily to pulmonary embolism in 14% of cases.

Tow and Simon[52] also have analyzed the anatomical locations of pulmonary embolization in the Urokinase Pulmonary Embolism Trial, expressing their results as the percentage of *patients* having emboli in various locations (Table 3). This analysis indicates that equal numbers of patients have emboli involving right and left lower lung vessels, while somewhat fewer patients have emboli in the right upper and middle lung, and the smallest percentage demonstrates involvement of the left upper lung. Important from both diagnostic and pathophysiologic standpoints was the bilateral and multiple nature of embolic involvement in these patients.

The likelihood that pulmonary embolization will produce pulmonary hypertension depends largely on the total volume of embolized thrombotic material and whether it is fragmented in transit through the right heart to be disbursed in the large distribution volume of multiple smaller vessels or remains relatively intact to occlude major proximal vessels. The age and degree of organization of the thrombus are important factors in this regard. In 54 autopsy patients with pulmonary embolism, Smith et al.[13] found embolus obstruction of the large elastic pulmonary arteries in 20 cases, or 37%. The thromboemboli in these cases were large enough to have permitted pulmonary embolectomy had the diagnosis been made antemortem. Angiographic observations made in the Urokinase Pulmonary Embolism Trial revealed that a considerably higher percentage of patients had emboli involving the large pulmonary arteries (Table 3, Tow and Simon), undoubtedly reflecting the fact that these data are from living patients soon after embolization and before endogenous lysis and distal migration of the thrombus had occurred. Seventy-four percent of the patients had involvement of the intermediate pulmonary arteries. Thus, embolic material is present in major pulmonary vessels in one-third to three-

TABLE 3
Anatomical Locations of Pulmonary Emboli

Location	Vessel Analysis Embolized Vessels (%)		Patient Analysis Patients Having Emboli (%)
	UPET[51]	Smith et al.[13]	Tow and Simon[52]
Right lower lung	23	28	63
Left lower lung	20	22	63
Right upper lung	15	4	52
Right middle lung	8	14	45
Left middle lung	8	—	39
Left upper lung	8	10	31
Right intermediate artery	6	—	74
Left intermediate artery	5	—	
Right pulmonary artery	4	8	46
Left pulmonary artery	2	4	
Main pulmonary artery	<1	10	4
Right lung	56	54	—
Left lung	44	36	—
Upper lobes	22	14	—
Middle lobes	17	14	—
Lower lobes	43	50	—
Lobar arteries	31	—	—
Segmental arteries	52	—	—
Bilateral	—	—	67
Multiple	—	—	93

quarters of patients with thromboembolism depending on the study methods employed.

Although embolic distribution data are important to our understanding of the pathogenesis of thromboembolic pulmonary hypertension, the degree of obliteration of the total pulmonary vascular cross-sectional area is a more important causal factor. Accurate measurements of cross-sectional obliteration are very difficult to achieve in living patients. The objective analysis of angiographic abnormalities employed in the Thromboyltic Trials[53] is a useful method to assess the extent of embolization in a reproducible manner, taking into account the differing occlusive potentials of angiographic filling defects and arterial obstructions. Utilizing a maximum severity index value of 18, this method demonstrated an average value of 9.29 for the 147 pulmonary embolism patients analyzed, suggesting that approximately 50% of the segmental vessels were potentially or actually underperfused because of clot. This estimation of embolic perfusion abnormality in living patients is surprisingly similar to the postmortem results of Smith et al.[13] who measured an average reduction of 59% in the pulmonary arterial vascular volume utilizing injection methods. The distribution of severities of angiographic vessel involvement among the Thrombolytic Trial patient population is presented in Table 4. These angiographic estimates of obstruction differ considerably from the mean lung scan perfusion deficit of only 25%, or one-half of one lung.[52] The latter technique, of course, measures capillary rather than arterial perfusion and did agree rather well with a subjective angiographic estimate of overall perfusion deficit from the same study. In a subset of the Trials' patients free from coexisting cardiopulmonary disease, Sharma et al.[54] observed a 36% reduction in pulmonary−capillary blood volume following 2 weeks of heparin therapy. Immediate post-embolic measurements were not performed.

Since the terms massive and submassive commonly are used in clinical discussion, their precise quantitative definitions, as employed

TABLE 4
Angiographic Severity of Pulmonary Embolism*

Number of Segmental Arteries Involved	Percent of Patients
< 0.5	12
0.5−8.9	36
9.0 +	52

*From data in reference 53. Here and in Table 6, involvement of all segmental arteries would yield a value of 18.

in the Thrombolytic Trials, warrant emphasis. In these studies, "massive" pulmonary embolism was liberally defined as the presence of obstruction or significant filling defects involving only 2 or more lobar pulmonary arteries or an equivalent amount of emboli in other vessels.[18] The term was not meant to imply hemodynamic or clinical information about the patient. Submassive embolism was the presence of obstruction or filling defects in at least one segmental pulmonary artery with the sum of defects being less than that for massive embolism. Utilizing these definitions, the massive pulmonary embolization population, in whom thromboembolic pulmonary hypertension might reasonably be anticipated, comprised 60% of the patients studied (Table 5).[18,19] The extent to which this patient material is representative of the general population of thromboembolic disease is unknown, but a suspicion is not unwarranted that some bias may have existed toward the inclusion of massive embolism patients in the latter phases of the Thrombolytic Trial.

Information is limited concerning the anatomical locations and massivity of pulmonary emboli in chronic recurrent thromboembolic pulmonary hypertension. Often referred to as multiple or microembolism, this condition always involves repeated embolization which usually occludes the small muscular pulmonary arteries or arterioles[55] but can obstruct both right and left main pulmonary arteries.[32,37] Repeat embolization and subsequent organization over months to years ultimately produce significant vascular obstruction and secondary thromboembolic pulmonary hypertension.[29]

Pathology of Thromboembolic Pulmonary Hypertension

A detailed description of the pathology of thromboembolic pulmonary hypertension has been presented elsewhere,[13,33,35,56] and also is discussed in Chapter 11. The pathologic hallmark of thromboembo-

TABLE 5
Angiographic Massivity of Pulmonary Embolism*

	Submassive		Massive	
	n	(%)	n	(%)
UPET	70	(44)	90	(56)
USPET	60	(36)	107	(64)
	130	(40)	197	(60)

*From data in references 18, 19. See text for definition of massive and submassive.

lism is the marked heterogeneity of gross and histological findings caused by variations in embolus size and age, and the recurrent nature of the embolic process. Morrell and Dunnill[15] found fresh emboli in 59% of cases and organizing emboli, fibrous bands and webs of organized emboli, and intimal fibrosis from chronic emboli each in about a third of cases, attesting to the high incidence of recurrence. In a small fraction of cases with massive pulmonary embolism and acute pulmonary hypertension, a large gelatinous thromboembolism straddles the main trunk bifurcation or occludes one or both main pulmonary arteries with little change apparent in the underlying vessel wall. Occasionally the main pulmonary arteries are the site of thrombosis secondary to prior thromboembolism with gradual obliteration of the pulmonary vasculature and severe pulmonary hypertension.[57]

Although many emboli lodged in large elastic pulmonary arteries undergo nearly complete lysis, others organize and recanalize leaving a residue of fibrous trabeculae, varying degrees of luminal obstruction, medial hypertrophy, intimal fibrosis, and atherosclerotic plaques similar to those caused by pulmonary hypertension per se. The majority of thromboemboli are incompletely occlusive, with fresh thrombi being more occlusive but less likely to have attachment to the vessel wall.[13]

Extension distally from the elastic into the smaller muscular arteries may occur by direct continuity or embolic fragmentation. In the average case, distal thromboemboli appear older, suggesting recurrence, and are organized with varying degrees of shrinkage, underlying fibroelastic intimal thickening, and recanalization. When pulmonary hypertension develops, small muscular arterial vessels less than 100 μm in diameter frequently are seen.[58] Bronchial to pulmonary arterial collaterals may develop by neovascular formation through vessels having the appearance of enlarged capillaries in areas of healed infarction and at sites of organizing thromboemboli. These collaterals may have significant survival value in some patients.[13]

Although the clinical distinction between primary pulmonary hypertension and recurrent thromboembolic pulmonary hypertension may be difficult or impossible, these rare causes of obliterative pulmonary hypertension have significantly different pathological characteristics.[33,35] In the typical case of thromboembolic pulmonary hypertension, recurring embolic episodes produce gradual occlusion of the muscular pulmonary vessels and arterial thrombi of varying ages are present with several stages of organization and recanalization. Eccentric pads of intimal fibroelastosis develop with slight medial hypertrophy, rare arteritis, and no plexiform lesions or fibrinoid necrosis (Figure 4). Primary pulmonary hypertension characteristically exhibits

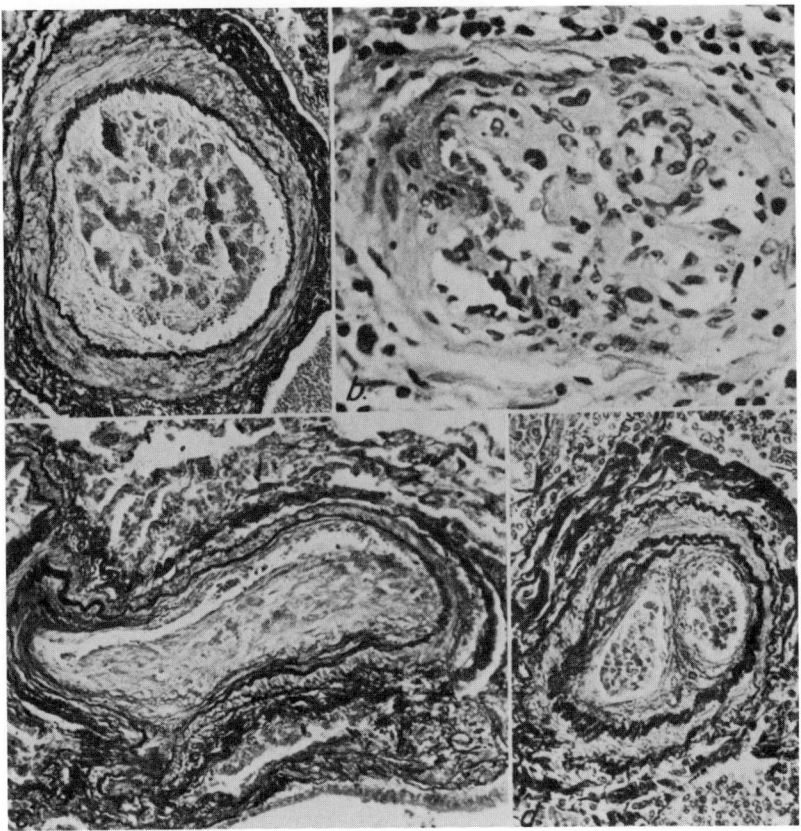

Figure 4. Recurrent pulmonary thromboembolism in a 20-year-old woman; photomicrographs showing thrombi of varying ages in the muscular pulmonary arteries. Elastic-van Gieson stain in a, c, and d; hematoxylin and eosin stain in b. a) Recent unorganized occlusive thrombus, and medial hypertrophy of artery, × 75. b) Recent organizing thrombus with early recanalization, × 380. c) Organized mural thrombus resulting in slit-like lumen, × 100. d) Old organized recanalized thrombus with fibrous septum crossing the lumen, × 200. (Reproduced with permission from Reference 55 and the American Heart Association, Inc.)

medial hypertrophy of muscular arteries, "onion-skin" concentric intimal fibrosis, plexiform lesions, fibrinoid necrosis, and pulmonary arteritis (Figure 5). In some cases of primary pulmonary hypertension, thromboembolism may coexist, requiring great care by the pathologist to establish the correct diagnosis (See Chapter 11).

The cardiac response to thromboembolic pulmonary hypertension reflects the acute or chronic nature of the underlying pulmonary

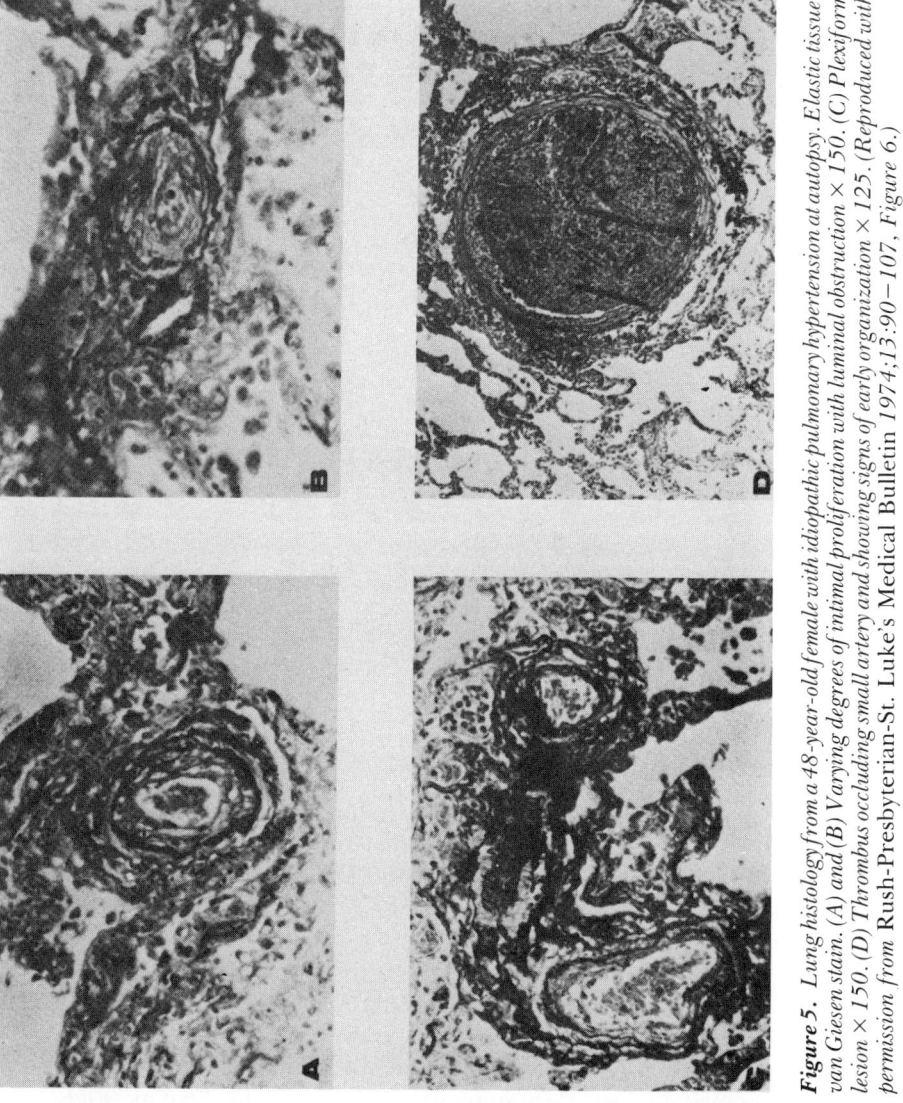

Figure 5. Lung histology from a 48-year-old female with idiopathic pulmonary hypertension at autopsy. Elastic tissue–van Giesen stain. (A) and (B) Varying degrees of intimal proliferation with luminal obstruction × 150. (C) Plexiform lesion × 150. (D) Thrombus occluding small artery and showing signs of early organization × 125. (Reproduced with permission from Rush-Presbyterian–St. Luke's Medical Bulletin 1974;13:90–107, Figure 6.)

vascular obstruction. In acute thromboembolic pulmonary hypertension, hypertrophy is absent unless secondary to preexisting cardiopulmonary disease. Right ventricular and atrial dilatation are the rule with rapid elevation of ventricular filling pressures, tricuspid regurgitation, and systemic venous hypertension. In chronic thromboembolic pulmonary hypertension, however, elevation of pulmonary pressure is gradual and progressive, producing both right ventricular enlargement and compensatory hypertrophy (Figure 6). Filling pressures ultimately increase as ventricular diastolic compliance declines, and tricuspid regurgitation and severe systemic venous congestion are present in the end stage of the disease. Increased right ventricular myocardial blood flow demand caused by severe pulmonary hypertension may exceed the limits of autoregulatory vasodilatation in the presence of coexisting coronary atherosclerosis, increased right ventricular myocardial vessel compression, or systemic hypotension.[59]

THE PATHOGENESIS OF THROMBOEMBOLIC PULMONARY HYPERTENSION

Pulmonary arterial obstruction, preexisting cardiopulmonary disease, and pulmonary vasoconstriction are the primary pathogenetic factors responsible for thromboembolic pulmonary hypertension.

Vascular Obstruction

Most investigators agree that the mechanical effects of embolic obstruction are primarily responsible for the increased pulmonary vascular resistance that produces thromboembolic pulmonary hypertension.[16,19,60,91] Numerous animal and human studies have demonstrated that acute occlusion of more than 50% of the pulmonary vasculature is required to produce pulmonary hypertension. In clinically occurring thromboembolism, however, a considerably smaller percentage of occlusion is sufficient to elevate the pulmonary arterial pressure.

McIntyre and Sasahara[20] observed that only 30% or more of the pulmonary vasculature need be obstructed by pulmonary embolism to produce pulmonary hypertension in patients without preexisting cardiopulmonary disease. Very limited experimental data are available relating the amount of embolic obstruction to elevations in pulmonary artery pressure in human thromboembolic pulmonary hypertension.[20] Analysis of subgroup data from the Urokinase Pulmonary Embolism

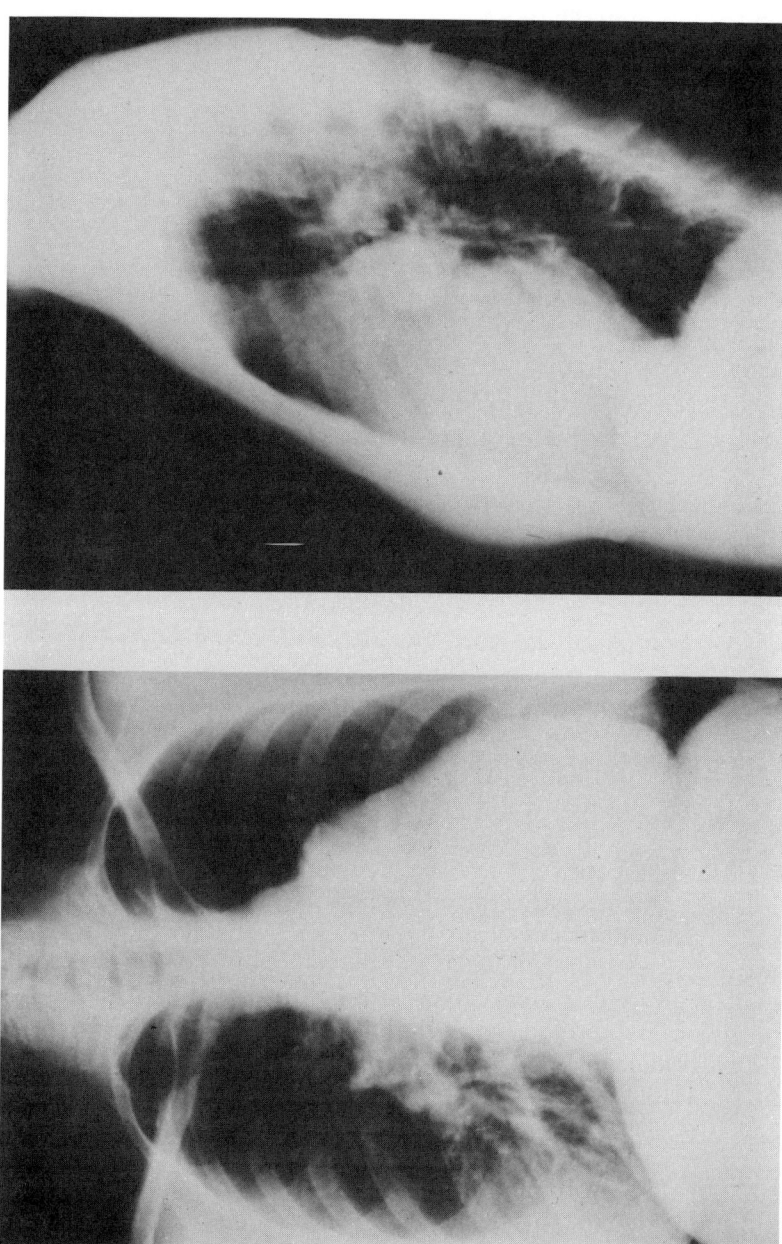

Figure 6. Chest x-ray, PA and lateral, of a 29-year-old female patient in the author's series with a 4-year history of severe progressive idiopathic pulmonary hypertension. Note the marked prominence of the central pulmonary arteries and right ventricular enlargement. At autopsy lesions of both primary and thromboembolic pulmonary hypertension were found.

Trial is of some value in this regard. Mean angiograpic severity indices, lung scan defects, and pulmonary artery pressures from various subgroups are presented in Table 6. It is of interest that a relatively small difference was observed in mean pulmonary artery pressures between subgroups with the least and the most pulmonary obstruction as judged by angiography and lung scanning. These data suggest a rather flat slope, approximating 10 mm Hg for each 20% perfusion defect, for the relationship between pulmonary artery pressure and vascular obstruction within the range of available mean values. Obviously, large numbers of individual data points are needed in patients without preexisting cardiopulmonary disease to determine the nature of this important relationship over the range of values occurring in human thromboembolic pulmonary hypertension.

Preexisting Cardiopulmonary Disease

Rosenow has estimated that 25–50% of patients with pulmonary embolism have preexisting cardiopulmonary disease,[16] and the Urokinase Pulmonary Embolism Trial demonstrated such conditions in 35% of patients.[62] The status of right ventricular function primarily determines the extent to which pulmonary artery pressure can be elevated in acute and chronic thromboembolic pulmonary hypertension. When preexisting cardiopulmonary disease has already produced pulmonary hypertension or right ventricular hypertrophy, significant further elevation of pulmonary artery pressure can be sustained acutely. Without right ventricular hypertrophy, however, pulmonary artery pressures rarely exceed twice normal values before right ventricular failure supervenes. Thus, the presence or absence of preexisting cardiopulmonary disease may influence the hemodynamics of thromboembolic pulmonary hypertension nearly as much as the extent of underlying embolic vascular obstruction. This fact was clearly demonstrated in the Urokinase Pulmonary Embolism Trial where the presence or absence of preexisting cardiopulmonary disease was associated with differences in mean pulmonary artery pressure almost as great as those observed between groups with massive and submassive pulmonary embolism.[62] Conversely, of course, severe coexisting cardiopulmonary disease may account for circulatory failure out of proportion to the extent of embolic involvement. Myocardial infarction is a primary offender in this regard, particularly if the right ventricle is involved.

TABLE 6
Relationship Between Pulmonary Vascular Obstruction and Pulmonary Arterial Pressures[*]

Subgroup	Angiographic Severity Index	Lung Scan Defect (%)	Pulmonary Artery Mean (mm Hg)
Shock, pre-treatment	13	38	37
Massive, pre-teatment	13	33	29
Heparin, post-treatment	8	22	25
Urokinase, post-treatment	5	21	21
Submassive, pre-treatment	4	18	23

[*]From data in references 18 (Tables A 2.1 – .3) and 53 (Figure 3).

Vasoconstriction

Whether mechanical obstruction of the pulmonary vessels produces all of the increase in pulmonary resistance following embolization is widely debated. Much of the confusion concerning possible humoral-reflex mechanisms appears to relate to species differences. The human pulmonary circulation, unlike that of the dog or cat, appears to be unresponsive to serotonin, a powerful pulmonary vasoconstrictor released from platelet thrombi.[60] Other potentially vasoactive substances are released during platelet degranulation including histamine, adenine nucleotides, catecholamines, prostaglandins, and thromboxanes which may produce pulmonary arterial smooth muscle constriction.[63] Bradykinin and vasoactive fibrinopeptides from the breakdown of fibrinogen and fibrin may contribute to pulmonary vascular changes, and diffuse pulmonary vasoconstriction does occur when the pulmonary arterioles are embolized, but not following occlusion of larger vessels where most human emboli lodge.[9] Secondary hypoxemia probably produces modest elevations of pulmonary artery pressures as the result of arteriolar vasoconstriction, and increased pulmonary vascular tone has been postulated in chronic thromboembolic pulmonary hypertension on the basis of a decline in total pulmonary vascular resistance following vasodilator therapy.[64] The transient nature of symptoms, sometimes lasting only a few minutes, and the occasional discordance between symptomatology and angiographic severity tend to support the presence of humoral-reflex vasoconstriction in some cases of human thromboembolic pulmonary hypertension. The consensus is, however, that these vasoconstrictor mechanaisms only reinforce the mechanical effects of pulmonary emboli which are primarily responsible for thromboembolic pulmonary hypertension.[61]

Experimental Studies

In general, experimental studies of pulmonary hypertension have produced more questions than answers concerning the pathogenesis of this complex condition. For obvious reasons, studies in humans are severely limited, and animal models have utilized several different species and a variety of embolic materials whose physicochemical properties may influence pathophysiological responses. Although over a decade ago, Bloor and associates[65] demonstrated the importance of using awake, trained animals in studying experimental pulmonary embolism, most investigators still employ anesthetized animals.

In recent years, major attention has been directed to the role of platelets and vasoactive substances in the pathogenesis of pulmonary hypertension. Utilizing glass bead emboli in anesthetized dogs, Mlczoch et al.[66] demonstrated that pulmonary hypertension and hypoxia were significantly reduced by platelet depletion or inhibition, and suggested that platelet-inhibiting drugs might be useful in human pulmonary microembolism. Chesebro et al.[67] recently have reported shortened platelet survival in patients with cardiac failure and suggest that this abnormality may explain the predisposition to thromboembolism in such patients. Kohanna and Salzman,[68] however, have challenged the concept of platelet aggregate microemboli in thromboembolic disease based on two newer methods for measuring platelet aggregates in vivo.

Platelet release of thromboxane A_2 may play a role in pulmonary hypertension and lung edema. Exploring this hypothesis in an isolated rabbit lung model of the adult respiratory distress syndrome, Heffner et al.[69] produced pulmonary hypertension by perfusions of human platelets and acetyl glyceryl ether phosphorylcholine, a potent platelet activator. Their studies suggested that pulmonary hypertension resulted from thromboxane A_2 released from platelets. McDonald et al.[70] reported that thromboxane may be synthesized by sources other than platelets and postulated that leukocytes exposed to activated complement may damage vascular endothelial cells stimulating the synthesis of thromboxane A_2 which causes pulmonary vasoconstriction. These observations are particularly important since Weir et al.[71] demonstrated previously that circulating platelets are not necessary for hypoxic pulmonary vasoconstriction in the dog.

The role of prostaglandins in the pulmonary circulation is controversial and has attracted much attention in recent years. It appears that the prostaglandins are protective in the normal lung, where prostaglandin antagonists increase pulmonary vascular resistance and pressure.[72] Although some disagreement persists, prostaglandin inhibitors such as indomethacin have been shown to significantly attenuate the increase in pulmonary artery pressure in experimental microembolism in both dogs and sheep,[73] suggesting the synthesis of a pulmonary vasoconstrictor prostaglandin following microembolism.

Further studies are needed to resolve existing discrepancies and to extend the usefulness of experimental models of thromboembolic pulmonary hypertension. Nonetheless, sufficient data are available to warrant clinical studies of inhibitors of platelet function and of prostaglandin synthesis in patients highly predisposed to thromboembolic pulmonary hypertension.

The Natural History of Thromboembolic Pulmonary Hypertension

Little is known about the natural history of untreated thromboembolic pulmonary hypertension although it can be assumed that such patients share the high rate of fatal recurrent thromboembolism reported in Barritt and Jordan's control group with untreated pulmonary embolus.[8] Most natural history data are obtained from patients treated with anticoagulants, and the advent of thrombolytic therapy may alter these data considerably.[74]

The Heterogeneity of Thromboembolic Pulmonary Hypertension

When defined as the existence of a mean pulmonary artery pressure exceeding 20 mm Hg, thromboembolic pulmonary hypertension is, in fact, several entities whose clinical presentation, pathophysiology, and prognosis differ, but that share the common features of systemic venous thrombosis and embolization of thrombotic material to the pulmonary arteries. Unfortunately, quantitative descriptors such as massive, submassive, multiple, and micro have gained widespread usage in depicting clinical presentations of pulmonary embolism. These descriptors, although convenient, are unreliable in predicting the extent of embolic pulmonary vascular occlusion or the degree of pulmonary hypertension since the consequences of thromboembolism are a complex function of the several variables discussed previously.

The Clinical and Hemodynamic Course of Thromboembolic Pulmonary Hypertension

Massive pulmonary embolism usually implies the catastrophic condition resulting from sudden embolic occlusion of the main pulmonary artery or one or both of its primary branches. Fortunately, this occurs in a small percentage of large vessel emboli (Table 3). Pulmonary vascular resistance rises abruptly, acute thromboembolic pulmonary hypertension occurs, right ventricular output falls as filling pressures rise, tachypnea, systemic hypotension and cyanosis ensue, and death usually results from ventricular arrhythmias. In the absence of preexisting right ventricular hypertrophy, even massive pulmonary embolic obstruction rarely produces severe pulmonary hypertension since the normal right ventricle dilates and fails at systolic pressures above 50 to 60 mm Hg and pulmonary artery mean pressures above 35 to 40 mm Hg. Death in such patients often occurs within 1 to 2 hours,[75] even before therapy is initiated (Figure 7).

More frequently, patients with an initially massive clinical presentation demonstrate rapid improvement with persistent mild to moderate systemic hypotension and a subsequent course similar to that of submassive thromboembolism in which lobar or segmental pulmonary arteries are usually involved. The time course of the rise and return toward normal of pulmonary artery pressures in massive pulmonary embolism can be relatively short, over 30 minutes to a few hours,[9,76] and is attributed to lysis of emboli, distal migration with enlargement of the pulmonary vascular cross-sectional area, revascularization of the lung by blood forced past the embolus, and opening of new vessels in unoccluded areas of the lung.[9] In their long-term follow-up of patients with acute massive pulmonary embolism, Riedel et al.[29] observed pulmonary artery mean pressures of greater than 30 mm Hg acutely and a return to normal values in most patients when reexamined approximately 2 months and 4 years later. Thus, in the majority of cases, acute severe thromboembolic pulmonary hypertension is relatively transient and reversible. Usually, pulmonary vascular resistance, flows, and arterial pressures return to normal within 2 to 8 weeks as long as recurrent thromboembolism is prevented.

As stated earlier, the term massive does not necessarily imply occlusion of proximal pulmonary arteries or profound hemodynamic derangement. As defined in the Thrombolytic Trials, massive pulmonary embolus indicated obstruction or filling defects involving 2 or more lobar pulmonary arteries or an equivalent amount of emboli in other vessels.[18] Sixty percent of patients entering the Trials had massive embolization (Table 5), but only 12% of the massive subgroup had clinical evidence of circulatory collapse (Table 7). The mean pulmonary artery pressure in patients with shock was 37 mm Hg compared to 26 mm Hg in patients without shock, and pressures fell insignificantly during 24 hours of heparin therapy.[77] This relatively low incidence of systemic hypotension in massive pulmonary embolism is due to the liberal definition of angiographic massivity in the Urokinase Pulmonary Embolism Trial, and underscores the importance of clearly defining the meaning of "massive" when describing the pathophysiology and natural history of thromboembolic pulmonary hypertension.

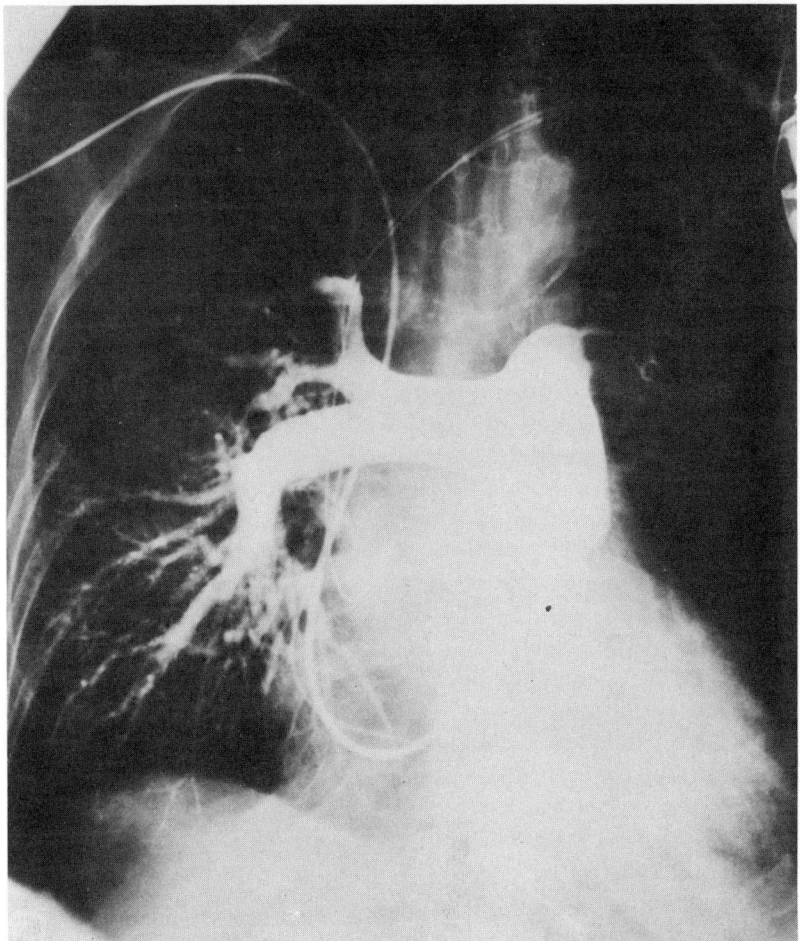

Figure 7. Main pulmonary artery opacification in a 66-year-old female patient from the author's series with a history of refractory ventricular arrhythmias and serial electrophysiological studies via the femoral veins 3 months prior to admission for chest pain, sudden dyspnea and mild hypotension 2 days prior to angiography. Total obstruction of the left intermediate pulmonary artery is present with lobar and segmental artery involvement of the right lung. PA mean pressure was 32 mm Hg and RA mean pressure was 5 mm Hg. Patient died with recurrent ventricular tachycardia 4 hours after thrombolytic therapy was begun. (Courtesy of M.D. Bogdonoff, M.D., Department of Diagnostic Radiology, Rush-Presbyterian-St. Luke's Medical Center.)

Submassive pulmonary embolism usually produces modest degrees of thromboembolic pulmonary hypertension initially, with an average mean pulmonary artery pressure of only 23 mm Hg observed in the Urokinase Pulmonary Embolism Trial (Table 6). Somewhat paradoxi-

TABLE 7
Relationship of Shock to Massivity in Pulmonary Embolism*

Clinical Shock	Angiographic Involvement		Totals
	Submassive n (%)	Massive n (%)	n (%)
Absent	127 (98)	174 (88)	301 (92)
Present	3 (2)	23 (12)	26 (8)
Totals	130	197	327

*From data in references 18 (Table V.2) and 19 (Table 1).

cally, pulmonary hypertension resolves more gradually in this subgroup, probably because multiple smaller emboli are less susceptible to endogenous lysis. As in all forms of thromboembolic pulmonary hypertension, the clinical and hemodynamic course of submassive pulmonary embolism is strongly influenced by the presence or absence of preexisting cardiopulmonary disease [20] which may result in long-lasting pulmonary hypertension and circulatory embarrassment despite modest embolic involvement.

The symptomatology in the submassive subgroup also is strongly influenced by the presence or absence of associated pulmonary infarction which occurs in about 10% of pulmonary embolism patients,[13,78] and is more common in submassive than massive embolism. Other than influencing clinical presentation and creating potential confusion in diagnosis, the development of pulmonary infarction is of little importance to the severity or resolution of thromboembolic pulmonary hypertension.

Little information is available concerning the hemodynamic course of thromboembolic pulmonary hypertension in submassive pulmonary embolism beyond 24 hours, but pressures usually return to normal in 2 to 4 weeks. Riedel et al.[29] suggest that most patients with isolated subacute or recurrent submassive pulmonary embolism have normal or borderline pulmonary artery pressures when first reexamined at least 2 months following their most recent clinical episode, although a smaller percentage had significant persistent pulmonary hypertension and showed further progression when studied from 4 to 6 years later. No factors were identified that allowed early prediction of those patients likely to develop persistent thromboembolic pulmonary hypertension in these subgroups. It seems most probable, however, that the total sum of thromboembolic recurrences before and after diagnosis primarily influences the hemodynamic course of submassive pulmonary embolism.

The hemodynamic course of chronic, recurrent thromboembolic pulmonary hypertension is poorly defined since the disease is rarely appreciated in its initial stages. Following repeated embolic episodes, pulmonary vascular resistance rises progressively, pulmonary arterial pressure may achieve near systemic levels, and chronic right heart failure develops. The central pulmonary arteries become dilated and there is marked attenuation of the peripheral branches, clearly evident on chest x-ray, but not distinguishable from other forms of chronic pulmonary hypertension. Riedel et al.[29] observed a mean pulmonary artery pressure of 55 mm Hg on initial measurement in 13 patients with chronic thromboembolic pulmonary hypertension and modest progression on reexamination of 7 patients an average of 3 years later. Over two-thirds of these patients were dead within 3 years of initial study and one-third had fresh emboli at autopsy. Steele et al.[36] reported similar outcomes in their autopsy series of 32 patients with idiopathic pulmonary hypertension due to thromboembolism. The median intervals from onset of symptoms and diagnosis to death were 6 and 2 years, respectively. Since these patients frequently are untreated, recurrent acute pulmonary embolism is a very common cause of death.

The Course of Pulmonary Vascular Obstruction in Thromboembolic Pulmonary Hypertension

The pathological changes that occur following thromboembolism have been discussed above. The lungs have extraordinary ability to dispose of thromboemboli and removal occurs primarily by fibrinolysis (Figure 8). Sautter et al.[79] observed angiographic resolution of a massive pulmonary embolus in 24 hours. However, most serial studies suggest that the rate of resolution of emboli during heparin treatment is minimal in the first 3 to 6 days following embolization and moderate or complete within 7 to 21 days.[80,81] Results from the Urokinase Pulmonary Embolism Trial showed only slight improvement in angiographic severity after 20 hours of heparin therapy,[18] the longest interval assessed angiographically in these studies. Older emboli appear to lyse more slowly, and removal is influenced by coexisting disease and the severity of the embolic process.[46]

Serial lung scan assessment of thromboembolic pulmonary vascular obstruction indicates that approximately 50% of the ultimate improvement in perfusion is achieved within 1 week following initiation of

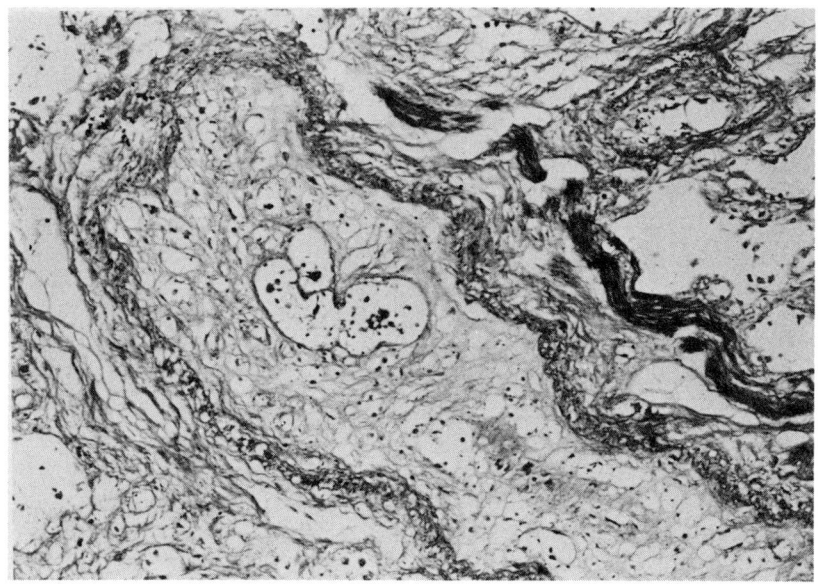

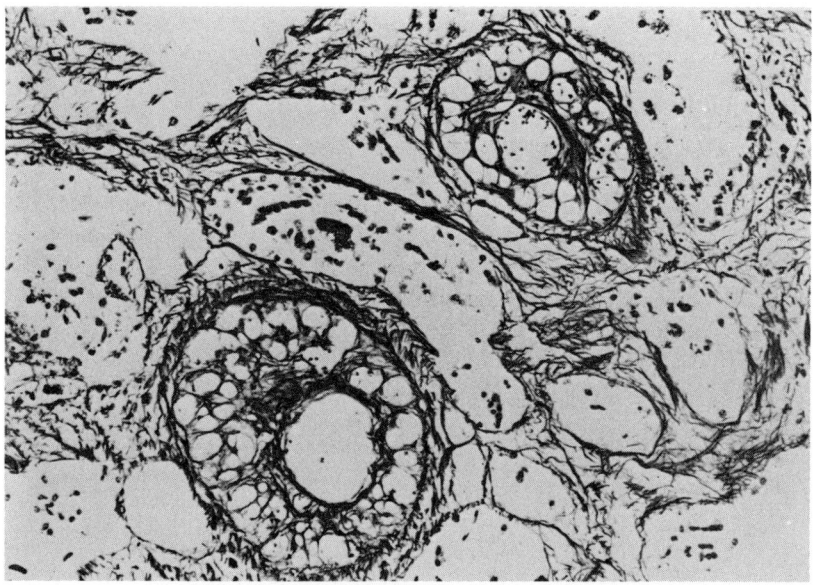

Figure 8, a and b. Various stages of organization and resolution of recanalizing thromboemboli. (Courtesy of J. Coon, M.D., Ph.D., Department of Pathology, Rush-Presbyterian-St. Luke's Medical Center.)

heparin therapy, and maximum improvement occurs by 3 months[18] (Figure 9). Although baseline postembolic values were not measured, Sharma et al.[54] demonstrated that pulmonary capillary perfusion was significantly impaired in heparin treated patients at 2 weeks and remained unchanged at 1 year.

The Prognosis of Thromboembolic Pulmonary Hypertension

Death from thromboembolic pulmonary hypertension is uncommon with proper therapy. Mortality occurs primarily in patients with

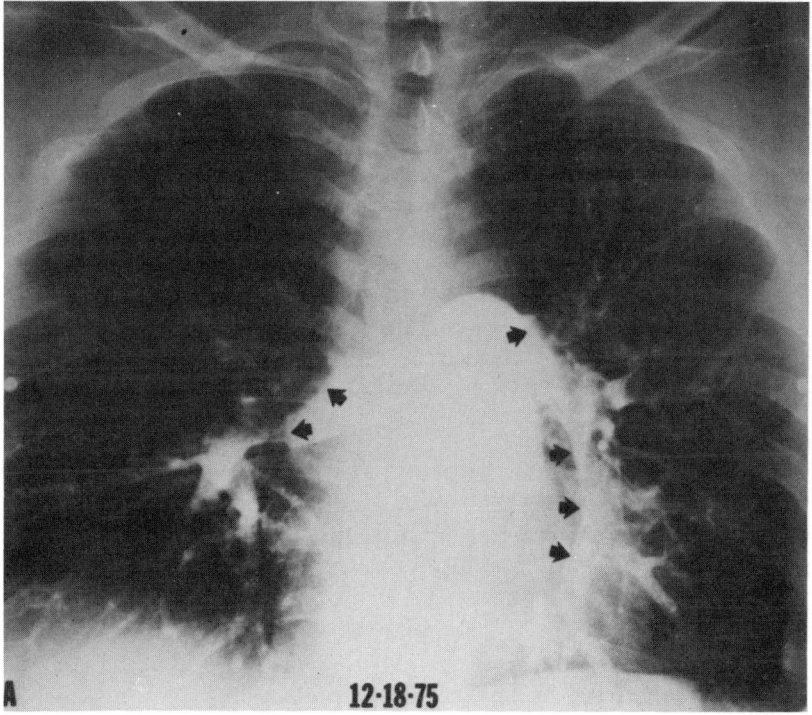

Figure 9 a. 48-year-old male with history of foot trauma admitted for right ileofemoral thrombophlebitis. Initial pulmonary angiogram obtained after circulatory collapse occurred following 1 week of heparin therapy for phlebitis. Treatment consisted of vasopressors, respirator therapy, and intraluminal inferior caval interruption. (Reproduced with permission from Internat Angiology 182;1:149–153, Figure 4.)

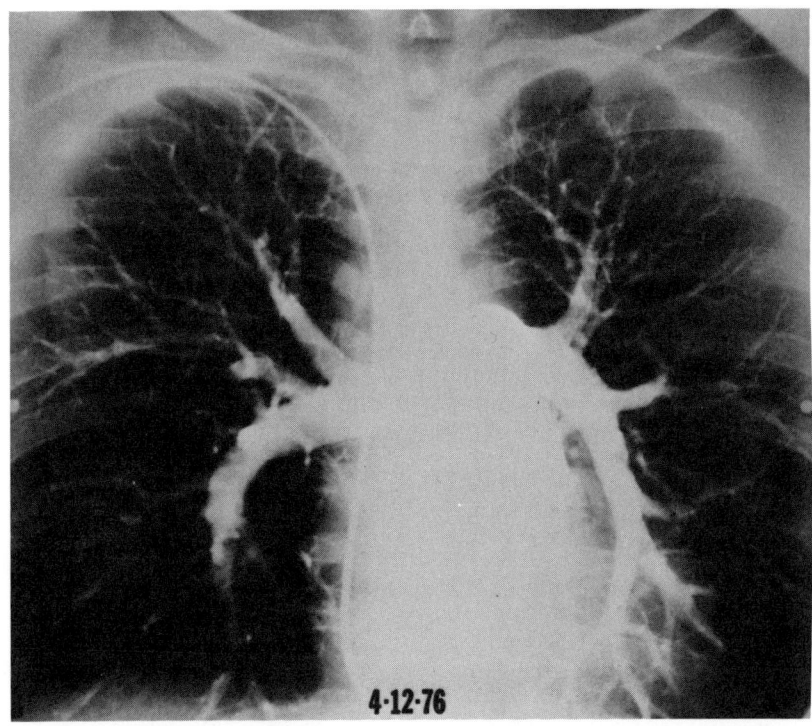

Figure 9 b. Same patient following 4 months of warfarin therapy and complete resolution of thrombophlebitis. The angiogram is markedly improved. (Reproduced with permission from Internat Angiology *1982;1:149–153, Figure 4.)*

massive acute embolization before therapy can be initiated or in chronic unrecognized thromboembolic pulmonary hypertension. When recurrent thromboembolism is prevented, fatality from thromboembolic pulmonary hypertension usually results from exacerbation of preexisting cardiopulmonary disease or as a consequence of complications of therapy. In the Urokinase Pulmonary Embolism Trial, approximately 60% of patients had thromboembolic pulmonary hypertension on entry, 35% had preexisting cardiopulmonary disease, and 6% had malignant neoplasms. There was an overall mortality rate of 8% within 2 weeks following initiation of therapy. At one year 80% of the patients were known to be alive, 7% were lost to follow-up, and 13% had died.[18]

THE DIAGNOSIS OF THROMBOEMBOLIC PULMONARY HYPERTENSION

Differential Diagnosis

Accurate diagnosis represents one of the major continuing challenges of thromboembolic pulmonary hypertension. It is well documented that many of the pathophysiologic consequences of pulmonary embolism are nonspecific derangements of circulatory and respiratory function that can be caused by many cardiac and pulmonary conditions. When encountered in its classical form in a predisposed patient, acute pulmonary hypertension due to massive pulmonary thromboembolism is rarely a diagnostic problem. In such cases, attention should be directed to the exclusion of other conditions mimicking massive thromboembolism and to urgent therapy. In terms of the numbers of patients at risk, the greatest diagnostic challenge is posed by transient, mild, or moderate pulmonary hypertension caused by submassive thromboembolism. It is this subgroup that forms a large reservoir of misdiagnosed and undiagnosed patients in whom multiple episodes of pulmonary embolism occur, ultimately resulting in sudden death or chronic thromboembolic pulmonary hypertension. It is also the subgroup for whom excellent diagnostic tools exist and therapy is highly effective once the condition is suspected. Silent thromboembolism leading to irreversible pulmonary hypertension is a rare, but frustrating, diagnostic problem in which the etiology is usually not apparent to even the most skilled clinician. Efforts are directed toward the differential diagnosis of pulmonary hypertension rather than of acute or subacute cardiorespiratory symptoms, treatment has limited value, and the available diagnostic tools are either inaccurate or pose considerable risk to the patient.

Table 8 contains a listing of types of embolic materials and other disease states that should be considered in the differential diagnosis of thromboembolic pulmonary hypertension. Equally important is the clinician's inclusion of *thromboembolism* in the differential diagnosis of each of the conditions listed. The advent of thrombolytic therapy for major pulmonary embolism, the significant risks of caval interruption and pulmonary embolectomy, and the dangers of erroneously omit-

TABLE 8
Differential Diagnosis of Thromboembolic Pulmonary Hypertension

Massive Thromboembolism
Acute myocardial infarction
Aortic dissection
Pericardial tamponade
Pneumothorax

Submassive Thromboembolism
Pneumonia
Atelectasis
Neoplasm
Chronic obstructive pulmonary disease
Pleurisy

Chronic Recurrent Thromboembolism
Primary pulmonary hypertension
Pulmonary veno-occlusive disease
Cardiac disease, especially mitral stenosis and congenital heart disease
Sickle-cell disease
Collagen-vascular disease

Type of Emboli
Fat and marrow
Tumor, including right atrial myxoma
Trophoblastic tissue
Amniotic fluid
Air
Foreign bodies
Parasites

ting treatment accentuate the importance of accurate diagnosis in managing patients suspected of having thromboembolic disease.

The diagnostic procedures most frequently employed in suspected thromboembolic pulmonary hypertension include history, physical examination, chest x-ray, electrocardiogram, arterial blood gases, lung scanning, and pulmonary angiography. An extensive literature is available describing the sensitivity, specificity, and risks of these diagnostic aids.[2,6,18,19,23,37,52,82] They will be discussed here primarily in terms of their diagnostic accuracy and value in patient management.

History and Physical Examination

Except when assessing a patient with obvious acute severe thromboembolic pulmonary hypertension, the clinician's index of suspicion for thromboembolism is generally too low. Unfortunately, neither history nor physical examination has particular sensitivity or specificity for moderate acute or chronic thromboembolic pulmonary hypertension. Clinically apparent thrombophlebitis, which occurs only in one-third of patients, and the signs and symptoms of pulmonary infarction, which occurs only in 10−20% of patients, too often are sought before the diagnosis of pulmonary embolism is actively pursued. As observed in the Cooperative Thrombolytic Trials, dyspnea is the most common symptom of pulmonary embolism, followed by pleuritic pain and apprehension. Rales, cough, and a loud pulmonary second sound are noted in about one-half of patients, whereas tachycardia, gallop, rhythm, fever, hemoptysis, pleural friction rub, and phlebitis are more frequently absent than present in patients with documented pulmonary embolism. When present, pleural pain and hemoptysis suggest less severe pulmonary vascular obstruction, while a loud pulmonary second sound, right ventricular S_3 gallop, cyanosis, and syncope suggest massive embolism. Because the classic clinical findings of pulmonary embolism are frequently absent or may reflect nonembolic cardiac and pulmonary disease, history and physical examination have minimal diagnostic accuracy. Their greatest value relates to predisposing factors and early detection of deep venous thrombosis, especially when noninvasive screening methods for this condition are employed in predisposed patients. In the rare individual with chronic, silent thromboembolic pulmonary hypertension, history and physical examination primarily are useful in establishing the diagnosis of pulmonary hypertension, per se, and only rarely suggest a history of recurrent pulmonary embolism.

Electrocardiography and Chest X-ray

Abnormalities of the electrocardiogram and chest x-ray are of little value in diagnosing pulmonary embolism because they also are highly nonspecific. The classical electrocardiographic findings of acute right heart strain are observed in only a minority of patients with thromboembolic pulmonary hypertension, although the chronic changes of right ventricular hypertrophy often are the clinician's first clue to the presence of chronic pulmonary hypertension. The electrocardiogram, although abnormal in nearly 90% of patients with pulmonary embolism, is highly nonspecific. T-wave inversion is the most common abnormality and is seen in 40% of patients. The primary value of the electrocardiogram is in the differential diagnosis of acute myocardial infarction whose clinical presentation is often easily confused with that of massive thromboembolic pulmonary hypertension.

Consolidation and elevation of the ipsilateral hemidiaphragm, seen in about 40% of patients, are the most common radiographic findings of pulmonary embolism. Although these changes are not specific for pulmonary embolic disease, they are most important factors in limiting the value of lung scanning. The electrocardiogram and chest x-ray usually have very little diagnostic accuracy for pulmonary embolism, but are essential components of patient evaluation in order to define the value of subsequent lung scanning and to detect the presence of possible myocardial involvement.

Arterial Blood Gases

Arterial blood gases are the most used diagnostic aids employed in the evaluation of suspected pulmonary embolism. Although originally introduced as a screening test that, when normal, tended to exclude the diagnosis, arterial blood gas measurements commonly are used to support the diagnosis when abnormal. Unfortunately, neither conclusion is reliably accurate. Approximately 12% of patients with pulmonary embolism will have arterial oxygen tensions above 80 mm Hg, resulting in a sensitivity of approximately 88% for arterial hypoxemia in the detection of pulmonary embolism. Since hypoxemia is very common in many forms of cardiopulmonary disease, it has little specificity for pulmonary embolism. In fact, McNeil and associates[22] found that arterial blood gases were not useful in identifying young patients with pulmonary embolism or in distinguishing such patients from those with other diseases. In 97 young patients with pleural pain, the mean arterial oxygen tension was *higher* in those who had pulmonary embolism than in those who did not. On the other hand, the finding of a significant reduction in arterial oxygen tension compared to recently normal values should be considered important supporting evidence in the diagnostic evaluation of patients suspect for thromboembolism. The potential hazards of arterial entry in patients about to be anticoagulated, especially when punctured in the commonly used femoral arterial location, must be considered before requesting this relatively inaccurate screening test.

Lung Scanning

Pulmonary scintigraphy is the most valuable screening tool available for the diagnosis of pulmonary thromboembolism. The degree of controversy surrounding the diagnostic accuracy of lung scanning is attested to by the recent decision of the National Institutes of Health to fund a major cooperative trial assessing the sensitivity and specificity of this technique in the diagnosis of pulmonary embolism. Initial optimism concerning the diagnostic value of perfusion lung scanning was tempered by the experience gained in the Thrombolytic Trials[5,18,19] and, more recently, by the correlative studies of McNeil and associates[6,22] and Hull and associates.[23] Lung scanning has its greatest value when completely normal in the presence of a normal chest x-ray. Under these circumstances, pulmonary thromboembolism is essentially excluded, only rare instances having been reported of pulmonary embolism with negative lung scans. The sensitivity of lung scanning is extremely high, virtually all patients with pulmonary embolism being detected by this screening technique. Unfortunately, however, an abnormal perfusion scan does not necessarily reflect pulmonary thromboembolism. Any preexisting lung disease may cause perfusion defects and even when these defects are matched by x-ray abnormalities, the so called indeterminate scan, 25% of such patients may have pulmonary embolism.[6] In fact, as noted above, approximately 40% of patients with pulmonary emboli had consolidation on chest x-ray in the Thrombolytic Trials.[18]

When lung scans are interpreted critically according to anatomic subdivisions and the number and bilateral distribution of defects, diagnostic accuracy is improved. A previously published analysis[83] of the sensitivity, specificity, and diagnostic accuracy of various lung scanning criteria is presented in Table 9. Forty percent of these patients having perfusion scans and 60% of the patients having ventilation-perfusion scans had thromboembolism, an unusually high incidence of disease in unselected populations and a factor that improves the diagnostic accuracy of any screening test. Given a patient population whose incidence of thromboembolic disease is similarly high, ventilation-perfusion mismatched defects of multiple segmental or greater extent appear to have a 91–95% true positivity for thromboembolism (Table 9, Criteria A-C) (Figure 10). When positivity is limited to these highly specific criteria, however, the sensitivity of lung scan-

TABLE 9

Sensitivity, Specificity and Diagnostic Accuracy of Lung Scanning*

Lung Scan Abnormality	Sensitivity	Specificity	Positivity True	Positivity False	Negativity True	Negativity False	Error
Ventilation-Perfusion Mismatch Defects:							
A. Multiple Lobe or Lung	56	95	95	5	59	41	28
B. Multiple Lobe, Lung or Segmental	88	90	93	7	83	17	11
C. Multiple Segmental	31	95	91	9	48	52	43
Perfusion Defect(s):							
D. Multiple Lobe or Lung	52	92	81	19	74	26	24
E. Multiple Lobe, Lung or Segmental	86	70	66	34	88	12	24
F. Multiple Segmental	33	78	50	50	64	36	40
G. Any Abnormality	100	2	40	60	100	0	59
H. Single Lobe, Lung or Segmental	7	89	30	70	59	41	44
Combination of Criteria:							
I. Criteria B. and D.	76	92	86	14	85	15	14
J. Criteria B. and E.	86	79	73	27	89	11	18

*From data in references 6 and 84. All values are percentages. Incidence of pulmonary embolism in patient population: 60% for ventilation-perfusion scans; 40% for perfusion scans and combination criteria (see text). (Reproduced with permission from Reference 83.)

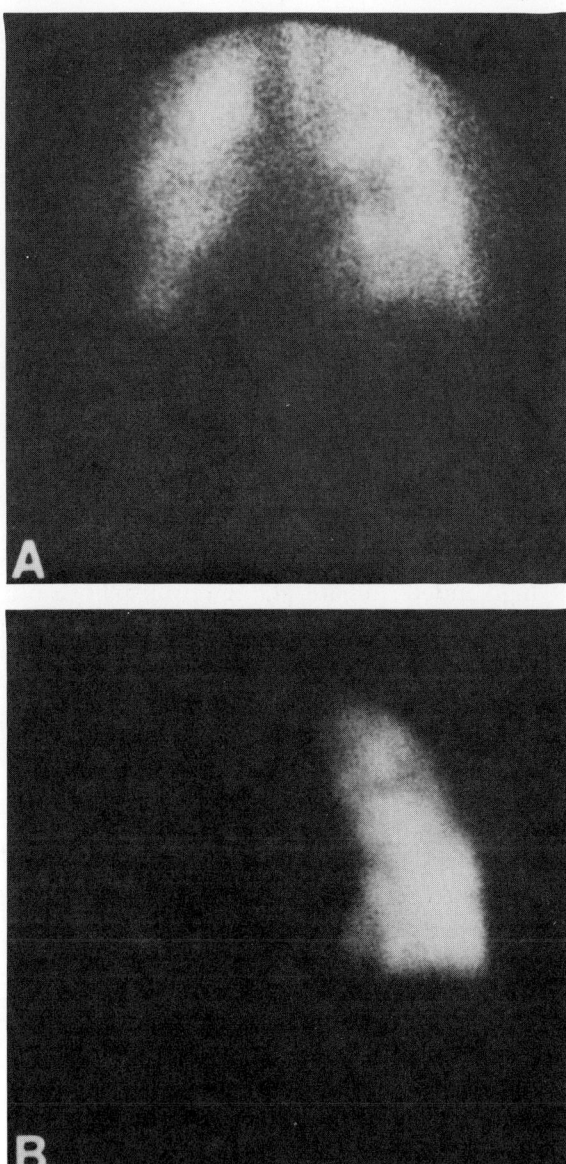

Figure 10. Lung scans from patient illustrated in Figure 7. (A) Posterior ventilation study demonstrates abnormalities in the lower lungs bilaterally. (B) Absent perfusion of left lung with small segmental and subsegmental defects in the right lung. (Courtesy of David L. Turner, M.D., Department of Diagnostic Radiology, Section of Nuclear Medicine, Rush-Presbyterian-St. Luke's Medical Center.)

ning decreases significantly. Although unnecessary treatment due to false positivity is reduced to 5–10%, false *negativity* occurs at a rate of 17–52%, inviting the withholding of therapy unless angiographic validation is sought.

The study of Hull et al.[23] produced very similar estimates of the accuracy of segmental ventilation-perfusion mismatched defects in diagnosing thromboembolism. In addition, their study offers valuable new information concerning the predictive accuracy of lung scanning for "venous thromboembolism," the presence of thrombosis in either the pulmonary arteries or deep leg veins, or both. Ninety-one percent of patients with segmental or greater ventilation-perfusion mismatched defects and adequate pulmonary angiograms had thromboembolism in the pulmonary arteries or deep leg veins. This diagnostic concept, including both the pulmonary arteries and deep leg veins, is particularly relevant to thromboembolic pulmonary hypertension in which recurrent embolism from deep venous thrombosis has such etiologic and therapeutic importance.

It is common practice for lung-scanning experts to interpret scans according to high, indeterminate, and low probability for thromboembolism. In the Urokinase Pulmonary Embolism Trial, significant interinterpreter disagreement occurred on the probability of thromboembolism. Sixteen percent of patients with high-probability *perfusion* scans had normal pulmonary angiograms, and 17 of 18 patients with low-probability scans had massive or submassive emboli by angiography.[5] The caution suggested by these findings has now been extended to ventilation perfusion scanning by Hull et al., who recommend that therapeutic decisions be made on the basis of lung scanning, only in patients with segmental or larger perfusion defects that ventilate normally, a finding in only 25% of their patient population. Pulmonary angiography and venography are required in the remaining patients with perfusion lung scan abnormalities to confirm or exclude the presence of thromboembolism[23] (Figures 11 and 12).

The diagnostic accuracy of lung scanning decreases as the anatomic size of the perfusion defect decreases (Table 9, Criterion G). This is especially pertinent to the use of lung scanning to detect thromboembolism in chronic, obliterative pulmonary hypertension. In patients with the clinical diagnosis of chronic idiopathic pulmonary hypertension studied by Wilson et al.,[37] perfusion lung scanning proved useful in identifying thromboembolism when defects were large, multiple, and asymmetrical. In those patients in whom angiography excluded embolism, lung scans were normal. In approximately one-third of cases, however, scans were diffusely abnormal with small, multiple

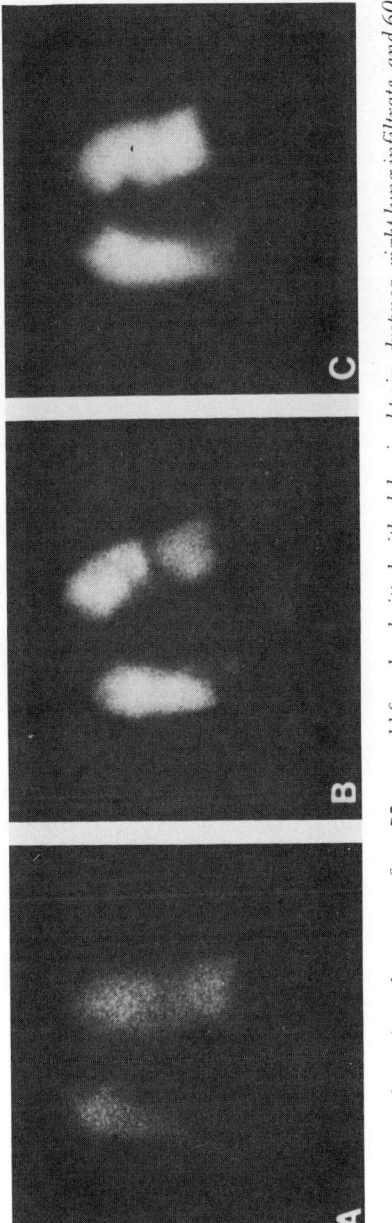

Figure 11. Indeterminate lung scans from 53-year-old female admitted with abdominal pain, dyspnea, right lung infiltrate, and 60 pound weight loss on steroids for severe rheumatoid arthritis. Hypotension, new infiltrates, left lower lobe consolidation, and dyspnea developed prior to lung scan. (A) Posterior ventilation study reveals normal right lung and large defect in left lower lung. (B) Posterior perfusion study reveals multiple segmental defects in both lungs. (C) Posterior perfusion study performed 4 months later reveals nearly completely normal perfusion. (Courtesy of David L. Turner, M.D., Department of Diagnostic Radiology, Section of Nuclear Medicine, Rush-Presbyterian-St. Luke's Medical Center.)

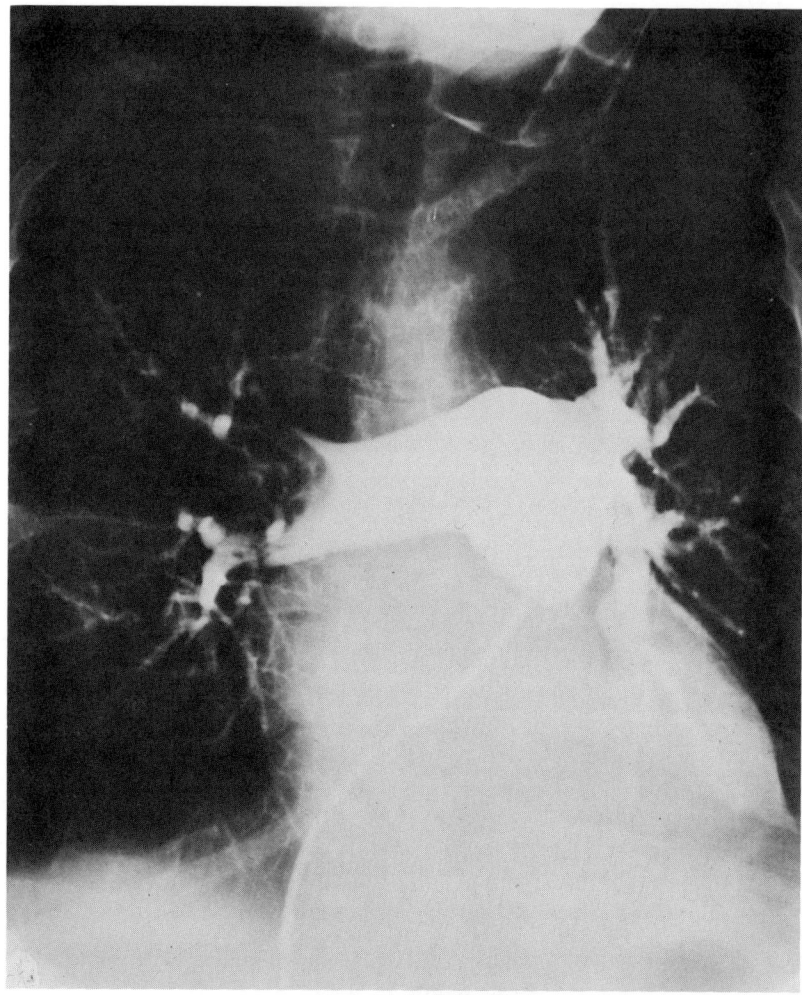

Figure 12. Pulmonary angiogram from patient illustrated in Figure 11, demonstrating a massive thromboembolism in the right pulmonary artery with extension to the right upper lobe. Multiple filling defects appear in the right lower lobe with probable involvement of the left lower lobe. An inferior vena caval study was normal. (Courtesy of M. D. Bogdonoff, M.D., Department of Diagnostic Radiology, Rush-Presbyterian-St. Luke's Medical Center.)

ill-defined defects. Angiography revealed minor nonspecific abnormalities consistent with small vessel occlusion, and thromboembolism was neither confirmed nor excluded. Thus, lung scanning appears useful in approximately two-thirds of patients with unexplained chronic obliterative pulmonary hypertension, but is uninformative for the remaining one-third for whom more definitive diagnostic methods are required.

Is lung scanning accurate in detecting recurrent thromboembolism? From several viewpoints, the precise delineation of embolic recurrence has importance equal to accurate diagnosis of the initial episode. Recurrence is virtually essential to the pathogenesis of thromboembolic pulmonary hypertension and therefore its detection has both diagnostic and therapeutic implications. Furthermore, embolic recurrence is usually accepted as conclusive evidence of failure of medical therapy and an indication for surgical intervention, whose mortality and morbidity far exceed those of anticoagulation.

The reported incidence of recurrent thromboembolism varies considerably. Twenty-three percent of the heparin treated patients in the Thrombolytic Trials were diagnosed as having recurrent embolization with 2 weeks of treatment, and 40% of these had inferior vena caval ligation. The signs and symptoms of recurrence may also be caused by the delayed effects of an earlier embolus, its thrombotic extension, or fragmentation and distal migration of the original embolus.[3,84,85] Lung scanning is of little value in distinguishing these mechanisms from true embolic recurrence and may falsely suggest recurrence when varying rates of embolic resolution produce changes in the regional distribution of pulmonary vascular resistance.[86] In the Thrombolytic Trials, 15% of the patients demonstrated post-treatment *worsening* of lung scans despite *reduction* of angiographic severity. The tendency of emboli to fragment and migrate distally was as common in patients receiving heparin as in those given urokinase (Figure 13).

In summary, lung scanning is a safe, relatively inexpensive, and valuable technique for screening patients suspect for acute and chronic thromboembolic pulmonary hypertension. When rigid interpretation criteria are applied, the diagnostic accuracy of positive tests is enhanced, but sensitivity decreases significantly. Lung scanning is of limited value in documenting true recurrence, especially during the process of resolution of a recent thromboembolism. Further studies are needed to determine whether the diagnostic accuracy of lung scanning can be improved by inhalation "hot spot" imaging with cyclotron produced $^{15}O_2$-labeled carbon dioxide,[87] or conventionally available radioiodinated methyl iodide gas.[88]

Pulmonary Angiography

When performed within 72 hours of the suspected embolic episode, pulmonary angiography has extremely high sensitivity, specificity, and

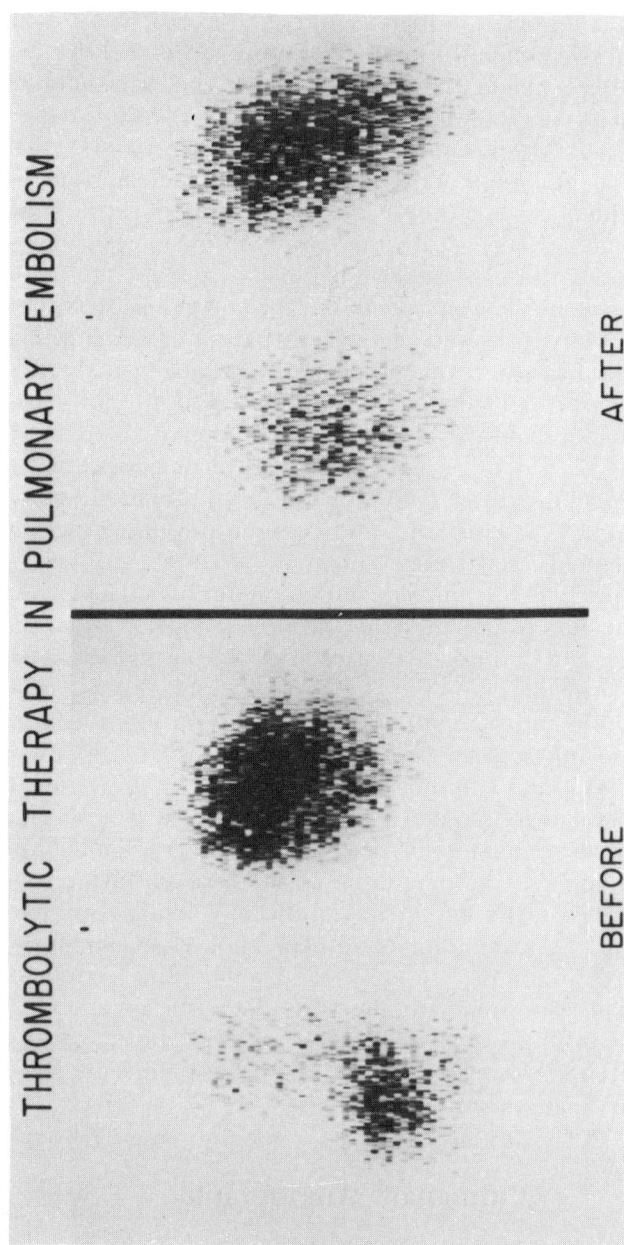

Figure 13. Anterior perfusion lung scans before and after thrombolytic therapy was begun suggesting recurrent embolization in association with a new clinical episode. (Reproduced with permission from Reference 83.)

predictive accuracy, and is the only definitive method available for diagnosing thromboembolic pulmonary hypertension. Limited autopsy correlations in close proximity to angiography are available, but the data indicate a high degree of diagnostic accuracy.[5,82,89] Patients with negative pulmonary angiograms have a very low risk of subsequent pulmonary embolism.[90]

The indications for pulmonary angiography differ somewhat in acute massive, moderate submassive, and chronic thromboembolic pulmonary hypertension. The angiographic signs of thromboembolism are quite uniform, however, and can be classified according to their respective diagnostic specificities. Filling defects and vessel cutoffs are the only findings generally considered reliable evidence of emboli. Less specific signs such as vessel pruning, oligemia, asymmetrical filling, and prolongation of arterial opacification are supportive of the diagnosis, but also are observed with chronic pulmonary and cardiac diseases, for which both pulmonary angiography and lung scanning are less accurate. In chronic recurrent thromboembolic pulmonary hypertension, pulmonary angiography shows smooth convex bordered occlusions, stenoses, intravascular webs or strands, and bronchial arteriography has been recommended in studying these patients.[91] In patients suspects of having acute massive thromboembolic pulmonary hypertension, pulmonary angiography is indicated to determine the degree and type of vascular obstruction before embarking on aggressive management such as thrombolytic therapy, inferior vena caval ligation, or pulmonary thromboembolectomy. In submassive moderate thromboembolic pulmonary hypertension, pulmonary angiography is primarily indicated as a definitive diagnostic tool rather than as a guide to the selection of therapeutic alternatives. In a minority of patients with chronic idiopathic pulmonary hypertension, pulmonary angiography may be the only diagnostic procedure available during life to establish an embolic etiology. Given the importance of pulmonary angiography in the diagnosis of thromboembolic pulmonary hypertension, it is fortunate that equivocal angiograms are obtained in only 15–20% of patients and are usually correctly interpreted by experienced angiographers. In the Thrombolytic Trials, for example, the angiographic panel disagreed with the angiographer performing the study in less than 4% of cases. Interpanel disagreement was less than 6%, compared with 67% disagreement among interpreters of lung scanning data.

Subselective angiograms with oblique views greatly enhance angiographic specificity (Figure 14). Magnification and subtraction angiography have similar value but are time consuming, expensive, and often

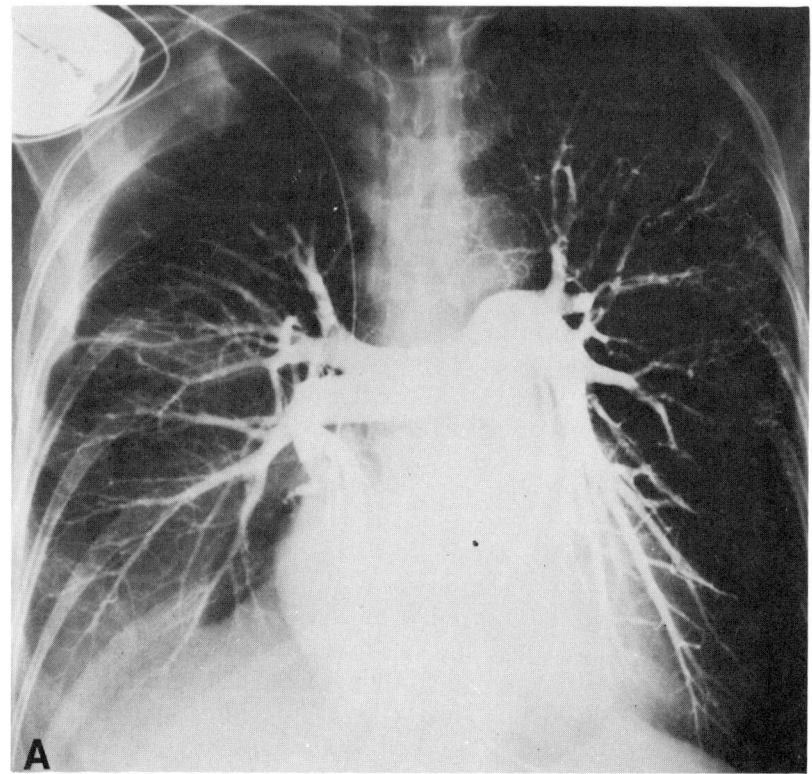

Figure 14 a. Main pulmonary artery opacification showing possible involvement of the segmental arteries of the right lower lobe. *(Courtesy of M.D. Bogdonoff, M.D., Department of Diagnostic Radiology, Rush-Presbyterian-St. Luke's Medical Center.)*

lack reproducibility. Wilson and Bynum have made an important contribution to the technique of pulmonary angiography in the form of a balloon-tipped catheter permitting subselective stop-flow filming with minute volumes of contrast material[92] (Figure 15). This technique has greatly reduced angiographic inaccuracy while increasing patient safety, especially in the presence of severe thromboembolic pulmonary hypertension where larger volumes of contrast material are especially hazardous. The use of this technique usually clarifies the question of "small vessel" emboli (Figure 16), but where such methods fail, management is best guided by the presence or absence of deep venous thrombosis in the pelvis or lower extremities as determined by venography or appropriate non-invasive techniques. When recurrent thromboembolism is suspected, comparison of post-recurrence and

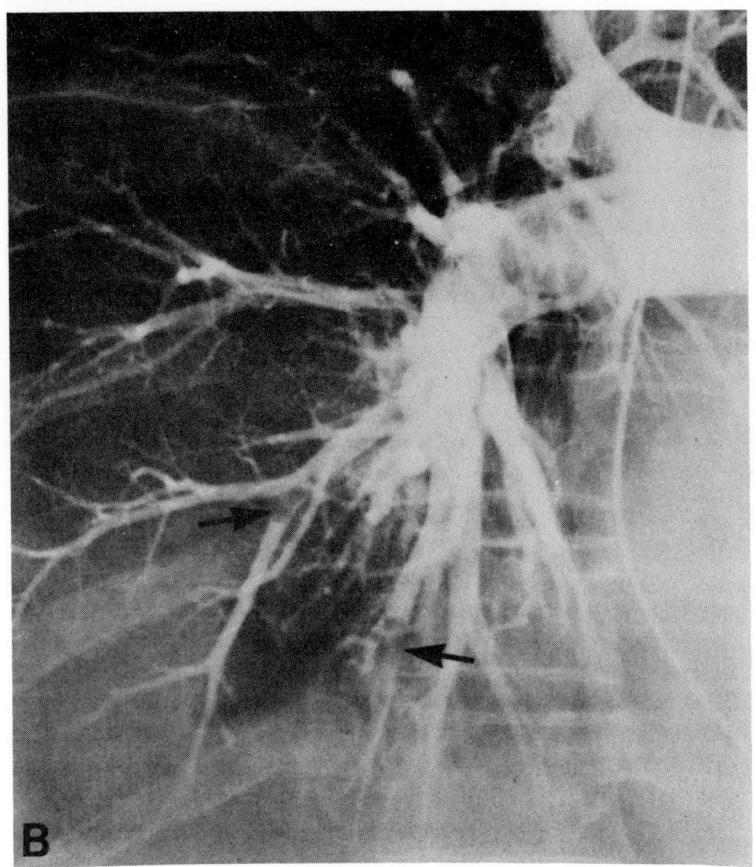

Figure 14 b. Selective right pulmonary artery opacification with patient in moderate right anterior obliquity. Multiple filling defects are demonstrated in the right lower lobe vessels. (Courtesy of M.D. Bogdonoff, M.D., Department of Diagnostic Radiology, Rush-Presbyterian-St. Luke's Medical Center.)

baseline angiograms is the only method allowing reliable distinction between true and spurious recurrent embolization.[3,17,85,86] The therapeutic implications of this distinction are most important.

Pulmonary angiography can be performed percutaneously from the femoral vein or preferably, by venous cutdown or percutaneous entry from the arm. Concurrent heparinization for suspected pulmonary embolus is not a contraindication to carefully performed angiography. The arm approach allows better control of bleeding in anticoagulated patients, somewhat greater ease in performing multiple subselective

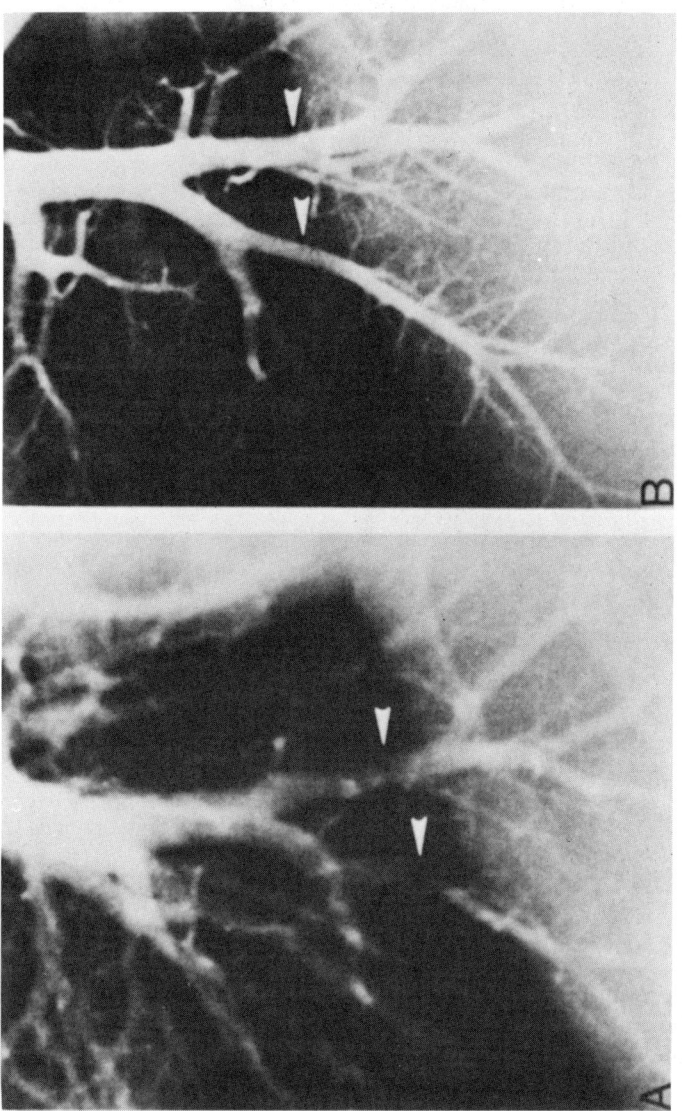

Figure 15. Probably abnormal angiogram found to be normal on balloon-occlusion study. (A) Selective right lower lobe injection by standard techniques, showing 2 probable filling defects (arrows). (B) Balloon-occlusion angiogram with no abnormalities, demonstrating that "filling defects" were artifacts caused by crossing of small vessels (arrows). (Reproduced with permission from Reference 92, Figure 4.)

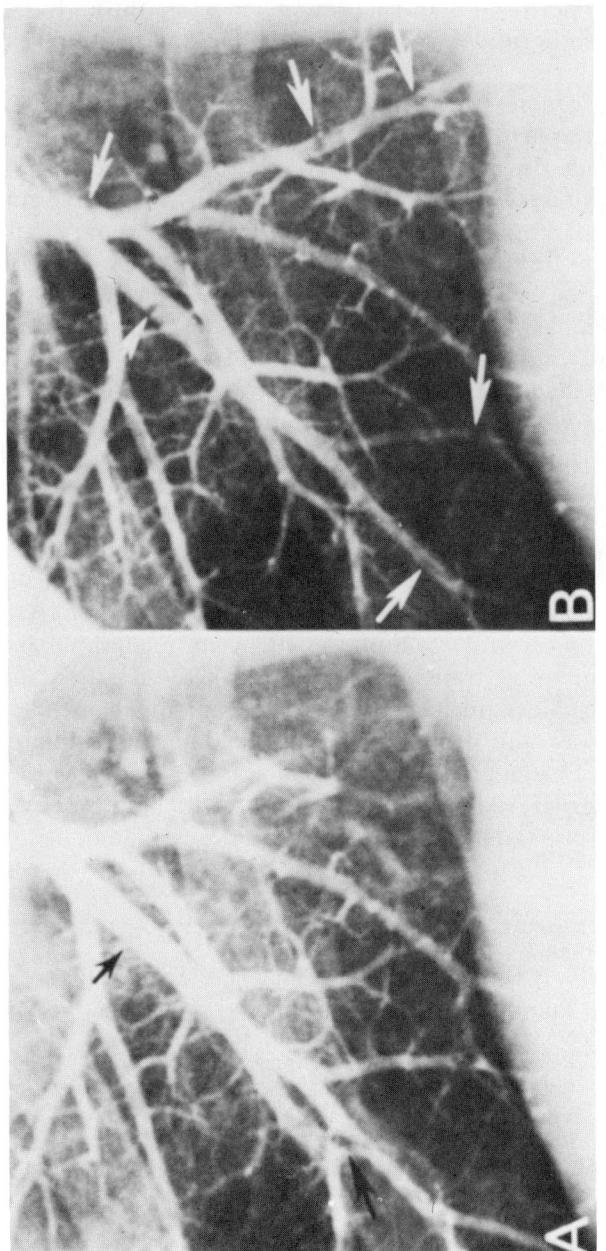

Figure 16. Multiple small emboli diagnosed by balloon-occlusion angiography. Both A and B show multiple small emboli in subsegmental vessels (arrows). A standard pulmonary angiogram was normal. (A) Early stage of a balloon-occlusion injection of contrast material in the right lower lobe. (B) Later state of the same injection from a slightly different angle. (Reproduced with permission from Radiology 1979;133:518–520, Figure 1.)

injections when required, and may reduce the risk of ventricular arrhythmia and perforation during catheter passage through the right ventricle. The inferior vena cava and both iliac and femoral veins can be examined during the same procedure (Figure 17), and the potential of dislodging venous thrombi through the transfemoral route is obviated when the arm is used. Careful hemodynamic measurements should be made during all pulmonary angiogram procedures, since the circulatory responses to thromboembolism are invaluable guides to assessing the pathophysiologic consequences of pulmonary embolization and the presence of preexisting cardiopulmonary disease.

In some patients with suspected thromboembolic pulmonary hypertension, pulmonary angiography is absolutely or relatively contraindicated by those conditions listed in Table 10. Severe pulmonary hypertension is usually aggravated by pulmonary angiography and special precautions are required when the procedure is considered essential to patient management. Acute right ventricular failure, systemic hypotension, cyanosis, and ventricular arrhythmias can be reduced by the administration of oxygen, small hand injections of contrast material during cinefluoroscopy, and opacification of the pulmonary vasculature on an individual, subselective lobar basis preferably utilizing balloon occlusion techniques. Femoral partial cardiopulmonary bypass has been used successfully to support patients during pulmonary angiography. Temporary transvenous pacing can reduce the danger of complete heart block during catheterization of patients with left bundle branch block and proper radiation shielding can minimize fetal exposure when angiographic confirmation is required because of the fetal and maternal risks of unnecessary anticoagulation. As in virtually all diagnostic procedures, the contraindications to pulmonary angiog-

TABLE 10
Relative Contraindications to Pulmonary Angiography
- Known allergic sensitivity to contrast material
- Severe pulmonary hypertension
- Recent myocardial infarction
- Left bundle branch block
- Ventricular arrhythmias
- Pregnancy
- Right-sided bacterial endocarditis
- Inadequate patient cooperation
- Severe hypoxemia

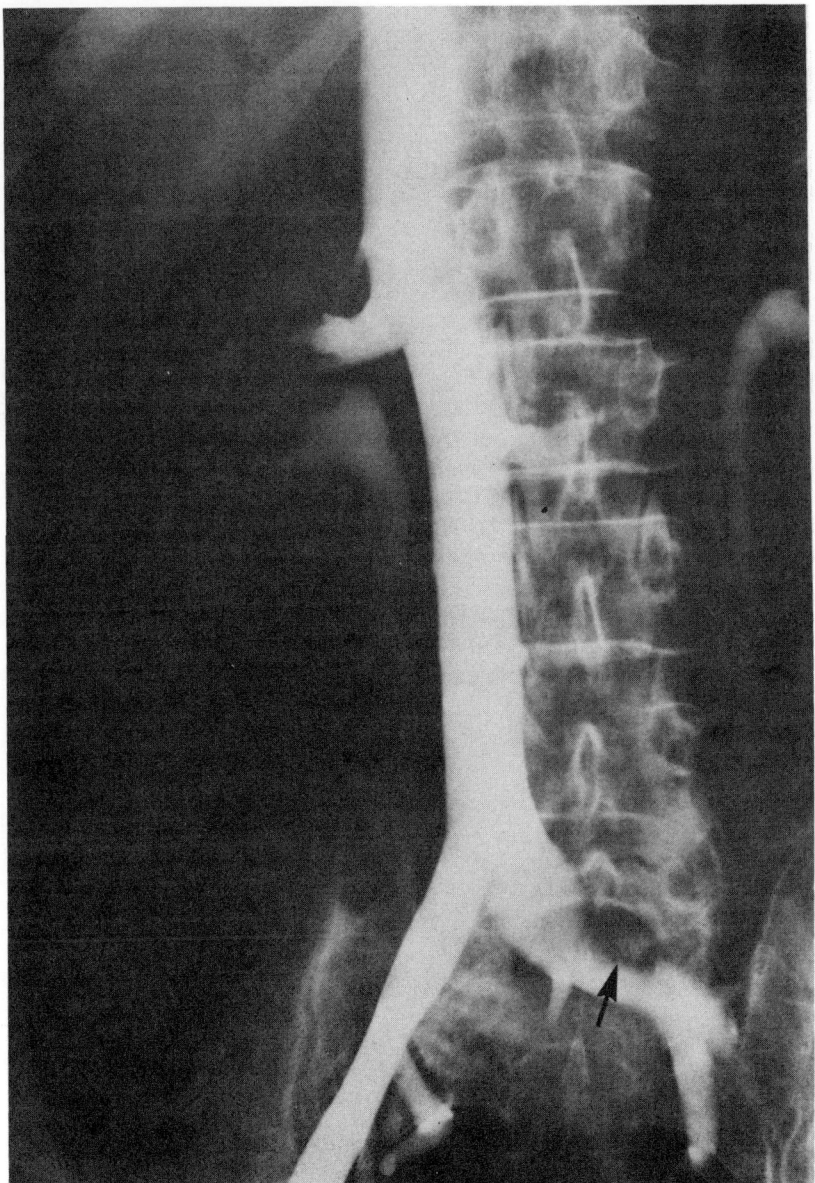

Figure 17. An inferior vena cavagram demonstrating a large filling defect in the left iliac vein. (Courtesy of M. D. Bogdonoff, M.D., Department of Diagnostic Radiology, Rush-Presbyterian-St. Luke's Medical Center.)

raphy must be considered on an individual basis, weighing the hazards of angiography against those of inappropriate therapy.

The vast majority of complications caused by pulmonary angiography can be avoided or successfully managed by an experienced angiographic team, proper pre-medication, and monitoring during the procedure. These risks can be divided into those related to contrast material and to right heart catheterization. The most important complications of pulmonary angiography are listed in Table 11 and have been significantly overestimated by most practitioners. The Steering Committee for the Thrombolytic Trials examined over 2,000 pulmonary angiograms reported by 6 centers. Mortality and morbidity data, including those reported from the Trial, are presented in Table 12. A mortality rate of less than 0.2% occurred in the studies with a morbidity rate of approximately 1%. The risks of pulmonary angiography have been significantly overestimated by most practitioners who are not aware of the excellent safety record of this definitive diagnostic test when it is performed by experienced angiographers. The practitioner's failure to incorporate this knowledge into his decision-making process undoubtedly results in suboptimal manangement for many patients with thromboembolic pulmonary hypertension.

Diagnosis of Deep Venous Thrombosis

Deep venous thrombosis of the lower extremities is often evident on careful physical examination, but more commonly requires laboratory testing for its detection and quantification. Several methods are available including invasive and non-invasive techniques.

TABLE 11
Complications of Pulmonary Angiography
- Death
- Allergic reactions to contrast material
- Myocardial perforation with or without pericardial tamponade
- Ventricular arrhythmias
- Bleeding
- Atrial arrhythmias
- Infection
- Pyrogenic reactions

TABLE 12
Mortality and Morbidity of Pulmonary Angiography

	Number of Pulmonary Angiograms Performed	Cardiac Perforations	Serious Complications	
			Arrhythmias	Death
Pre-UPET Analysis*	2347	15	8	5
UPET Experience†	310	1	5	0
Totals:Number	2657	16	13	5
%	100	0.6	0.5	0.19

UPET = Urokinase Pulmonary Embolism Trial
* = 93, † = 18

Contrast Venography

Contrast venography is the definitive standard by which all other techniques are judged. The anatomy of the venous system of the lower extremity is complex and subject to considerable distortion in the presence of disease. Contrast venography must be properly performed with adequate filling of the superficial, deep, and muscular veins to assure accurate interpretation (Figure 18). The procedure is relatively expensive, frequently painful, and is not suitable for serial evaluation. In addition, venography requires a significant volume of contrast material with potentially adverse hemodynamic effects, occasional sensitivity reactions, and rare precipitation or aggravation of phlebitis. The procedure is rarely indicated at the time of acute pulmonary thromboembolism and never as a substitute for pulmonary angiography to confirm the diagnosis of embolism. Its primary indication is in guiding surgical management such as inferior vena caval interruption and pulmonary embolectomy, in which the source of emboli should be clearly demonstrated.[91]

Non-invasive Methods

None of the currently available non-invasive methods for detecting deep venous thrombosis has equal sensitivity for thrombi above and below the knee. Venous Doppler studies are inexpensive and highly accurate for deep venous thrombosis in the thigh when performed by expert technicians. The Doppler technique is most suited to repeated studies and should be readily available in most institutions. Impedance plethysmography is commonly used in conjunction with the Doppler examination and provides information concerning iliac vein thrombosis (Figure 19). In the most recent studies of Hull et al.,[23] impedance plethysmography compared quite favorably with contrast venography in the diagnostic assessment of deep venous thrombosis. Using venography as the standard, impedance plethysmography had an 86% sensitivity and a 97% specificity for proximal deep venous thrombosis. The observed insensitivity was due primarily to small non-occlusive proximal venous thrombi. In the population studied by Hull et al., a positive impedance plethysmogram had a 97% predictive accuracy for proximal deep venous thrombosis, but was less accurate in diagnosis of thrombi below the knee.

Fibrinogen scanning is based on the incorporation of ^{125}I-labeled fibrinogen into developing thrombus. The technique is best used in prospective studies in high risk patients and is the only non-invasive procedure with sensitivity for deep venous thrombosis below the knee.

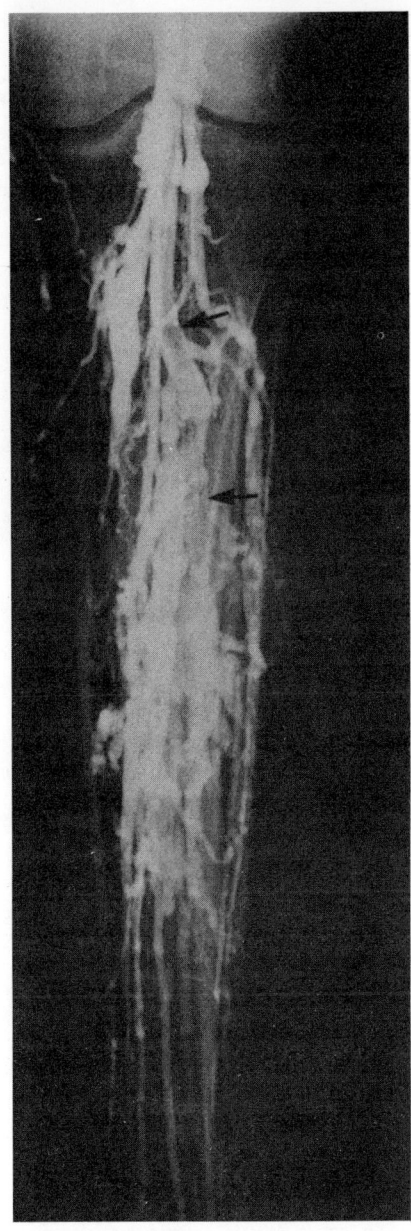

Figure 18. Contrast venogram of the lower extremity demonstrating considerable distortion of the venous anatomy and a large filling defect in the popliteal vein. (Courtesy of M.D. Bogdonoff, M.D., Department of Diagnostic Radiology, Rush-Presbyterian-St. Luke's Medical Center.)

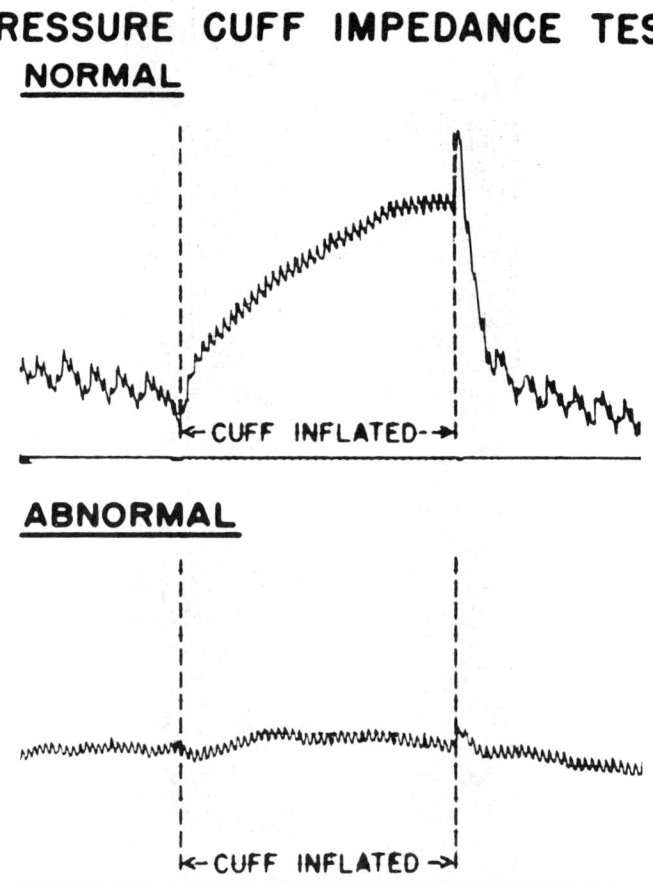

Figure 19. The effect of cuff-pressure on the impedance phlebogram. Top panel: Normal response. The venous outflow within 3 seconds of cuff release exceeds 75% of the total venous volume increase during cuff inflation. Bottom panel: Flat response characteristic of venous thrombosis. Note that a fall in electrical impedance (ordinate) is indicated by an upward deflection. (Reproduced with permission from Reference 99, Figure 2.)

Lower extremity surgery or inflammation may produce false positivity, and anticoagulant therapy must be delayed 6 to 24 hours in order to obtain valid results. Radionuclide venography can be used in patients with allergic sensitivity to contrast media or in combination with perfusion lung scanning by injection of radioactive macro-aggregates into the dorsal veins of the foot. The test is unreliable for detecting thrombi below the knee.

Thus a wide variety of methods is available for detecting deep venous thrombosis, an important pathogenetic factor in thromboembolic pulmonary hypertension. Great skill is required in their application, but hopefully they will receive wider use as additional prospective studies document their diagnostic accuracy. Reliable non-invasive diagnostic methods are essential to any strategy for the prevention or early detection and treatment of deep venous thrombosis.

From this impressive array of diagnostic techniques, what strategy should the clinician pursue to exclude thromboembolism when confronted with a patient having pulmonary hypertension? Except in cases of acute, massive thromboembolic pulmonary hypertension and circulatory failure, a deliberate, step-wise evaluation scheme is most likely to yield successful results. Depending upon the patient's clinical presentation, an appropriate differential diagnosis should be constructed and all non-embolic forms of pulmonary hypertension should be carefully considered. If this search is unsuccessful in clarifying etiology, the patient should have a multiple view perfusion lung scan whose interpretation is guided by a high quality chest x-ray and ventilation study. If these studies are normal, an embolic source can probably be excluded. If segmental or greater multiple mismatched perfusion defects are observed, a diagnosis of thromboembolic pulmonary hypertension may be warranted from these studies alone, although some investigators believe that only pulmonary angiography is definitive in determining the presence or absence of pulmonary emboli.[83] If the criteria for high probability for pulmonary emboli are not met, such patients should have pulmonary angiography. When this invasive procedure is performed, careful hemodynamic studies should be obtained and extreme caution exercised during contrast injection, particularly in patients with severe pulmonary hypertension. Balloon occlusion segmental arteriography is recommended in such cases. Concurrently, non-invasive tests for deep venous thrombosis should be performed, and contrast venography is recommended if the clinical presentation suggests the need for surgical intervention in patients with pulmonary hypertension.

THE TREATMENT OF THROMBOEMBOLIC PULMONARY HYPERTENSION

Prevention and Treatment of Deep Venous Thrombosis

Since nearly all cases of thromboembolic pulmonary hypertension represent complications of deep venous thrombosis, the prevention and early treatment of deep venous thrombosis provide a major opportunity for effective intervention. Methods of prevention relate directly to Virchow's pathogenetic triad, and are primarily based upon the reduction of coagulability, venous stasis, and, to a much lesser extent, the avoidance of vascular injury.

Prophylactic Anticoagulation

Subcutaneous low-dose heparin has become the mainstay of prevention. Since the clotting cascade represents a biological amplifier with multiplication of effect at each step, far less heparin is required to prevent thrombosis than to treat it. Ten to fifteen thousand units of heparin in 24 hours is extremely effective in preventing deep venous thrombosis and pulmonary embolism, with reductions as great as two-thirds reported in some studies.[94]

Based largely on the results of the International Multicentre Trial,[43] the Council on Thrombosis of the American Heart Association recommends that 5,000 units of heparin be given subcutaneously 2 hours before and every 12 hours following surgery in hemostatically competent patients over the age of 40 undergoing abdominal, thoracic, or pelvic surgery.[95] Prophylaxis is continued until the patient becomes ambulatory. These recommendations reflect the observation that venous thrombosis usually begins during surgery or 24 to 48 hours thereafter. This approach has been disappointing in hip surgery which is frequently post-traumatic and nonelective. Oral anticoagulants have provided significant benefit in this setting.[46] Although the data for low-dose heparin and oral anticoagulation in acute myocardial infarction are controversial, many centers routinely employ low-dose heparin in such patients.

Prevention of Venous Stasis

Without doubt, early ambulation of high risk patients is the best way to prevent venous stasis. Other worthwhile approaches include leg elevation and avoidance of the dependent position, active and passive leg exercise, properly fitted and applied elastic stockings,[96] and, in some studies, intermittent compression of the legs by pneumatic devices.[97]

Treatment of Deep Venous Thrombosis

When preventive measures fail, deep venous thrombosis should be treated with therapeutic doses of heparin followed by oral anticoagulation as described below. Hull et al.[98] have reported that long-term adjusted low-dose heparin is as effective as coumadin in preventing recurrent venous thromboembolism and is associated with fewer bleeding complications. Sharma et al.[99] have reported more rapid and adequate resolution of deep venous thrombosis with thrombolytic than with conventional heparin therapy. A greater incidence of bleeding was observed in the thrombolytic group, however, and others have cautioned that lytic therapy may liberate segments of thrombi causing embolization and sudden death.[100] No advantage over anticoagulant therapy has been reported for defibrinating agents, dextran infusion, or antiplatelet agents in the treatment of deep venous thrombosis.

The choice of therapy in thromboembolic pulmonary hypertension must be individualized and is dictated by the clinical presentation and pathophysiologic factors specific to each patient. For *convenience*, therapy will be discussed within the broad context of the three most common clinical presentations: acute massive thromboembolic pulmonary hypertension with circulatory collapse, submassive thromboembolic pulmonary hypertension with or without circulatory decompensation, and chronic thromboembolic pulmonary hypertension.

The Treatment of Acute Massive Thromboembolic Pulmonary Hypertension

Although the majority of such patients probably die before therapy can be initiated, the practitioner may encounter this dramatic condition in hospitalized post-surgical and other high risk patients. The first goal of therapy is restoration and stabilization of adequate circulation and tissue oxygenation. Intravenous fluids are indicated to raise right ventricular filling pressures and output, together with a vasopressor agent such as dopamine. Oxygen should be administered and other agents such as antiarrhythmics and digitalis may be indicated in some patients. Large dose heparin, 15,000 units, should be administered intravenously in an effort to reduce the action of thrombin in platelet degranulation with secondary release of vasoactive and bronchoconstrictor substances.

Continued therapy should be directed to the reduction of embolic pulmonary vascular obstruction and to the prevention of recurrent thromboembolism. Measures chosen depend on the severity of persisting circulatory failure, the availability of experienced personnel and facilities for further diagnostic studies and possible surgical intervention, and the patient's suitability for thrombolytic therapy.

Pulmonary Embolectomy

This heroic and sometimes lifesaving procedure has a mortality rate of 40–100% (Table 13), and is indicated only when massive thromboembolic obstruction of major pulmonary arteries has been documented and cardiopulmonary arrest has occurred.[85] Although some enthusiasm persists for this technique, particularly when rapidly mobilized portable cardiopulmonary bypass facilities are available,[101] pulmonary embolectomy undoubtedly will be replaced by thrombolytic therapy in most documented instances of massive thromboembolic pulmonary hypertension with shock.[18,85] Transvenous extraction of pulmonary emboli[102] is occasionally employed. In virtually all patients having pulmonary embolectomy, inferior vena caval ligation is indicated since recurrent embolism is common and anticoagulation must be discontinued for the embolectomy procedure. Although surgical removal of proximal thrombus may well reduce the incidence of late chronic thromboembolic pulmonary hypertension, no data are available in this regard.

Thrombolytic Therapy

The commercially available thrombolytic agents streptokinase and urokinase stimulate plasminogen circulating and within the thrombus matrix, activating clot lysis. In properly selected patients, these agents can achieve remarkable reduction in pulmonary vascular thromboembolic obstruction (Figure 20) and may reduce the frequency of chronic post-embolic pathologic changes that contribute to persistent thromboembolic pulmonary hypertension in some patients.[74] When compared to heparin, 12 or 24 hour infusions of these thrombolytic agents clearly speed the rate of resolution of pulmonary emboli and the return toward normal of right ventricular hemodynamics.[18,19] Sharma et al.[54] have found that post-embolic permanent defects in pulmonary capillary blood volume are significantly reduced by thrombolytic therapy compared to conventional anticoagulation. The salutary effects of thrombolytic therapy appear to be most likely when therapy is begun within 5 days of the embolic event and involvement is of major degree.

It is generally agreed that thrombolytic therapy should be considered in patients with documented massive thromboembolism with

TABLE 13
Complications of Therapy

Type of Therapy	Mortality (%)	Morbidity (%)	Recurrent Embolism	
			Fatal (%)	Total (%)
Alterations in Hemostais				
Acute Heparinization	1.2	13	} 0–3	2–23
Chronic Anticoagulation+	1.2	4		
Thrombolytic Therapy	1	17	1	8
Inferior Vena Caval Interruption				
External	15	10–50	0–2	0–50
Intracaval—Umbrella	0.5	10	0.8	3
—Balloon	0	3	0	1
—Filter	3.5	15	0	2
Pulmonary Embolectomy	40–100	—	—	—

References: see text, † = per patient-year.

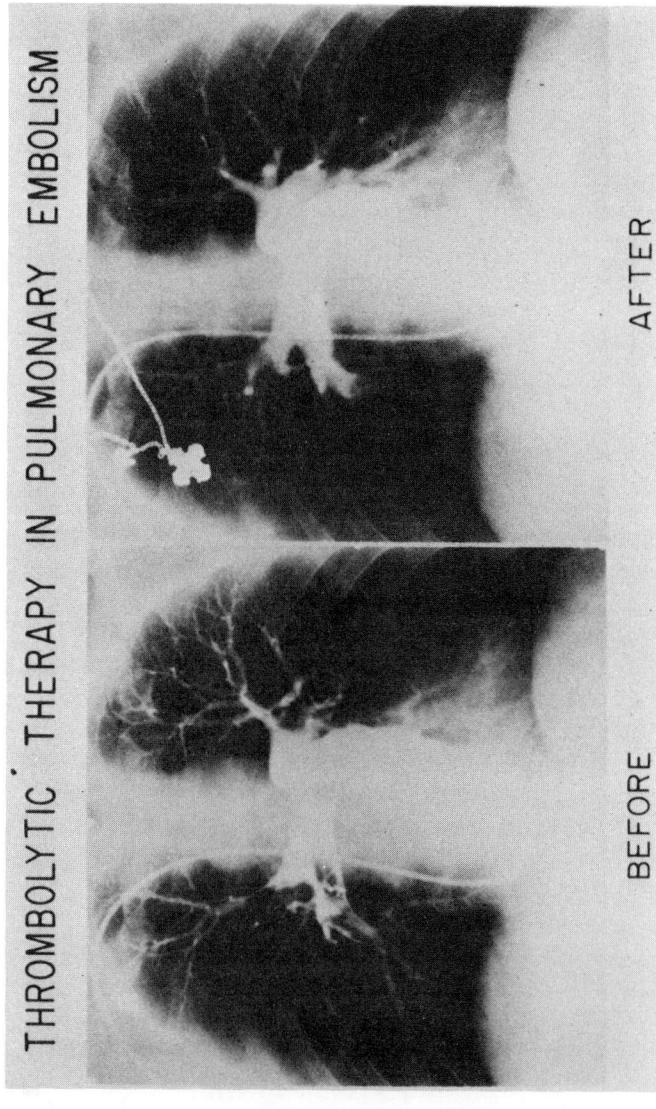

Figure 20. Pulmonary angiograms obtained at the times of scanning shown in Figure 13, demonstrating fragmentation of proximal emboli and distal migration in the right lower lobe. Significant lysis of thromboembolic material has occurred during thrombolytic therapy. (Reproduced with permission from Reference 83.)

shock, and those experienced in the use of these agents urge their consideration in massive thromboembolism without shock as well as submassive thromboembolism with circulatory failure due to preexisting cardiopulmonary disease.[18,19,74,103] While streptokinase is antigenic, urokinase is considerably more expensive, and the selection of agent should be made on an individual basis.

Thrombolytic agents should not be employed in the presence of active bleeding, a history of cerebrovascular accident, transient ischemic attacks, intracranial or intraspinal surgery within 2 months, or intracranial neoplasm. Relative contraindications include severe renal or hepatic failure, diastolic hypertension above 100 mm Hg, hemostatic incompetence, trauma, surgery, or closed biopsies within 2 weeks, and recent closed chest cardiopulmonary resuscitation.[74] Insufficient experience is available to judge the safety of these agents during pregnancy. These contraindications existed in 13% of 2,049 patients considered ineligible for the Urokinase Pulmonary Embolism Trial.[18]

Thrombolytic agents are administered by a standard dosage, constant infusion protocol after anticoagulants have been stopped. Urokinase may be given for 12 to 24 hours in a dose of 4,400 CTA units per pound body weight per hour; streptokinase is usually given for 24 hours in a dose of 100,000 units per hour after a 30-minute loading dose of 250,000 units.[46] Monitoring of therapy is done with thrombin times, and the thrombolytic state can be reversed by stopping the drug and by administering epsilon aminocaproic acid.[103] Thrombolytic agents must be followed by conventional heparin and oral anticoagulant therapy as used in other forms of thromboembolism.

When invasive procedures are avoided, bleeding complications occur in 5–7% of patients receiving thrombolytic therapy, about the same as with anticoagulant therapy. In the Thrombolytic Trials[18,19] therapy was associated with fatal bleeding in approximately 1% of patients and produced major bleeding in an additional 17% (Table 13). As experience increases in the use of these potent agents, it is likely that the complication rate will decrease further and that their value in preventing the long-term complication of thromboembolic pulmonary hypertension will be more widely established.

The Treatment of Submassive Thromboembolic Pulmonary Hypertension

Acute heparinization is the keystone of adequate therapy for most patients with submassive thromboembolic pulmonary hypertension, when administered with adequate intensity and duration. Heparin and oral anticoagulation are usually sufficient to prevent recurrence while the body's endogenous lytic system clears thromboemboli from the pulmonary vessels. When circulatory decompensation occurs with submassive thromboembolism, significant preexisting cardiopulmonary disease is usually present. Some experts have advocated thrombolytic therapy, as discussed above, to shorten the period of decompensation and enhance the potential for recovery.[103]

Guidelines for anticoagulation in thromboembolism are well documented in the literature,[10,46,85,94,98] and will not be extensively discussed here. Certain issues warrant emphasis, however, including adequate dosage, method of administration, and complication rates. As indicated above, large doses of heparin should be given during the first 24 hours after diagnosis, even in suspected cases while awaiting diagnostic confirmation. Initial doses of 15,000 units and up to 60,000 units in the first 24 hours are commonly recommended to minimize platelet degranulation. Thereafter, heparin therapy should be continued for 7 to 10 days at rates of 1,000 to 1,500 units per hour by constant infusion which appears to reduce total dosage and complication rates when compared to intermittent bolus administration.[10,11]

Disagreement persists concerning the need for laboratory monitoring of heparin therapy, but the Urokinase Pulmonary Embolism Trial experience[18] strongly supports the value of dosage control in preventing complications. The partial thromboplastin time is the most commonly used test, and 1½–2 times baseline values are recommended to assure adequate anticoagulation. Hemoglobin and platelet counts should be obtained periodically during treatment.

Oral anticoagulation, usually with warfarin, should be started after 48 hours of heparin and requires up to 7 days to produce sufficient inhibition of hepatic synthesis of Vitamin-K dependent clotting factors and fibrin formation. Prothrombin activities should be kept between 20% and 30% to optimize the relationship between reduced recurrence rates and bleeding complications.[104] Care must be exercised to avoid other drugs known to potentiate or decrease warfarin's action. The duration of oral anticoagulation is controversial, but 3 months seems a reasonable minimum. The need for additional therapy should be based upon the continued presence of factors predisposing to venous thrombosis or the existence of chronic thromboembolic pulmonary hypertension where prolonged oral anticoagulation appears to significantly prolong survival.[36]

Although highly effective in preventing and treating thromboembolic pulmonary hypertension, anticoagulation involves greater hazard than generally appreciated (Table 13). In 9 well conducted clinical studies involving acute heparinization of more than 800 patients, fatal bleeding averaged 1.2% and major hemorrhage requiring transfusion and cessation of therapy was observed in an additional 13% of patients.[8,10,11,18,41,105-108] Jick and associates have reported bleeding as frequently as 50% in women over age 60[108] and observed that heparin is the second most common drug associated with in-hospital death.[109] Heparin can produce a reversible thrombocytopenia, and allergic reactions have been observed. Fortunately, protamine sulfate neutralizes heparin stoichiometrically and is the treatment of choice when overdosage occurs.

The rate of fatal bleeds in chronic oral anticoagulation averaged 1.2% per patient-year of treatment in two careful studies of over 600 patients anticoagulated following prosthetic valve replacement.[12,110] Non-fatal bleeding, usually cerebrovascular, averaged an additional 4% per patient-year of treatment. Thus, according to these studies, acute heparinization followed by 6 months of oral anticoagulation, a typical course of therapy for thromboembolism, exposes patients to a 1.8% mortality from bleeding. In addition to these serious complication rates, anticoagulation is not totally effective in preventing recurrent pulmonary embolism which has been reported in 2-23% of patients on therapy,[11,18,19] with fatal recurrence in 0-3%.[11,18,105] The teratogenic effects of coumarin drugs are well known and substitution by adjusted low-dose heparin is probably desirable during pregnancy. Vitamin K_1 reverses the effects of coumarin drugs in 4 to 6 hours, and fresh frozen plasma provides more rapid treatment of overdosage.

The Treatment of Chronic Thromboembolic Pulmonary Hypertension

Chronic Oral Anticoagulation

Chronic oral anticoagulation should be started when the diagnosis of recurrent thromboembolism is established, and should probably be offered to most patients with idiopathic pulmonary hypertension, since thromboembolism appears to play an etiologic role in many patients.[36,38] Steele's recent report[36] is most encouraging in this regard. Chronic anticoagulation was associated with a nearly four-fold greater percent survival at 3 and 5 years than with no anticoagulation.

Vasodilator Therapy

Vasodilator therapy has been assessed with conflicting results in chronic thromboembolic pulmonary hypertension.[64,111] Although some patients with primary pulmonary hypertension experience short-term reduction in pulmonary vascular resistance, only occasionally have vasodilators produced long-term beneficial effects. Thromboembolic pulmonary hypertension appears to share this disappointing response. Some patients are made worse when systemic effects predominate,[111] but others appear to enjoy some improvement in exercise tolerance, especially with nitrates.[64]

Inferior Vena Caval Interruption

Contraindications to anticoagulation, bleeding complications, and recurrent embolization despite adequate anticoagulation are commonly cited indications for interruption of venous return from the pelvis and lower extremities. Less frequently, septic emboli from pelvic disease and the performance of pulmonary embolectomy are additional indications. Although inferior vena caval interruption may be required as adjunctive therapy in any form of thromboembolic pulmonary hypertension, its discussion seems most appropriate in relation to chronic recurrent thromboembolic pulmonary hypertension. The primary goal of inferior vena caval interruption is the prevention of recurrent embolism, the central pathogenetic factor in chronic thromboembolic pulmonary hypertension.

Caval interruption is rarely required in today's therapy of pulmonary embolism. Rosenow has estimated that the procedure is done in about 2% of patients with proven pulmonary embolic disease.[16] In such cases it undoubtedly plays a major role in preventing early recurrence and further exacerbation of acute thromboembolic pulmonary hypertension, allowing valuable time for endogenous thrombolysis and restoration of pulmonary hemodynamics to occur.

In those patients subjected to caval interruption, an embolic source below the interruption site must be established by contrast venography since a small percentage of recurrent emboli arise from sources above the pelvis and will not be prevented by caval interruption.

Two methods are commonly employed to interrupt the inferior vena cava. The direct surgical approach, transabdominal or retroperitoneal, has an average operative mortality of 15%,[105,107,112,113] and significant morbidity for venous stasis occurs in 10–50% of survivors.[107] This approach is favored with septic emboli from the pelvis. Reported late recurrences following caval interruption average 6%, different series varying from 0–50%.[83,112] One to 2% of patients have fatal recurrence despite caval interruption[105,113] (Table 13). Other external procedures include suture plication or the use of a serrated clip. These procedures enjoy somewhat lower rates of operative mortality and venous complications but about the same recurrence rate.[112]

The transvenous method for caval interruption is of greater importance to the patient with chronic thromboembolic pulmonary hypertension since general anesthesia is avoided. The most commonly used transvenous devices are the Mobin-Uddin umbrella,[114] the Greenfield filter,[115] and the Hunter-Sessions intracaval balloon.[116] The techniques have nearly comparable results (Table 13), although the numbers of implanted Greenfield filters and Hunter balloons are small in comparison to the Mobin-Uddin umbrella. Certain important differences in design and technique exist among these devices. Particularly attractive in the Hunter balloon (Figure 21) are the built-in provision for venography to insure accurate placement, the absence of perforating structures, its adaptability to varying caval dimensions, and the ability to continue heparinization throughout the procedure.[116] The balloon has been used in 130 patients to date with no in-hospital recurrence, 2 late recurrences, and no late worsening of lower extremity swelling when compared to pre-occlusion edema.[117] The balloon deflates gradually over 6 to 18 months and the balloon remnant remains encapsulated within an occlusive vena caval fibrous scar (Figure 22).

In at least one series, inferior vena caval interruption has been performed prophylactically with the Greenfield filter in patients with chronic pulmonary hypertension.[118] Eighty-three percent of these patients had embolic pulmonary vascular obstruction on pulmonary angiography and none had embolic deaths due to filter malfunction when followed an average of 23 months. It seems unlikely that caval interruption will assume an important role in the management of chronic thromboembolic pulmonary hypertension as thrombolytic therapy and anticoagulation are used more effectively. In selected cases, however, transvenous caval interruption, preferably with continuous anticoagulation, may offer important advantages to the seriously ill patients. In those unable to tolerate anticoagulation, these techniques offer the only reasonable approach to therapy.

Pulmonary thromboendarterectomy for chronic obstruction of major pulmonary arteries represents another aggressive surgical approach to the management of disabling chronic thromboembolic pulmonary hypertension and cor pulmonale. In carefully selected patients with

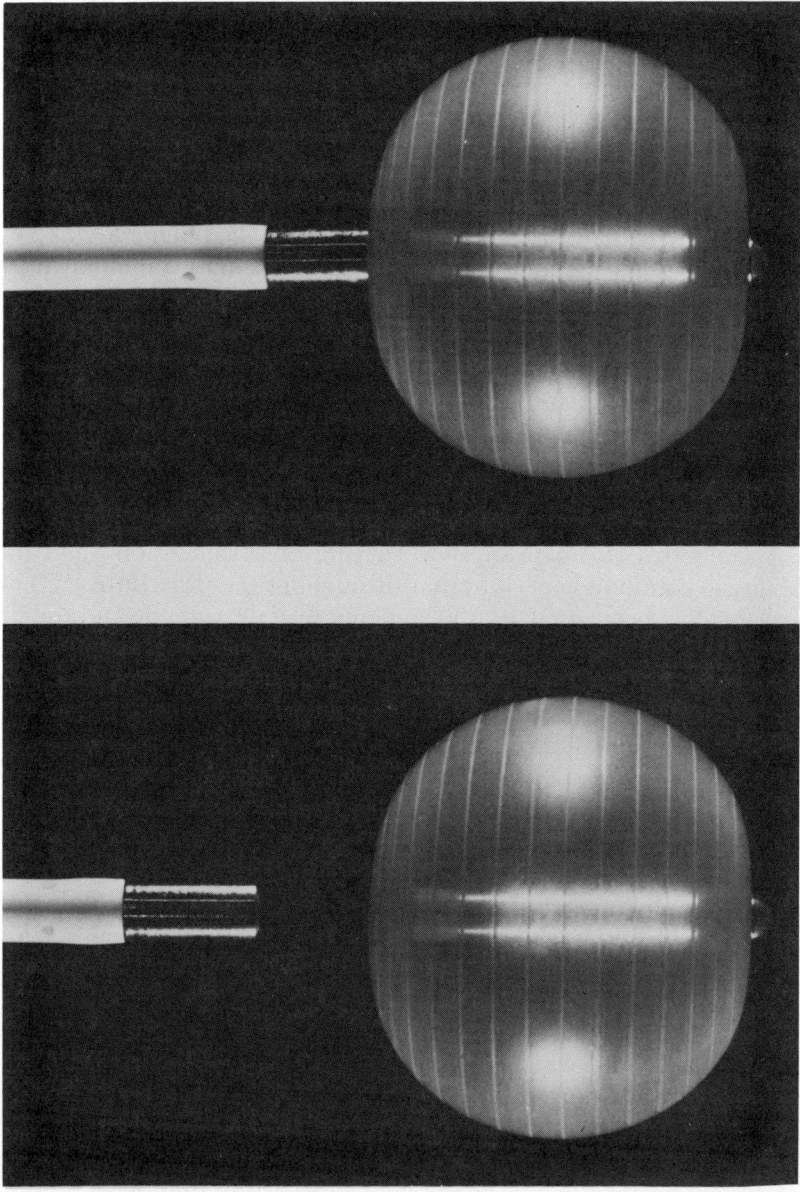

Figure 21. The Hunter-Sessions Balloon. *(Top)* Catheter tip with balloon attached and *(bottom)* separated. Note the side holes in the outer catheter for injection of contrast material and intravenous infusion. (Reproduced with permission from Reference 116, Figure 2.)

Thromboembolic Pulmonary Hypertension

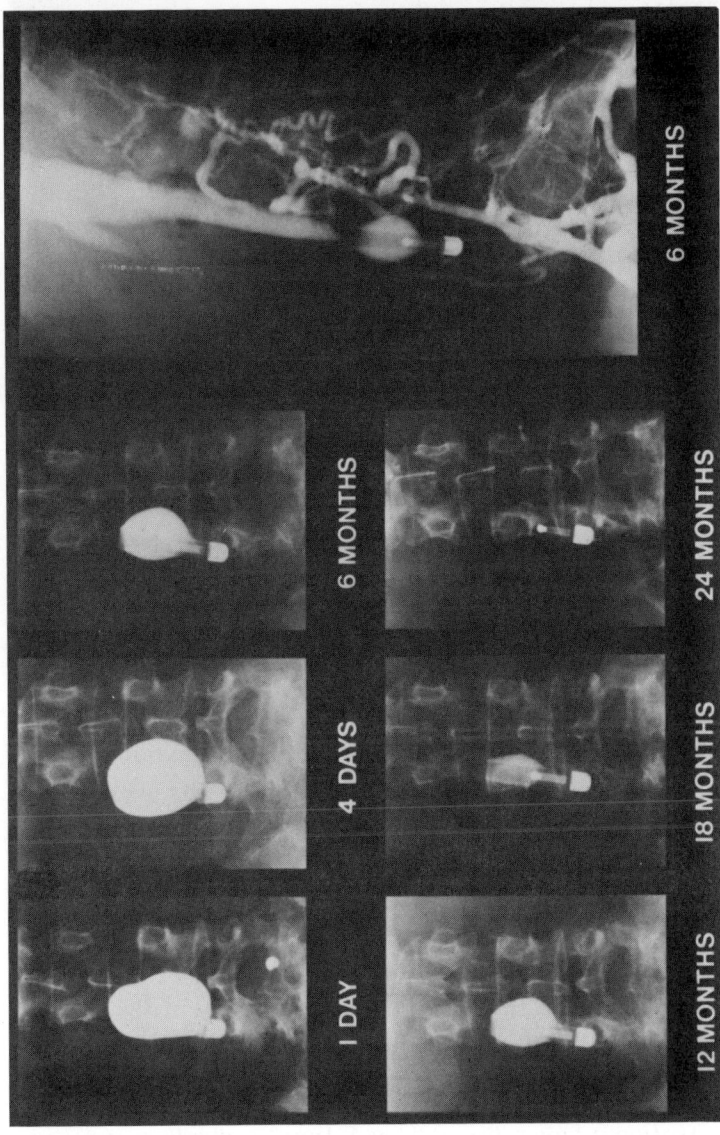

Figure 22. The Hunter-Sessions Balloon. Sequence of x-rays shows gradual deflation of the balloon. Rounding of balloon on day 4 occurs as I.V.C. accommodates to lateral pressure of the balloon. Venogram at six months shows collapsing balloon with patent I.V.C. above. (Reproduced with permission from Reference 116, Figure 6.)

severe symptoms, surgical removal of organized thrombi and occluding membranes may produce remarkable symptomatic relief.[119] A recent review of this procedure presents results in 36 collected cases, and suggests that sustained symptomatic improvement has occurred in 25 of the 27 long-term survivors.[120] In a more recent report on their own experience with this procedure, Moser et al.[57] conclude that thromboendarterectomy is beneficial in selected patients with extensive chronic large vessel pulmonary arterial obstruction, a rare but operable form of thromboembolic pulmonary hypertension.

Symptomatic Treatment

Chronic oxygen therapy, limitation of physical activity, avoidance of sudden postural changes, and conventional treatment for chronic cor pulmonale may provide symptomatic relief in patients with end stage chronic thromboembolic pulmonary hypertension. The long-term prognosis in these patients is extremely poor, death usually occurring within a few years of the onset of symptoms.

SUMMARY

Pulmonary hypertension secondary to venous thromboembolism is one of the most common forms of cardiopulmonary disease. In most cases, the condition is acute and transient. Ultimate outcome depends on proper diagnosis and application of highly effective methods of treatment to prevent embolic recurrence, the primary pathogenetic factor in thromboembolic pulmonary hypertension.

Methods of prevention and early detection of deep venous thrombosis are available, high risk patient populations have been identified, and new forms of therapy are available, some of which require further evaluation. Improved techniques for the diagnosis of pulmonary embolism are urgently needed.

Further reduction in the morbidity and mortality of thromboembolic pulmonary hypertension will depend on the practitioner's ability to recognize predisposing factors, initiate effective preventive measures, and apply the results of available diagnostic tests to ensure effective treatment only when indicated. Improvements in anticoagulant management and the use of thrombolytic therapy have significantly improved the prognosis of thromboembolic pulmonary hypertension.

Acknowledgment: The author wishes to acknowledge the invaluable assistance of Ms. Misette D. Boksa and Ms. Martha A. Campe in the preparation of this chapter.

REFERENCES

1. LeQuesne LP: Diagnosis and prevention of postoperative deep-vein thrombosis. *Ann Rev Med* 1975;26:63–74.
2. Modan B, Sharon E, Jelin N: Factors contributing to the incorrect diagnosis of pulmonary embolic disease. *Chest* 1972;62:388–393.
3. Hirsh J, Gallus AS: Diagnosis of venous thromboembolism: Limitations and applications. In: Madden JL, Hume M, eds. *Venous Thromboembolism: Prevention and Treatment.* New York: Appleton-Century-Crofts, 1976: 183–213.
4. Robin ED: Overdiagnosis and overtreatment of pulmonary embolism: The emperor may have no clothes. *Ann Intern Med* 1977;87:775–781.
5. Bell WR, Simon TL: A comparative analysis of pulmonary perfusion scans with pulmonary angiograms. *Am Heart J* 1976;92:700–706.
6. McNeil BJ: A diagnostic strategy using ventilation-perfusion studies in patients suspect for pulmonary embolism. *J Nucl Med* 1976;17:613–616.
7. Virchow R: Die verstopfung der lungenarterie und inhr folgen. *Beitr Exp Pathol Physiol* 1846;2:227–380.
8. Barritt DW, Jordan SC: Anticoagulant drugs in the treatment of pulmonary embolism—a controlled trial. *Lancet* 1960;1:1309–1312.
9. Alpert JS, Irwin RS, Dalen JE: Pulmonary hypertension. *Curr Probl Cardiol* 1981;5:1–39.
10. Salzman EW, Deykin D, Shapiro RM, Rosenberg R: Management of heparin therapy. Controlled prospective trial. *N Engl J Med* 1975;292: 1046–1050.
11. Glazier RL, Crowell EB. Randomized prospective trial of continuous vs. intermittent heparin therapy. *JAMA* 1976;236:1365–1367.
12. Isom OW, Dembrow JM, Glassman E, Pasternack BS, Sackler JP, Spencer FC: Factors influencing long-term survival after isolated aortic valve replacement. *Circulation* 1974;49(Suppl II):154–162.
13. Smith GT, Dexter L, Dammin GJ: Postmortem quantitative studies in pulmonary embolism. In: Sasahara AA, Stein M eds. *Pulmonary Embolic Disease.* New York: Grune and Stratton, 1965;120–130.
14. Frieman DG, Suyemoto J, Wessler S: Frequency of pulmonary thromboembolism in man. *N Engl J Med* 1965;272:1278–1280.
15. Morrell MT, Dunnill MS: The postmortem incidence of pulmonary embolism in a hospital population. *Br J Surg* 1968;55:347–352.

16. Rosenow EC III, Osmundson PJ, Brown ML: Pulmonary embolism. *Mayo Clinic Proc* 1981;56:161–178.
17. Dalen JE, Alpert JS: Natural history of pulmonary embolism. *Prog Cardiovasc Dis* 1975;17:259–270.
18. The Urokinase Pulmonary Embolism Trial: A national cooperative study. *Circulation* 1973;47(Suppl II):1–108.
19. Urokinase-Streptokinase Pulmonary Embolism Trial, Phase 2 results, A cooperative study. *JAMA* 1974;229:1606–1613.
20. McIntyre KM, Sasahara AA. Hemodynamic and ventricular responses to pulmonary embolism. *Prog Cardiovasc Dis* 1974;17:175–190.
21. Schwartz WB, Gorry GA, Kassirer JP, Essig A: Decision analysis and clinical judgment. *Am J Med* 1973;55:459–472.
22. McNeil BJ: The value of diagnostic aids in patients with potential surgical problems. In, Bunker JP, Barnes BA, Mosteller F eds. *Costs, Risks and Benefits of Surgery*. New York: Oxford University Press, 1977.
23. Hull RD, et al.: Pulmonary angiography, ventilation lung scanning, and venography for clinically suspected pulmonary embolism with abnormal perfusion lung scan. *Ann Int Med* 1983;98:891–899.
24. Moser KM: Diagnosis and management of pulmonary embolism. *Hosp Prac* 1980;October:57–68.
25. Breckenridge RT, Ratnoff OD: Pulmonary embolism and unexpected death in supposedly normal persons. *N Engl J Med* 1964;270:298–299.
26. Gallus AS, Hirsh J: Prevention of venous thromboembolism. *Semin Thromb Hemostas* 1976;2:232–290.
27. Neu LT Jr, Waterfield JR, Ash CJ. Prophylactic anticoagulant therapy in the orthopedic patient. *Ann Int Med* 1965;62:463–467.
28. Dalen JE, Dexter L: Diagnosis and management of massive pulmonary embolism. *Disease-a-Month* 1967;August.
29. Riedel M, Stanek V, Widimsky J, Prerovsky I: Long term follow up of patients with pulmonary thromboembolism. *Chest* 1982;81:151–158.
30. Hall RJC, Sutton GC, Kerr IH. Long term prognosis of treated acute massive pulmonary embolism. *Br Heart J* 1977;39:1128–1134.
31. Fishman AP: *Pulmonary Diseases and Disorders*. New York: McGraw-Hill, 1980;1:863.
32. Owen WR, Thomas WA, Castleman B, Bland EF. Unrecognized emboli to the lungs with subsequent cor pulmonale. *N Engl J Med* 1953;249:919–926.
33. Harris P, Heath D: *The Human Pulmonary Circulation*. 2nd ed. Edinburgh: Churchill Livingstone, 1977:557.
34. Wood P: *Diseases of the Heart and Circulation*. 2nd ed. London: Eyre and Spottiswoode, 1956.
35. Wagenvoort CA, Wagenvoort N: Primary pulmonary hypertension. A pathologic study of the lung vessels in 156 clinically diagnosed cases. *Circulation* 1970;42:1163–1184.
36. Steele PM, Fuster V, Edwards WD: Idiopathic pulmonary hypertension: Correlation of pathological type, anticoagulant therapy and outcome in 120 patients. *J Am Coll Cardiol* 1983;1(2):735 (Abstract).

37. Wilson AG, Harris CN, Lavender JP, Oakley CM: Perfusion lung scanning in obliterative pulmonary hypertension. *Br Heart J* 1973;35:917–930.
38. Dexter L: Case records of the Massachusetts General Hospital—No. 43311. *N Engl J Med* 1957;257:235–241.
39. Moser, KM: Pulmonary embolism: Where the problem is not. *JAMA* 1976;236:1500.
40. Rossi EC, Green D, Rosen SJ, Spies SM, Yao JST: Sequential changes in Factor VIII and platelets preceding deep vein thrombosis in patients with spinal cord injuries. *Br J Haemat* 1980;45:143–151.
41. Emerson PA, Teather D, Handley AJ: The application of decision theory to the prevention of deep vein thrombosis following myocardial infarction. *Q J Med*, New Series 1974;43:389–398.
42. Kakkar VV, Howe CT, Flanc C, Clarke MB: Natural history of postoperative deep-vein thrombosis. *Lancet* 1969;2:230–232.
43. International Multicentre Trial: Prevention of fatal postoperative pulmonary embolism by low doses of heparin. *Lancet* 1975;2:45–51.
44. Gallus AS: Established venous thrombosis and pulmonary embolism. *Clin Hematol* 1981;10:583–611.
45. Moreno-Cabral R, Kistner RL, Nordyke RA. Importance of calf vein thrombophlebitis. *Surgery* 1976;80:735–742.
46. Bell WR, Simon TL: Current status of pulmonary thromboembolic diseases: Pathophysiology, diagnosis, prevention and treatment. *Am Heart J* 1982;103:239–262.
47. Bynum LJ, Wilson JE III: Lower extremity phlebography in the management of venous thromboembolism. *Am Rev Respir Dis* 1977;115 (Suppl):94 (Abstract).
48. Moser KM, Stein M, eds.: *Pulmonary Thromboembolism.* Chicago: Year Book, 1973;133–270.
49. Green D: Recurring pulmonary emboli, a clinical conference in pulmonary disease. *Chest* 1982;81:230–236.
50. Harris P, Heath D: *The Human Pulmonary Circulation.* 2nd ed. Edinburgh: Churchill Livingstone, 1977:550.
51. The Urokinase Pulmonary Embolism Trial: A national cooperative study. *Circulation* 1973;47(Suppl II)II-43.
52. Tow DE, Simon AL: Comparison of lung scanning and pulmonary angiography in the detection and follow-up of pulmonary embolism: The Urokinase-Pulmonary Embolism Trial Experience. *Prog Cardiovasc Dis* 1975;17:239–245.
53. Walsh PN, Greenspan RH, Simon M, et al.: An angiographic severity index for pulmonary embolism. *Circulation* 1973;47(Suppl II):101–108.
54. Sharma GVRK, Burleson VA, Sasahara AA: The effect of thrombolytic therapy in pulmonary-capillary blood volume in patients with pulmonary embolism. *N Engl J Med* 1980;303:842–845.
55. Edwards WD, Edwards JE: Clinical primary pulmonary hypertension. *Circulation* 1977;56:884–888.

56. Wagenvoort CA, Wagenvoort N: *Pathology of Pulmonary Hypertension.* New York, Wiley, 1977.
57. Moser KM, Spragg RG, Long WB, Utley JR: Chronic thrombotic obstruction of major pulmonary arteries: Results of thromboendarterectomy in 15 patients. *Am Rev Respir Dis* 1982;125(Suppl 2):87 (Abstract).
58. Harris P, Heath D: *The Human Pulmonary Circulation.* 2nd ed. Edinburgh, Churchill Livingstone, 1977:560.
59. Oldham HN, Jr, Cox JL, Pass HI, Wechsler AS, Sabiston DC Jr: Effects of pulmonary embolism on regional myocardial blood flow. *Surgery* 1974; 76:160–169.
60. Harris P, Heath D: *The Human Pulmonary Circulation.* 2nd ed. Edinburgh: Churchill Livingstone 1977:553.
61. Fishman AP: *Pulmonary Diseases and Disorders.* New York: McGraw Hill, 1980;1:814.
62. The Urokinase Pulmonary Embolism Trial: A national cooperative study. *Circulation* 1973;47(Suppl II):55–56.
63. Stein M, Hirose T, Yasutake T, Tarabeih A: Airway responses to pulmonary embolism—pharmacologic aspects. In, Moser KM, Stein M, eds. *Pulmonary Thromboembolism.* Chicago: Year Book, 1973:166–177.
64. Dantzker DR, Bower JS: Partial reversibility of chronic pulmonary hypertension caused by pulmonary thromboembolic disease. *Am Rev Respir Dis* 1981;124:129–131.
65. Bloor CM, Sobel BE, Henry PD: Autologous pulmonary embolism in the intact unanesthetized dog. *J Appl Physiol* 1970;29:670–674.
66. Mlczoch J, Tucker A, Weir EK, Reeves JT, Grover RF: Platelet-mediated pulmonary hypertension and hypoxia during pulmonary microembolism. *Chest* 1978;74:648–653.
67. Chesebro JH, Fuster V, Robertson JS, Dewanjee MK, Wahner HW, Burnett JC: Shortened platelet survival in cardiac failure: Predisposition to amrinone-induced platelet reduction. *Circulation* 1982:66(Suppl II):382 (Abstract).
68. Kohanna F, Salzman E: Circulatory platelet aggregation in thromboembolic disease? *Circulation* 1982;66(Suppl II):320 (Abstract).
69. Heffner JE, Shoemaker SA, Canham EM, et al.: Acetyl glyceryl ether phosphorylcholine-stimulated human platelets cause pulmonary hypertension and edema in isolated rabbit lungs. *J Clin Invest* 1983;71: 351–357.
70. McDonald JW, Ali M, Morgan E, Townsend ER, Cooper JD: Thromboxane synthesis by sources other than platelets in association with complement-induced pulmonary leukostasis and pulmonary hypertension in sheep. *Circ Res* 1983;52:1–6.
71. Weir EK, Mlczoch J, Seavy J, Cohen JJ, Grover RF: Platelet antiserum inhibits hypoxic pulmonary vasoconstriction in the dog. *J Appl Physiol* 1976;41:211–215.
72. Weir EK, Grover RF: The role of endogenous prostaglandins in the pulmonary circulation. *Anesthesiology* 1978;48:201–212.
73. Weidner WJ: Effects of indomethacin on pulmonary hemodynamics and extravascular lung water in sheep after pulmonary microembolism. *Prostaglandins and Medicine* 1979;3:71–80.

74. Sherry S, Bell WR, Duckert FH, et al: Thrombolytic therapy in thrombosis: A National Institutes of Health Consensus Development Conference. *Ann Int Med* 1980;93:141–144.
75. Dexter L: Natural history of pulmonary embolism. In, Sherry S, Brinkhous KM, Genton E, Stengle JM (Eds): *Thrombosis.* Washington, National Academy of Science, 1969;85.
76. Mangano DT: Immediate hemodynamic and pulmonary changes following pulmonary thromboembolism. *Anesthesiology* 1980;52:173–175.
77. The Urokinase Pulmonary Embolism Trial: A national cooperative study. *Circulation* 1973;47(Suppl II):Table A2.3:II–95.
78. Fishman AP: *Pulmonary Diseases and Disorders.* New York: McGraw-Hill, 1980;1:818.
79. Sautter RD, Fletcher FE, Ousley JL, Wenzel FJ: Extremely rapid resolution of a pulmonary embolus. *Dis Chest* 1967;52:825–827.
80. Dalen JE, Banas JS Jr, Brooks HL, Evans GL, Paraskos JA, Dexter L: Resolution rate of acute pulmonary embolism in man. *N Engl J Med* 1969;280:1194–1199.
81. Fred HL, Axelrod MA, Lewis JM, Alexander JK: Rapid resolution of pulmonary thromboemboli in man. *JAMA* 1966;196:1137–1139.
82. Dalen JE, Brooks HL, Johnson LW, Meister SG, Szucs MM, Dexter L: Pulmonary angiography in acute pulmonary embolism: indications, techniques, and results in 367 patients. *Am Heart J* 1971;81:175–185.
83. Messer JV: Pulmonary arteriography should be performed routinely in patients with suspected acute pulmonary emboli. In: Rapaport E, Ed. *Current Controversies in Cardiovascular Disease.* Philadelphia: W. B. Saunders, 1980:445–471.
84. McNeil BJ: Personal communication.
85. Sasahara AA: Therapy for pulmonary embolism. *JAMA* 1974;229:1795–1978.
86. Moser KM, Longo AM, Ashburn WL, Guisan M: Spurious scintiphotographic recurrence of pulmonary emboli. *Am J Med* 1973;55:434–443.
87. Nichols AB, Cochavi S, Hales CA, et al.: Scintigraphic detection of pulmonary emboli by serial positron imaging of inhaled ^{15}O-labelled carbon dioxide. *N Engl J Med* 1978;229:279–284.
88. Grossman, ZD, McAfee JG, Subramanian G, et al.: New method for detection of pulmonary emboli: Methyl iodide-131 and methyl iodide-123 inhalation "hot spot" imaging. *J Nucl Med* 1981;22:42–47.
89. Fred HL, Bruderi JA, Gonzalez DA, et al.: Arteriographic assessment of lung scanning in the diagnosis of pulmonary thromboembolism. *N Engl J Med* 1966;275:1025.
90. Cheely R, McCartney WH, Perry JR, et al.: The role of noninvasive tests versus pulmonary angiography in the diagnosis of pulmonary embolism. *Am J Med* 1981;70:17–22.
91. Johnsrude IS: Pulmonary embolism. *Curr Probl Diagn Radiol* 1982;11:4–60.
92. Wilson JE III, Bynum LJ: An improved pulmonary angiographic technique using a balloon-tipped catheter. *Am Rev Resp Dis* 1976;114:1137.
93. *Manual of Operations, Urokinase Pulmonary Embolism Trial.* National Heart Institute, October, 1968.
94. Thomas DP: Heparin in prophylaxis and treatment of venous thromboembolism. *Semin Hematol* 1978;15:1–17.

95. Council on Thrombosis of the American Heart Association: Prevention of venous thromboembolism in surgical patients by low-dose heparin. *Circulation* 1977;55:423A–426A.
96. Schurr JH, Ibrahim SZ, Faber RG, LeQuesne LP: The efficacy of graduated compression stockings in the prevention of deep venous thrombosis. *Br J Surg* 1977;64:371–373.
97. Collins REC: Physical methods of prophylaxis against deep venous thrombosis. In, Fratantoni J, Wessler S, Eds. *Prophylactic Therapy of Deep Vein Thrombosis and Pulmonary Embolism.* DHEW Publication No. (NIH) 76–866, 1975:158–182.
98. Hull R, Delmore T, Carter C, et al.: Adjusted subcutaneous heparin versus warfarin sodium in the long-term treatment of venous thrombosis. *N Engl J Med* 1982;306:189–194.
99. Sharma GVRK, O'Connell D, Belko JA, Sasahara AA: Thrombolytic therapy in deep vein thrombosis. In, Paoletti R, Sherry S, eds. *Thrombosis and Urokinase,* New York: Academic Press, 1977.
100. Goldsmith JC, Lollar P, Hoak JC: Massive fatal pulmonary emboli with fibrinolytic therapy. *Circulation* 1982;64:1068–1069.
101. Mattox KL, Feldtman RW, Beall AC Jr, DeBakey ME: Pulmonary embolectomy for acute massive pulmonary embolism. *Ann Surg* 1982;195:726–730.
102. Greenfield LJ, Zocco JJ: Intraluminal management of acute massive pulmonary thromboembolism. *J Thorac Cardiovasc Surg* 1979;77:402–410.
103. Bell WR, Meek AG: Guidelines for the use of thrombolytic agents. *N Engl J Med* 1979;301:1266–1270.
104. Coon WW, Willis PW III: Hemorrhagic complications of anticoagulant therapy. *Arch Intern Med* 1974;133:386–392.
105. Nabseth DC, Moran JM: Reassessment of the role of inferior vena cava ligation in venous thromboembolism. *N Engl J Med* 1965;273:1250.
106. Mant MJ, Thong KL, Birtwhistle RV, O'Brien BD, Hammond GW, Grace MG: Haemorrhagic complications of heparin therapy. *Lancet* May 28, 1977;1:1133–1135.
107. Silver D, Sabiston DC Jr: The role of vena cava interruption in the management of pulmonary embolism. *Surgery* 1975;77:1–10.
108. Jick H, Slone D, Borda IT, Shapiro S: Efficacy and toxicity of heparin in relation to age and sex. *N Engl J Med* 1968;279:284–286.
109. Porter J, Jick H: Drug-related deaths among medical inpatients. *JAMA* 1977;237:879–881.
110. Solomon NW, Stinson EB, Griepp RB, Shumway NE: Mitral valve replacement: long-term evaluation of prosthesis-related mortality and morbidity. *Circulation* 1977;56(Suppl III):II–94.
111. Dash H, Ballentine N, Zelis R: Vasodilators ineffective in secondary pulmonary hypertension. *N Engl J Med* 1980;303:1062–1063.
112. Bomalaski JS, Martin GJ, Hughes RL, Yao JST: Inferior vena caval interruption in the management of pulmonary embolism. *Chest* 1982;82:767–774.
113. McNamara MF, Creasy JK, Takaki HS, Conn J Jr, Yao JST, Bergan JJ: Vena caval surgery to prevent recurrent pulmonary embolism. *Proc Inst Med Chic* 1977;31:173-177.

114. Mobin-Uddin K, Utley JR, Bryant LR: The inferior vena cava umbrella filter. *Prog Cardiovasc Dis* 1975;17:391–399.
115. Greenfield LH, Zocco J, Wilk J, Schroeder TM, Elkins RC: Clinical experience with the Kim-Ray Greenfield vena caval filter. *Ann Surg* 1977;185:692–698.
116. Hunter JA, Dye WS, Javid H, Najafi H, Goldin MD, Serry C: Permanent transvenous balloon occlusion of the inferior vena cava. Experience with 60 patients. *Ann Surg* 1977;186:491–499.
117. Hunter JA: The management of acute pulmonary embolism. *Morbidity and Mortality Conference.* Rush-Presbyterian-St. Luke's Medical Center, Chicago, June 6, 1983.
118. Greenfield LJ, Scher LA, Elkins RC: KMA-Greenfield® filter placement for chronic pulmonary hypertension. *Ann Surg* 1979;189:560–565.
119. Sabiston DC Jr, Wolfe WG, Newland DH Jr, Wechsler AS, Crawford FA Jr, Jones KW: Surgical management of chronic pulmonary embolism. *Ann Surg* 1977;185:699–704.
120. Daily PO, Johnston CG, Simmons CJ, Moser KM: Surgical management of chronic pulmonary embolism. *J Thorac Cardiovasc Surg* 1980;79:523–531.

CHAPTER 6

ACUTE HYPOXIC PULMONARY HYPERTENSION

E. Kenneth Weir

PATHOPHYSIOLOGIC SIGNIFICANCE

"I hold this place to be one of the highest parts of land in the world, . . . I therefore persuade myself, that the element of the air is there so subtle and delicate, as it is not proportionable with the breathing of man, which requires a more gross and temperate air" (Joseph Acosta, 1604).[1] While the discomfort of hypoxia has been well described for centuries, the fact that a fall in alveolar oxygen tension can give rise to pulmonary hypertension has been known only since 1946.[2] The pulmonary vascular pressor response to hypoxia has two components: acute and chronic. The acute phase involves vasoconstriction, predominantly of the small pulmonary arteries, which starts within a minute of the onset of hypoxia. The chronic phase involves not only an element of vasoconstriction but also morphologic changes in the small arteries, especially hypertrophy of the smooth muscle of the media and distal extension of the smooth muscle into the smaller, usually nonmuscular arterioles. These changes are discussed in Chapters 10 and 11. Pulmonary hypertension can result in right heart failure in patients with chronic bronchitis or chronic mountain sickness and is clearly deleterious in these instances. This provokes the teleologic question, "is there a physiologic advantage in the development of hypoxic pulmonary hypertension?"

In the fetus, oxygenation and loss of carbon dioxide is achieved through the placenta, and the blood flow through the uninflated lungs is similar on an ml/g basis to that of other organs. The pulmonary vascular resistance, which is high in comparison to the neonatal value, is maintained in part by vasoconstriction and in part by medial hypertrophy. If a pregnant ewe is exposed to hyperbaric oxygen, pulmonary vascular resistance falls markedly while systemic vascular resistance is relatively unchanged.[3] At birth there is a rapid decline in pulmonary vascular resistance, which is caused more by the change in oxygen and carbon dioxide tensions than by the mechanical expansion of the lungs.[4,5] These observations indicate that the high pulmonary vascular resistance which reduces pulmonary blood flow in utero is associated with the low tissue oxygen level. It could be that the pulmonary vascular response to hypoxia in the adult is merely the extrapolation of a mechanism primarily concerned with the control of blood distribution in the fetus.

The hypoxic pressor response does, however, offer several possible advantages to a neonatal or adult animal. Constriction of arteries supplying an area of consolidated or atelectatic lung reduces the shunt of poorly oxygenated blood to the systemic side.[6] If the hypoxic portion is increased to involve most of both lungs, redistribution of flow becomes less effective, and there is a greater rise in pulmonary arterial pressure. Vasodilator agents which prevent localized hypoxic pulmonary vasoconstriction cause systemic hypoxemia in animal models of pneumonia and atelectasis.[7-10] Similarly, in patients with chronic obliterative pulmonary vascular disease, the administration of vasodilators causes an increase in the perfusion of lung units with low ventilation-perfusion ratios.[11] When both lungs are hypoxic, pulmonary hypertension may be beneficial as it improves perfusion of the lung apices and the recruitment of alveolar capillaries (Figure 1),[12,13] thus increasing the surface area available for gas exchange. Consequently, in the face of pathology causing localized hypoventilation, or in the presence of generalized hypoxia, pulmonary vasoconstriction may be advantageous.

ALTERED VASCULAR TONE IN RESPONSE TO CHANGES IN OXYGEN TENSION

When some parts of the systemic circulation, such as the coronary and cerebral vascular beds, are perfused with hypoxemic blood (arterial $PO_2 < 40$ mm Hg), local mechanisms induce vasodilatation.[14] The renal vessels are less responsive. The local systemic vascular effect is modified by reflexes associated with chemoreceptor stimulation and the central pressor effect of hypoxia (Figure 2). It has been suggested

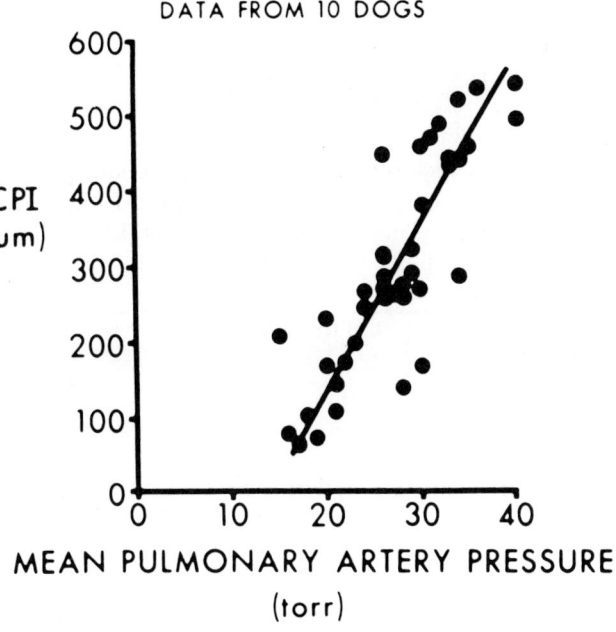

Figure 1. There is a strong positive correlation ($P < 0.001$) between mean pulmonary artery pressure and capillary perfusion index (CPI). (Reproduced with permission from Reference 12.)

that the local systemic vasodilatation caused by hypoxia is the result of ATP depletion,[15] but more recent work indicates that ATP supplies are adequate to support contraction down to a PO_2 of 8 mm Hg and probably less.[16] Increased adenosine formation may be partly responsible, as adenosine deaminase has been found to reverse the depression in isometric force which the transition from normoxia to anoxia induces in systemic arterial strips.[17] It is important to note that the complete restoration of force despite continued anoxia, suggests that ATP is not a limiting factor in terms of the strength of contraction. Adenosine also seems to play a part in the coronary vasodilatation observed during hypoxemia.[18] Tissue levels of adenosine increase markedly in the lungs of dogs exposed to hypoxia and adenosine infusions inhibit hypoxic pulmonary vasoconstriction.[19] However, the vasodilator effect of endogenous adenosine is over-ridden in the pulmonary vasculature during hypoxia.

In contrast to the systemic vasculature, when the pulmonary circulation is perfused with hypoxemic blood, or the lungs are ventilated with hypoxic gas mixtures, local mechanisms cause vasoconstriction. The reason for the disparity is unknown and remains the focus of intensive

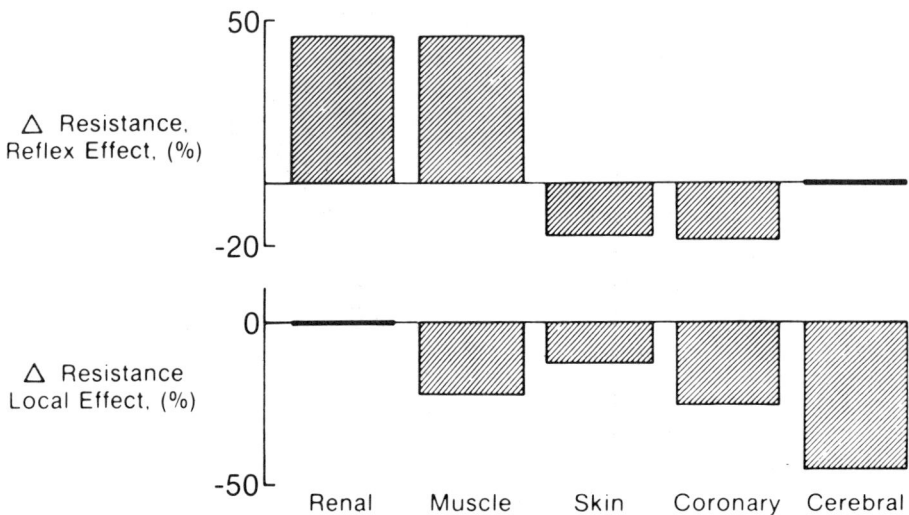

Figure 2. The systemic vascular response to hypoxemia depends on reflex effects of chemoreceptor stimulation (top) and local dilator effect of hypoxia (below). The values for reflex effects are responses to maximal chemoreceptor stimulation during normotension in anesthetized, ventilated dogs; the values for local effects are responses at an arterial PO_2 of 30 mm Hg. (Reproduced with permission of the American Heart Association, Inc., from Reference 14.)

investigation. It is tempting to consider that the high oxygen environment of the adult lung vessels, relative to the systemic vessels, might be responsible for the different reactivity. However, the pulmonary vasculature of the fetus is as hypoxic as the systemic vasculature and yet behaves entirely differently in response to changes in blood oxygen tension,[3] as discussed earlier. In a teleologic sense, it is not surprising that the mechanisms relating oxygen tension to vascular tone should be different in the systemic and pulmonary circulations. On the systemic side, vasodilatation increases blood flow and oxygen supply to hypoxic tissue. In the lungs, tissue hypoxia is seldom a metabolic problem. Consequently, it makes sense that blood should be diverted away from poorly ventilated alveoli in order to pick up oxygen elsewhere and avoid a shunt of unsaturated blood.

PHYLOGENY

Although the mechanism by which changes in oxygen tension alter pulmonary vascular tone is not understood, many characteristics of acute hypoxic pulmonary vasoconstriction have been described. A pulmonary pressor response to hypoxia, or its equivalent, is present in fish,[20] amphibia,[21] reptiles,[22] birds,[23] and mammals. Hypoxic pulmonary vasoconstriction can be demonstrated in virtually all mammalian species, both common, cattle,[24] cats,[2] dogs,[7-10] and uncommon, llamas[25] and coati mundi.[26] It occurs in the fetal,[3,27,28] neonatal,[29,30] and adult mammal.[7-10] While the pulmonary vascular resistance of the normoxic lung is relatively high in the neonate, the percentage increase in pulmonary arterial pressure and resistance stimulated by hypoxia increases with age. This increase in reactivity to hypoxia has been correlated in the pig with the gradual peripheral extension of muscle in the maturing pulmonary vascular bed.[30]

SITE OF HYPOXIC PULMONARY VASOCONSTRICTION

Given this correlation between hemodynamic response and peripheral extension of muscle, it is reasonable to suppose that the small muscularized and partially muscularized pulmonary arteries might be a major site of hypoxic vasoconstriction. The majority of investigators have in fact concluded that most of the increase in pulmonary vascular resistance caused by hypoxia occurs at this level (Figure 3).[31-37] It has also been suggested that interstitial cells in the alveolar septa might contract in response to hypoxia.[38] However, while these workers reported that human, rat, and bovine parenchymal strips contract in vitro when made hypoxic, others have noted relaxation in canine parenchymal strips.[39,40] Recent observations in the isolated, perfused pig lung support the contention that alveolar vessels constrict during hypoxia.[41] Pulmonary veins make only a small contribution to the increase in pulmonary vascular resistance induced by hypoxia.[42,43]

More direct evidence of the anatomic distribution of hypoxic vasoconstriction may be obtained by pressure measurement using micropuncture techniques. Preliminary micropuncture evidence suggests that during hypoxia the major locus of increased resistance is between arteries and capillaries, but that some of the increase occurs across the capillary and the venous segments[44] (Figure 4). Recent studies using laser technology have allowed visualization of the small arteries (30–200μ) in the bullfrog lung.[45] When localized hypoxia is introduced, these arteries can be seen to constrict, and flow velocity as measured by a laser Doppler microscope is decreased.

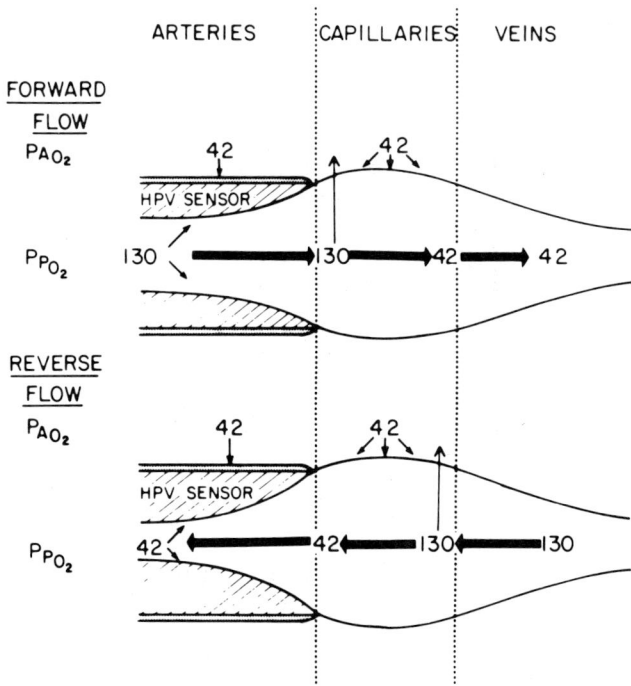

Figure 3. *A sensor region for hypoxic pulmonary vasoconstriction is hypothesized in the wall of small muscular pulmonary arteries that is influenced directly by the oxygen tensions of both the alveolar gas and the pulmonary artery blood. With forward flow (upper diagram), the influence of perfusate oxygen tension is consistent with this concept, and the final response reflects both the alveolar PO_2 of 42 and the perfusate PO_2 of 130 mm Hg. When flow is reversed, the perfusate PO_2 of 130 is reduced by equilibration with the alveolar gas in the pulmonary capillaries, and its tension becomes 42 mm Hg. The pre-capillary site of the sensor region is therefore identified by the abolition of perfusate influence on hypoxic pulmonary vasoconstriction when flow is retrograde. Reprinted by permission of the American Heart Association, Inc., from reference 37.*

FACTORS ALTERING THE PULMONARY PRESSOR RESPONSE TO HYPOXIA

Temperature: Severity and Duration of Hypoxia

The response is somewhat labile and can be influenced by many factors. While a reduction in body temperature increases normoxic

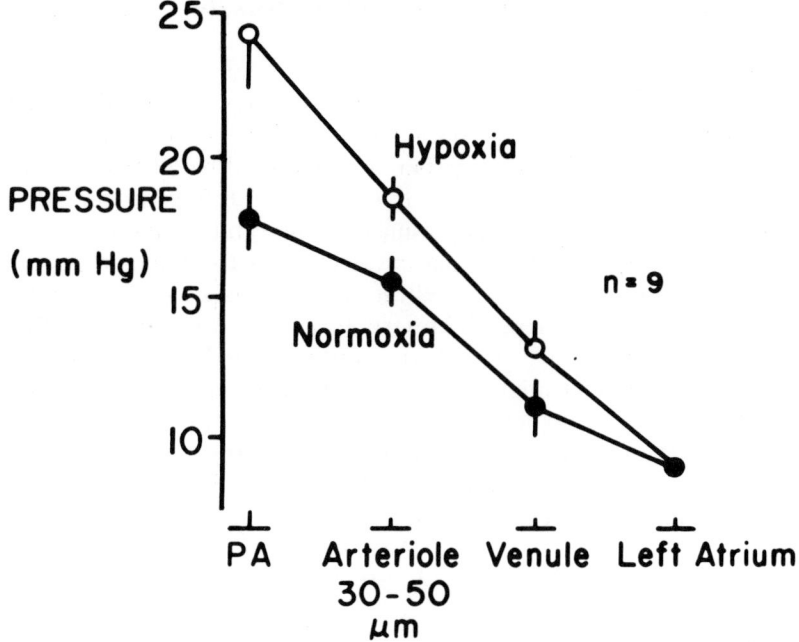

Figure 4. Micropuncture measurement of the pressure in the pulmonary microvasculature of the isolated cat lung, showing that hypoxic vasoconstriction affects all segments, but mainly the arteries. (Drawn from data in Reference 44.)

pulmonary arterial pressure and resistance in the anesthetized dog,[46] it diminishes hypoxic pulmonary vasoconstriction.[46–48] The severity of the hypoxic challenge is important. As the alveolar oxygen pressure is reduced from 670 to 60 mm Hg in the isolated pig lung, pulmonary arterial pressure gradually increases.[49] It remains constant between 60 and 30 mm Hg and then falls as alveolar oxygen is lowered further. A similar pattern has been reported in the anesthetized dog.[50] However, in the dog the vasoconstriction declines after the initial 5 minutes of hypoxia. It does not appear that the failure to maintain constriction is due to lack of ATP,[51] the production of dilator prostaglandins, or adrenergic-induced vasodilatation.[50] If the hypoxic challenge is continued until a steady-state is achieved, pulmonary vascular tone in the isolated dog lung returns to normoxic levels.[52] In the rabbit, cat, and ferret, hypoxic vasoconstriction reaches a steady-state plateau which is maximal at an inspired oxygen tension of 25 mm Hg.

Components of the Perfusate

The constituents of the fluid perfusing the lungs can alter the vascular reactivity to hypoxia. The importance of the perfusate is illustrated by the fact that fresh rat lungs perfused with old blood from earlier experiments have hypoxic pressor responses 10 times greater than fresh lungs perfused with old plasma.[53] Hauge and Melmon reported that the use of platelet-rich plasma enchances the hypoxic pressor response of the isolated perfused rat lung, in comparison to platelet-poor plasma.[54] However, McMurtry et al. were unable to confirm these findings in a similar preparation and suggested that the introduction of fresh plasma might have potentiated the response.[53] In the intact dog the prior depletion of circulating platelets by platelet antiserum increases, rather than reduces, the vasoconstriction stimulated by acute hypoxia.[55] The presence of red blood cells in the perfusate of isolate rat lungs prolongs the time during which the lung responds to hypoxia.[53] Polycythemia increases the severity of acute hypoxic pulmonary vasoconstriction in the anesthetized dog.[56] Consequently, it seems that red blood cells are more important than platelets in determining the strength of the pressor response to hypoxia. The number of circulating leukocytes does not seem to influence the response.[57]

Apart from formed elements in the perfusate, other components are also important. Isolated canine lungs are more responsive to hypoxia when perfused with plasma than when perfused with physiologic salt solution.[58] Blood glucose falls during the perfusion of isolated lungs and repletion of glucose levels reduces the reactivity to hypoxia, which is unchanged by the addition of sucrose. The glucose repletion does not alter the responsiveness to angiotensin II.[53] While this may appear to be a technical detail, it may be a clue to the mechanism of the interaction between oxygen tension and pulmonary vascular tone.

Many investigators have studied the interaction between hypoxic pulmonary vasoconstriction and changes in pH and carbon dioxide tension. It was found that the pressor response to hypoxia was potentiated by acidosis and diminished by alkalosis.[59,60] However, further dissection of the problem showed that the hypoxic pressor response in the dog is increased by hypercapnia but not by an increase in $[H^+]$, when the carbon dioxide tension is held constant.[61] On the reverse side, it was demonstrated that a decrease in $[H^+]$ reduces the hypoxic pressor response, while hypocapnia does not. In cattle, alkalosis achieved by infusion of sodium bicarbonate does not appear to reduce the pressor response.[62]

Environmental and Genetic Influences

It is well known that the pulmonary pressor response to hypoxia is largely intrinsic to the lungs as it has been demonstrated so consistently in isolated perfused lungs. However, the condition of the animal prior to the hypoxic challenge can alter the responsiveness of the pulmonary vasculature to hypoxia. For instance, lungs taken from rats exposed to simulated high altitude (4,270 m) for short (40 hours) or long (4–6 weeks) periods have decreased pressor responses to acute hypoxia.[63,64] It is likely that this reflects a non-specific decrease in reactivity to a range of vasoconstrictor stimuli.[63] Rats exposed to 100% oxygen for 48 hours also have reduced pressor responses to acute hypoxia.[65] The pressor response can be restored to control levels by meclofenamate, suggesting the possible involvement of a dilator prostaglandin-like substance. Dogs that are reared at higher altitudes (1,600 m) have more vigorous pressor responses to hypoxia than those from sea-level.[66] Cattle that are genetically prone to develop pulmonary hypertension show more marked acute hypoxic vasoconstriction than those who are not genetically susceptible.[67] This difference is in part the result of increased pulmonary vascular smooth muscle. The "susceptible" cattle have a greater pulmonary vascular resistance increase during acute hypoxia when pregnant, than post-partum.[68] However, the pulmonary vascular resistance attained in the anesthetized dog during hypoxia is less during the second or third trimester of pregnancy, than in the same dog post-partum.[69] In the blood of pregnant rats there is a circulating substance which reduces the pressor response to hypoxia when perfused in isolated lungs taken from non-pregnant rats.[70] These differences between cattle, dogs, and rats may be due to species variation, but could be secondary to differences in experimental technique.

Potential Experimental Artifacts

In addition to the influences mentioned already, there are several technical factors which can obscure the significance of experimentally-induced changes in the severity of hypoxic pulmonary vasoconstriction. When isolated perfused rat lungs are repetitively challenged with hypoxia, the magnitude of the response increases during the first few challenges and then declines.[71] Serial repetition of hypoxic challenges has been reported to increase the severity of the hypoxic pulmonary vasoconstriction in anesthetized dogs.[72] However, subsequent studies using intermittent unilateral hypoxia suggest that in some dogs time alone, following the induction of anesthesia and the initial hypoxic challenge, will increase the pressor response.[73] Several inhaled anesthetic agents, such as isoflurane and fluroxene, can inhibit hypoxic pulmonary vasoconstriction.[74] Very small amounts of endotoxin will completely ablate the hypoxic pressor response in the anesthetized dog,[75] although endotoxin does not appear to have an effect in the awake pig, or in the isolated rat lung. The action of endotoxin in the dog model is probably mediated through the formation of dilator prostaglandin-like substances.[76] A rise in blood flow through the lungs will attenuate the increase in pulmonary vascular resistance caused by hypoxia, probably because the dilated vessels have a poorer mechanical advantage.[77] When comparing the results of experiments in isolated perfused lungs, it is important to recognize that the pressor response to hypoxia is markedly decreased by pulsatile, as opposed to steady flow.[78] The use of glass in the circuit of an isolated lung perfused with blood will prevent the pressor response, possibly through the generation of bradykinin.[79] It can easily be appreciated that many factors have to be considered in the interpretation of experiments which examine the interaction between oxygen tension and pulmonary vascular reactivity.

THE MECHANISM OF ACUTE HYPOXIC PULMONARY VASOCONSTRICTION

The Stimulus for Vasoconstriction

The means by which a reduction in oxygen tension is sensed and by which it causes pulmonary vasoconstriction are unknown. In the third trimester fetus, pulmonary vascular tone is in part controlled by the oxygen tension of the pulmonary arterial blood.[3] The same is true of the collapsed, unventilated, but perfused lung of the adult cat.[80] More recent experiments, using antegrade and retrograde perfusion of the left lower lobe of the intact cat, suggest that the oxygen tension of the mixed venous blood is sensed upstream to the arteries exposed to alveolar gas.[81] The vasoconstriction elicited by marked pulmonary arterial hypoxemia can occur in the absence of alveolar hypoxia, or can be additive to the vasoconstriction induced by alveolar hypoxia. Other studies confirm the independent effects of hypoxemia and hypoxia.[82,83] While hypoxemia can stimulate pulmonary vasoconstriction and various constituents of the blood or perfusate can modulate the vasoconstriction, as discussed earlier, the sensing and transduction of the oxygen signal appears to occur in the lung.

Traditionally there have been two approaches to this problem. One hypothesis suggests that as the oxygen tension falls, a constrictor substance is released from storage or elaborated in the lung parenchyma and then acts on the pulmonary vessels. The second hypothesis suggests that the reduction in oxygen tension has a direct effect on the pulmonary vascular smooth muscle. In the case of the mediator hypothesis, the change in oxygen tension is thought to be sensed by the cell that elaborates or stores the vasoactive substance. The signal is then transmitted by the mediator to the pulmonary vascular smooth muscle. The direct effect hypothesis proposes that the oxygen tension is sensed in the smooth muscle cell itself. Both schools of thought accept that, at some stage, transmembrane calcium flux is involved. A variety of calcium channel blocking agents have been shown to prevent hypoxic pulmonary hypertension in the isolated lungs of rats[71] and pigs,[84] in the intact anesthetized dog,[85,86] and in both awake cattle[87] and man.[88] It is not apparent whether the calcium flux, which is susceptible to these blockers, occurs at the smooth muscle cell or some other cell, which then releases a vasoconstrictor mediator. The factors controlling the level of calcium in the smooth muscle cytoplasm will be discussed later.

Mediators

Proponents of a mediator substance have suggested that such a vasoconstrictor could be formed in mast cells, neuroepithelial bodies, or autonomic nerve endings. Given the recent evidence demonstrating the influence of endothelial cells on the tone of vascular smooth muscle, including rings of pulmonary artery,[89-91] endothelial cells should be added to the list. Possible contenders for the role of mediator have included histamine, norepinephrine, angiotensin II, 5-hydroxytryptamine, prostaglandins, and leukotrienes. The possibility that a mediator exists is supported by the observation that lymph collected from the thoracic duct of dogs during hypoxia causes the contraction of pulmonary artery strips, while lymph collected during normoxia does not.[92]

Histamine

The data concerning histamine have been reviewed in detail by Bergofsky.[93] Mast cells are found close to the small pulmonary arteries, they contain histamine, and they degranulate during hypoxia.[94] Despite these suggestive data, evidence has accumulated against histamine as the sole mediator of hypoxic pulmonary vasoconstriction and against mast cells as the source of any vasoconstrictor mediator. An H_1 receptor blocker, chlorpheniramine, which prevents the pulmonary vasoconstriction caused by histamine infusion in the anesthetized dog,[95] does not alter the pressor response to hypoxia.[96-98] The histamine content of the left ventricular blood has been noted to rise in hypoxic guinea pigs.[94] However, histamine levels increase in the systemic venous blood, rather than in the aortic blood during hypoxia in the dog.[99] This implies that the pulmonary release of histamine is small in the dog and that the systemic release of histamine cannot account for the pressor response to hypoxia observed in an isolated lung. The same group found that a dose of disodium cromoglycate (1 mg/kg iv), which will prevent the increase in systemic venous histamine, does not reduce the hypoxic pressor response in the dog.[100] Mast cell hyperplasia occurs in chronically hypoxic animals, but the pulmonary hypertension and right ventricular hypertrophy seem to precede the increase in the number of mast cells, rather than follow it.[101,102] This is in keeping with the observation that in cats the acute pressor response to hypoxia is inversely related to lung mast cell density.[103] The most convincing evidence against the role of mast cells is that mice which have no lung mast cells, develop the same severity of pulmonary hypertension during both acute and chronic hypoxia as control mice.[104] Lung histamine levels were the same in both strains, indicating a non-mast cell source. These experiments indicate that while histamine could contribute to, or modulate, hypoxic pulmonary vasoconstriction in some species, it is not the only mediator. Mast cells are evidently not an essential component of the response in all species.

Norepinephrine

The experimental data concerning norepinephrin also demonstrate variation between species but again allow the conclusion that norepinephrine is not the only mediator of hypoxic vasoconstriction. Dopamine beta-hydroxylase is contained in the vesicles of the adrenergic terminals and released along with norepinephrine. However, when hypoxia causes vasoconstriction in the perfused cat left lower lobe, there is no measurable increase in dopamine beta-hydroxylase to indicate norepinephrine release.[105] Results from the use of alpha-blocking agents have varied from species to species as shown in Table 1. It may be that the diminished vasoconstriction is in part due to the unopposed beta-adrenergic activity of catecholamines. Depletion of catecholamines by reserpine has failed to alter the pressor response to hypoxia in cats,[80] dogs,[114,115] or calves.[110] While alpha-receptors might be involved in the mechanism of hypoxic vasoconstriction in some species, they do not appear to be essential in all species.

Angiotensin II

Angiotensin II was found to augment the pulmonary hypertension stimulated by hypoxia in the isolated rat lung perfused with an albumin and salt solution.[116] However, subsequent experiments have shown that when the pulmonary pressor response to angiotensin II in the rat lung,[71] dog,[117] or fetal lamb[118] is blocked by saralasin, the pressor response to hypoxia is still intact. Similarly, when production of angiotensin II is prevented in the cat by inhibition of angiotensin-converting enzyme with captopril, hypoxic pulmonary vasoconstriction is unaffected.[119] Infused angiotensin II has no effect on pulmonary vascular resistance in the ferret, which has a strong pressor response to hypoxia.[120] These experiments make it unlikely that angiotensin II fulfills the role of mediator.

TABLE 1
Effect of Alpha-receptor Blockade on the Pulmonary
Pressor Response to Hypoxia

Species	Blocker	Hypoxic pressor response	Reference
Cat	Phenoxybenzamine	Diminished	106
Cat	Phenoxybenzamine	Diminished	80
	Dibenamine	Diminished	80
Cat	Phentolamine	Diminished	107
Ferrets	Phentolamine	Diminished	108
Dog	Phenoxybenzamine	Diminished	109
Calf	Phenoxybenzamine	No change	110
Dog	Phentolamine	No change	111
Dog	Phenoxybenzamine	No change	112
Fetal lamb	Phentolamine	No change	113
	Phenoxybenzamine	No change	113

5-hydroxytryptamine

5-hydroxytryptamine (5-HT) in some species is a potent pulmonary vasoconstrictor[32,121,122] and has been considered a possible mediator of the hypoxic pressor response. However, in man[123] and cattle[67] its pulmonary vascular effects are slight, and it causes relatively little contraction of isolated human pulmonary arteries.[124] Neonatal rabbits maintained in hypoxia have an increase in pulmonary neuroepithelial bodies and a depletion of 5-HT fluorescence in those bodies compared to normoxic controls.[125] Exposure to normoxia reverses these trends. Because neuroepithelial bodies contain a number of vasoactive substances, the significance of these findings is not yet clear. Evidence against the role of 5-HT as the only mediator of hypoxic pulmonary vasoconstrictor is strong. In both dogs[109] and cats[80] the pulmonary pressor response to 5-HT can be abolished or markedly diminished by lysergic acid diethylamide while the response to hypoxia is still unchanged. Another experiment indicates that infused 5-HT, like norepinephrine and histamine, may act on larger pulmonary vessels than hypoxia.[126] Finally, α-receptor blockers such as phentolamine[107] and phenoxybenzamine[105] can prevent hypoxic pulmonary vasoconstriction but have no significant effect on the pressor response to an infusion of 5-HT.

Cyclo-oxygenase Pathway

Most recent attention concerning mediators has been focused on the metabolites of arachidonic acid illustrated in Figure 5. In 1974 it was stated that prostaglandin-like activity could be detected in the venous effluent from perfused cat lungs during hypoxic ventilation. The addition of aspirin, which can inhibit cyclo-oxygenase, appeared to reduce the hypoxic pulmonary pressor response.[127] Taken at face value, these results would suggest that prostaglandin-like substances might mediate hypoxic pulmonary vasoconstriction. Unfortunately there were technical problems which make this interpretation dubious.[128,129] Also, in 1974, it was reported that two inhibitors of cyclo-oxygenase, meclofenamate and indomethacin, augmented rather than decreased the pulmonary vasoconstriction induced by hypoxia in the anesthetized dog.[130] This finding has been confirmed in several species using a variety of inhibitors[129,131–135] (Figure 6).

There are a number of possible ways to interpret the increase in the pulmonary pressor response to hypoxia observed in the presence of cyclo-oxygenase inhibitors. The effect of the inhibitors may not be

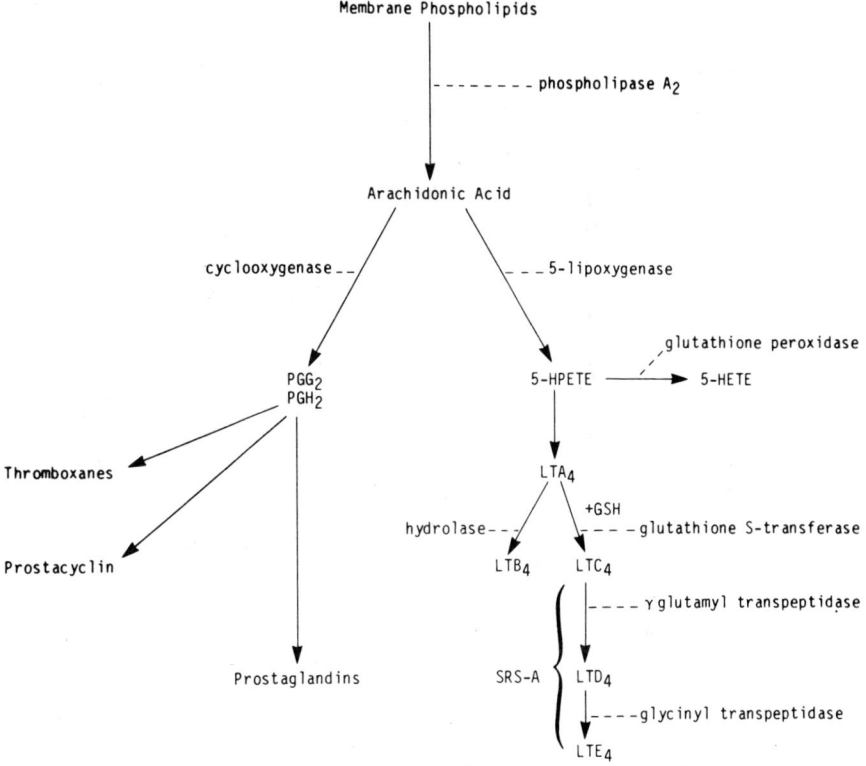

Figure 5. *The arachidonic acid cascade showing both cyclo-oxygenase and lipoxygenase pathways.*

specific for cyclo-oxygenase alone. Given the chemical dissimilarity of the agents used, it seems unlikely that they have a common action unrelated to their effect on cyclo-oxygenase. By blocking the cyclo-oxygenase pathway, the inhibitors may increase the availability of arachidonic acid to the lipoxygenase pathway. Some products of the lipoxygenase cascade (Figure 5) are pulmonary vasoconstrictors.[136,137] However, the effect of infusing arachidonic acid in the dog during hypoxia is to cause a significant decrease in pulmonary vascular resistance, not an increase.[138] Products of the cyclo-oxygenase pathway may act as modulators, rather than mediators, of the pressor response to hypoxia and reduce the severity of the pulmonary hypertension.[139] There is both "in vivo"[138] and "in vitro"[140] evidence that hypoxia increases prostacyclin production in the lungs of dogs. Consequently, inhibition of prostacyclin production seems the most likely explanation

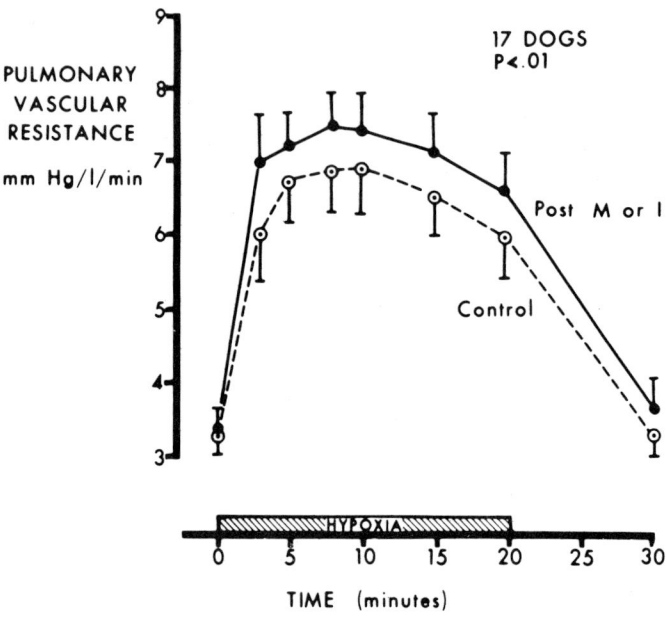

Figure 6. The pulmonary vascular resistance response to hypoxia is increased after meclofenamate (M) or indomethacin (I). (Reproduced with permission from Reference 129.)

of the increased pressor response caused by cyclo-oxygenase inhibitors. Differences in the synthesis or action of the modulating prostaglandins may account for the observed variation within a species of the strength of the pressor response to hypoxia.[141,142]

Lipoxygenase Pathway

As evidence has accumulated against cyclo-oxygenase products as possible mediators of hypoxic pulmonary vasoconstriction, so interest has turned to the leukotrienes, which are products of the lipoxygenase pathway (Figure 5).[143,144] The enzymes necessary for the formation and inactivation of leukotrienes have been demonstrated in the lung.[145] At present the data suggesting the involvement of leukotrienes depend on the use of blockers which are not necessarily specific. Ahmed and Oliver have concluded that in sheep, hypoxia causes mast cell degranulation[146] and the release of leukotrienes (SRS-A), which mediate pulmonary vasoconstriction.[143] Disodium cromoglycate (DSC) inhibited both hypoxic vasoconstriction and mast cell degranulation in the sheep.[146] However, if histamine release is a marker of degranulation, the dose of (DSC) which prevents histamine release in dogs is 8 times less than the dose required to prevent hypoxic vasoconstriction.[100] Similarly, a dose of DSC which "stabilizes" lung mast cells in the cat does not alter the pressor response to hypoxia.[147]

Disodium cromoglycate and the SRS-A antagonist, FPL-57231, are reported to be specific in that they inhibit the pressor response to hypoxia but not the response to bolus injections or brief infusions of tyramine, norepinephrine, histamine,[146] prostaglandin $F_2\alpha$, or histamine.[143] However, the dose of DSC given before the hypoxic response was measured on 85 mg/kg, compared to 24 mg/kg prior to the pharmacologic stimuli.[146] When a total of 30 mg/kg DSC was given during hypoxia,[143] no reduction of the hypoxic pulmonary hypertension was noted. Similarly, either 20 mg/kg or 34 mg/kg FPL-57231 was given before the hypoxic response was measured, but only 4 mg/kg prior to the phamacologic stimuli.[143] In view of these differences in dose, it is possible that neither DSC nor FPL-57231 are specific for hypoxic pulmonary vasoconstriction.

If leukotrienes mediate the pulmonary pressor response to hypoxia, then the administration of arachidonic acid might be expected to cause an increase in pulmonary vascular resistance during both normoxia and hypoxia. This increase in pulmonary vascular resistance should be unaffected, or possibly increased, by inhibitors of cyclo-oxygenase. In fact, the infusion of sodium arachidonate (1 mg/min) in the anesthetized dog during hypoxia causes marked pulmonary vasodilatation,[138] which can be prevented by pretreatment with the cyclo-oxygenase inhibitor, meclofenamate. Prostacyclin metabolites can be detected in the systemic arterial blood. A similar reduction in pulmonary arterial pressure, and identification of a prostacyclin-like substance, have been described following sodium arachidonate infusion in dogs during normoxia.[148] High infusion rates of arachidonic acid increase normoxic pulmonary vascular resistance, but decrease resistance when preconstriction has been induced by 15(S)-15-methyl prostaglandin $F_2\alpha$.[149] Both changes are prevented by pretreatment with indomethacin. These observations provide some evidence against a role for products of the lipoxygenase pathway as mediators of the pressor response to hypoxia in the dog, but further studies should be performed in other species.

Direct Effects of Changes in Oxygen Tension

Oxidative Phosphorylation

It has been proposed that hypoxic depression of oxidative phosphorylation may initiate pulmonary vasoconstriction by either a reduction in ATP production,[150] or a fall in the phosphate potential: [ATP]/[ADP] [Pi].[151] This ratio might fall without a decrease in the cellular concentration of ATP. ATP is normally produced in the course of glycolysis, the tricarboxylic acid (TCA) cycle (Krebs cycle, citric acid cycle), and electron transfer through the cytochrome chain which are shown in Figure 7. During hypoxia, electron transfer to oxygen is reduced and consequently NADH accumulates in the mitochondria and cytoplasm. Because of the NADH build-up, the TCA cycle slows down, ATP production is decreased and pyruvate is diverted to lactate. The rate of glycolysis is unchanged by hypoxia,[152,153] but lactate increases,[154] both because of the inhibition of the TCA cycle[155] and as a result of amino acid catabolism.[153] The high lactate production is not, itself, responsible for the pulmonary vasoconstriction as the high production rate is sustained for as long as 60 minutes after normoxia is restored,[153] while the pulmonary vascular resistance returns to normoxic levels within a few minutes.

The use of inhibitors at different stages in the metabolism of glucose provides some clues for the mechanism by which changes in oxygen tension may alter pulmonary vascular tone. Iodoacetate, an inhibitor of glycolysis, causes pulmonary hypertension in the anesthetized dog.[156] It also potentiates the pressor response to hypoxia in the perfused rat lung.[157] The potentiation can be overcome if glycolysis is bypassed by the addition of exogenous lactate and pyruvate. This observation suggests that the metabolic steps which alter pulmonary vascular tone are associated with the TCA cycle or electron transport system rather than glycolysis.

Fluoroacetate, an inhibitor of the TCA cycle (Figure 7), also causes pulmonary hypertension in the anesthetized dog,[156] while malonate, another TCA cycle inhibitor, potentiates the pressor response to hypoxia in the rat lung.[157] Inhibitors of the electron transport, such as cyanide,[158] azide, antimycin A, and rotenone, inhibit oxidative ATP production and induce transient pulmonary vasoconstriction.[150] These experimental results are all compatible with the hypothesis that a reduction in mitochondrial oxidative phosphorylation can cause pulmonary hypertension, possibly through a decrease in the phosphate potential: [ATP]/[ADP] [Pi][151,159] (Figure 8).

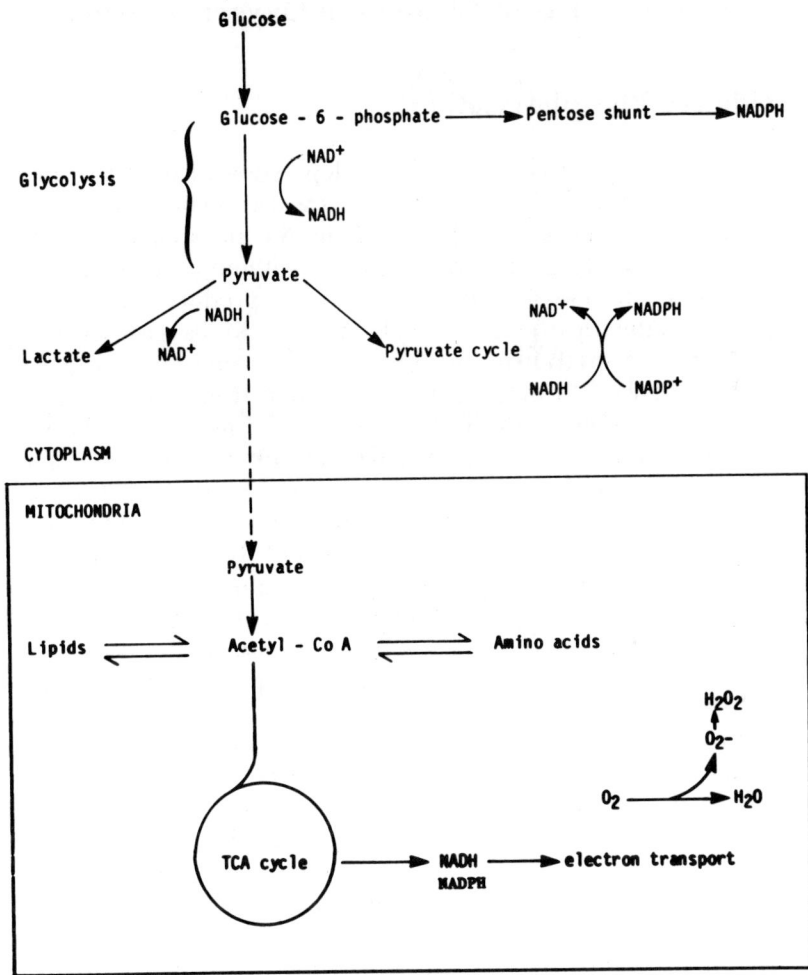

Figure 7. Glucose metabolism, indicating the sequence of glycolysis, tricarboxylic acid (TCA) cycle and electron transport system.

While the TCA cycle and electron transfer system may well be involved in the mechanism of hypoxic pulmonary vasoconstriction, some experimental data suggest that ATP per se may not be the critical factor. The vasoconstriction elicited by potassium chloride in the isolated pig lung is the same whether the $P_{I_{O_2}}$ is 10 or 100 mm Hg.[51] Consequently, even during severe hypoxia the supply of ATP is not reduced sufficiently to limit the ability of the smooth muscle to constrict. This does not preclude the possibility that a small decrease in ATP might alter some other energy-requiring process. In the isolated

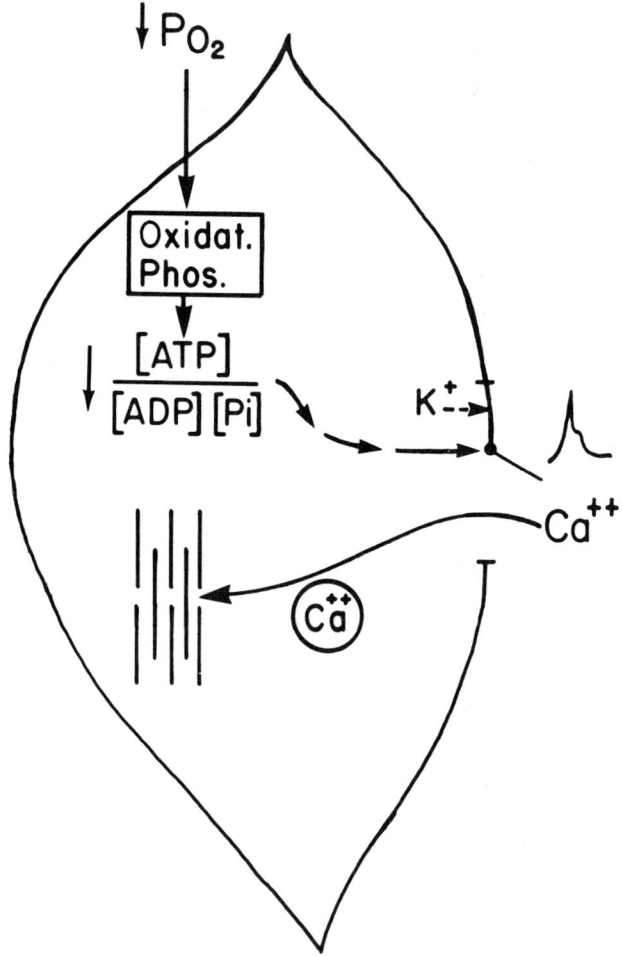

Figure 8. Working hypothesis for mechanism of hypoxic pulmonary vasoconstriction. It is proposed that hypoxia acts directly on smooth muscle of small, peripheral arteries reducing the rate of mitochondrial oxidative phosphorylation and the cytosolic [ATP]/[ADP] [Pi]. The decrease in phosphate potential (or change in level of some other metabolite) then leads to membrane depolarization, calcium influx, and contraction. Depolarization and calcium influx are allowed to reach a regenerative level because of low degree of K^+ conductance activation in the plasma membrane. (Reproduced with permission of the publisher from Reference 159. Copyright 1982 by Elsevier Science Publishing Co.)

trachealis smooth muscle of the dog, ATP levels are diminished after an hour of severe hypoxia.[160] The infusion of ATP in the perfused dog,[19] rat, or ferret lung[108] during normoxia causes an increase, rather than a decrease, in pulmonary vascular resistance, which runs contrary to the idea that ATP might maintain vasodilatation. However, during hypoxia ATP infusion does decrease pulmonary vasoconstriction in the anesthetized dog.[161] Carbon monoxide competes with oxygen to bind with cytochrome oxidase at the end of the electron transfer system. To the extent that it binds to cytochrome oxidase, ATP production falls,[162] but carbon monoxide reduces hypoxic pulmonary vasoconstriction rather than enhances it.[163]

The effect of acute hypoxia on cellular ATP levels in pulmonary vascular smooth muscle cells is unknown, however the ratio [ATP]/[ADP] [Pi] decreases both in isolated lung[164] and tumor[165] cells. While it is suggested that a reduction in this ratio may give rise to pulmonary vasoconstriction,[151,159] the converse is true in the coronary vasculature,[166] where several stimuli that reduce the phosphate ratio cause vasodilatation. As discussed at the start of this chapter, the responses of the pulmonary and systemic vasculatures to hypoxia are opposite and thus both could be linked to a reduction in [ATP]/[ADP] [Pi]. The reasons why a decrease in the phosphate ratio should have diametrically different effects in pulmonary and coronary vessels are not apparent, but could involve the concentration of free calcium in the cytoplasm of the smooth muscle near the contractile apparatus.

Cytoplasmic Calcium Concentration

The level of free cytoplasmic calcium is a balance between influx of calcium through the cell membrane, together with release from the cell membrane, the mitochondria, and the sarcoplasmic reticulum on the one hand, and extrusion of calcium through the cell membrane, together with uptake by the cell membrane, the mitochondria, and the sarcoplasmic reticulum on the other. Hypoxia alters several of these fluxes and the net result in the "compartment" associated with the contractile apparatus will determine the effect on smooth muscle tone. In the isolated perfused rat lung, the infusion of verapamil during hypoxic vasoconstriction causes rapid vasodilatation.[159] This is thought to indicate that transmembrane calcium flux is necessary to maintain hypoxic vasoconstriction. In the smooth muscle of the canine trachealis, hypoxia causes a release of intracellular calcium and, in the presence of normal extracellular calcium levels, an influx of calcium as well.[160] Although the net calcium flux is into the cell, there is a greater efflux of calcium from the cell during hypoxia than normoxia. This efflux, from a specific intracellular compartment, coincides with the increase in tension stimulated by hypoxia and suggests that in this preparation intracellular calcium stores play a part in the contraction. Studies on rat portal veins show that hypoxia for 30 minutes causes relaxation and a marked decrease in calcium-containing intramitochondrial granules.[167] In the rabbit aorta intracellular calcium is taken up by the mitochondria under normoxic, but not under hypoxic conditions.[168] These experiments, considered together, indicate an interaction between oxygen tension and the logistics of calcium handling by the smooth muscle cell, both at the cell membrane and in different compartments within the cell.

It is important to realize that the means by which calcium is sequestered varies in different smooth muscles. For example, in the rat aorta calcium is taken up by the mitochondria[168] and sarcoplasmic reticulum,[169] while in the longitudinal smooth muscle of the guinea pig ileum it is taken up primarily by the cell membrane.[169] Calcium sequestration by the sarcoplasmic reticulum of the aortic smooth muscle even varies between different genetic strains of the same species.[170] Rats which develop spontaneous systemic hypertension show reduced calcium uptake by the sarcoplasmic reticulum compared to control normotensive rats. It is possible that a difference of this nature could be responsible for determining susceptibility or resistance to hypoxic pulmonary hypertension.[171]

Vascular smooth muscle mitochondria contain considerably more calcium than mitochondria from other tissues, and the rate of calcium transport is high in pulmonary arterial mitochondria.[172] In uterine smooth muscle the calcium uptake of the mitochondria is much greater than that of the microsomes (plasmalemma and sarcoplasmic reticulum), and is probably responsible for uterine relaxation.[173] The sequestration of calcium by mitochondria from uterine, aortic, and umbilical arterial smooth muscle requires energy and is inhibited by azide.[170,174,175] Calcium efflux from systemic arterial smooth muscle cells is increased by inhibitors of mitochondrial respiration.[176] These observations suggest that mitochondrial calcium release, occurring as a result of a decrease in ATP or the phosphate ratio, might be responsible for some of the pulmonary hypertension caused by metabolic inhibitors and hypoxia.[150] However, the fact that verapamil rapidly inhibits this pulmonary vasoconstriction[159] indicates that at least some of the calcium flux stimulated by hypoxia also occurs across a cell membrane. In some respects this proposed effect of hypoxia on a combination of calcium stores resembles the action of norepinephrine, which initially releases calcium bound within the cell (mitochondria or sarcoplasmic reticulum) and also increases the calcium permeability of the cell membrane, thus sustaining the tonic phase of contraction.[177]

It is possible that the different responses of the pulmonary and systemic vasculatures to hypoxia reflect differences in calcium sequestration and release by the cell membrane, mitochondria, and sarcoplasmic reticulum. For instance, contraction of the canine coronary artery depends for a large part on extracellular calcium entering the smooth muscle cell,[177] while pulmonary arterial smooth muscle can contract in the virtual absence of extracellular calcium,[178] because of the intracellular calcium stored in the sarcoplasmic reticulum and mitochondria.

Redox Status of Pyridine Nucleotides (NADP) and Sulfhydryl Groups

As discussed above, mitochondrial uptake and release of calcium is an important control mechanism in the regulation of cytoplasmic calcium levels. Several groups have demonstrated that the oxidation-reduction state of the pyridine nucleotides controls calcium release in the mitochondria.[179-181] While the role of pyridine nucleotides has been questioned by some,[182,183] it appears that the NADPH/NADP$^+$ ratio is the determining factor, rather than the total NADH+NADPH/NAD$^+$+NADP$^+$ ratio.[184] The importance of the NADPH is that the retention of calcium by the inner mitochondrial membrane depends on the tight binding of MgADP, which in turn is dependent upon the reduced state of certain crucial sulfhydryl groups.[184-186] ATP is necessary for the intramitochondrial transhydrogenation[185,187] which maintains the supply of NADPH that is essential for maintaining glutathione and other sulfhydryl groups in a reduced state (Figure 9). The stoichiometry of this reaction is one high energy bond per NADPH formed,[187] and there has been found to be a fixed relationship between the amount of calcium transported into the mitochondrial matrix and the number of electrons flowing down the electron transfer system.[188] These observations provide a possible mechanism by which the phosphate ratio[151,159] may control intracellular calcium levels through the redox status of NADPH/NADP and GSH/

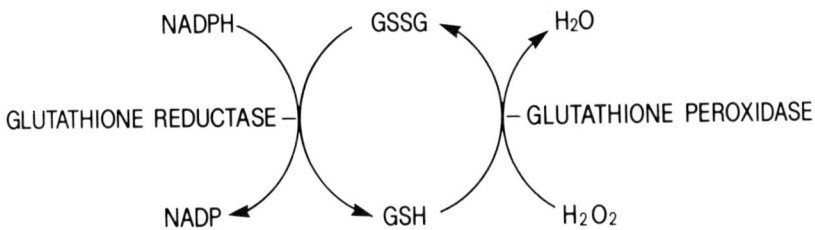

Figure 9. Control of glutathione redox status by supply of NADPH.

GSSG (oxidized glutathione/reduced glutathione). Recent information indicates that the reduced status of sulfhydryl groups also maintains intracellular calcium sequestration outside the mitochondria, including the endoplasmic reticulum.[189]

Oxygen Radicals

Oxygen can alter sulfhydryl redox status in two general ways. As illustrated in Figure 7, NADPH is formed at several points in the course of oxidative glucose metabolism, including the pentose shunt, the pyruvate cycle, and intramitochondrial transhydrogenation. NADPH is essential for the reduction of glutathione (Figure 9), which acts as the cell's main buffer to maintain the reduced status of sulfhydryl groups in membranes and enzymes. The alternative action of oxygen is mediated by the production of oxygen radicals. Radicals such as hydrogen peroxide are formed in the course of normal cellular oxidative metabolism (Figure 7) and the rate of production varies with the ambient level of oxygen in the tissue.[190-192] Figure 9 shows that hydrogen peroxide reduces the ratio GSH/GSSG, which is the opposite effect compared to the metabolism of oxygen associated with the production of NADPH.

The hypothesis that oxygen radicals might play a part in the control of pulmonary vascular tone is speculative, but there is some experimental evidence in support of the possibility. t-Butyl hydroperoxide, which is used because it crosses membranes more readily than hydrogen peroxide, causes oxidation of glutathione and the loss of calcium from cells.[189] The calcium loss can be prevented by pretreatment of the cells with the sulfhydryl reagent, dithiothreitol. t-Butyl hydroperoxide and other oxidants, diamide and 2-butanone peroxide, inhibit hypoxic pulmonary hypertension in the dog[193,194] (Figure 10). The pulmonary vasodilatation produced by diamide can be prevented by pre-incubation of the diamide with reduced glutathione or by pretreatment of the dog with the sulfhydryl reagent acetylcysteine. It seems clear that the vasodilatation induced by these oxidants is caused by the oxidation of sulfhydryl groups. However, the oxidation of sulfhydryl groups in this instance must have an effect in addition to the intracellular release of calcium, which would be expected to cause vasoconstriction, as discussed earlier. The mechanism of the vasodilatation might involve the depletion of a critical pool of calcium,[160,195] the inhibition of a sulfhydryl-containing enzyme,[196,197] or the alteration of leukotriene synthesis through the oxidation of glutathione (GSH) (Figure 5).[198]

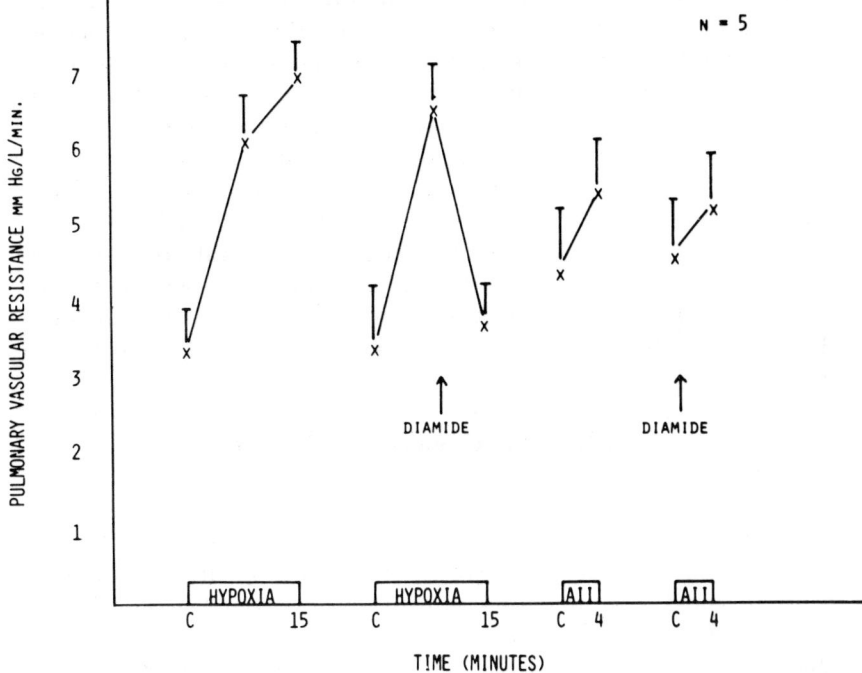

Figure 10. The administration of diamide (5 mg/kg, iv) to 5 anesthetized dogs during an hypoxic challenge (O_2:12%) or angiotensin II infusion (0.5 μg/kg/min) reduces only the pulmonary vascular resistance (PVR) response to hypoxia. $P < 0.01$ for the difference between the changes in PVR stimulated by 15 min of hypoxia, before and after diamide. (Reproduced with permission from Reference 194.)

It is not yet clear whether the release of intracellular calcium by oxygen radicals is a physiologic or a toxic event. Lipid peroxidation caused by oxygen radicals may increase the calcium permeability of cell membranes and the sarcoplasmic reticulum.[199,200] If oxygen radicals are found not to play a physiologic role in the control of the pulmonary vasculature, their formation in the course of lung metabolism and their ability to cause changes in calcium flux suggest that they could be involved in pathologic situations.[201]

Cytochrome P-450

It has been suggested that cytochrome P-450 might form part of the mechanism of hypoxic pulmonary hypertension, causing vasoconstriction when its heme binding site is unoccupied and vasodilatation when the site is occupied by oxygen.[163] Carbon monoxide (11.5%) and metyrapone ditartrate, which can both occupy the heme binding site of cytochrome P-450, inhibit hypoxic vasoconstriction in the isolated pig lung. Subsequent experiments on the relationship between oxygen tension and the rate of O-demethylation of p-nitroanisole by cytochrome P-450 from rabbit lungs, indicate that the reaction is 50% inhibited only at extremely low oxygen tensions: 4 mm Hg[202] and 0.3 mm Hg.[203] The fact that this cytochrome P-450 is not affected until such low oxygen tensions would indicate that it is not a mediator of hypoxic vasoconstriction, although other species of the same enzyme may have a different affinity for oxygen. The means by which the saturation of cytochrome P-450 causes vasodilatation is not apparent.

CLINICAL CORRELATIONS

The clinical significance of hypoxic pulmonary hypertension is easily appreciated in the setting of chronic hypoxic diseases, such as the lung disorders and hypoventilation syndromes described in Chapters 7 and 8. The hypoxic pulmonary vasoconstriction discussed in this chapter, which can be reversed by increasing the inspired oxygen, is an element in the pathophysiology of these conditions. However, in the later stages, when morphologic changes become marked, the vasoconstriction is relatively less important. High altitude pulmonary edema (HAPE) is a more acute condition in which hypoxic pulmonary hypertension is a major component of the disorder. Of 5 subjects susceptible to HAPE, 2 developed pulmonary hypertension (mean pulmonary arterial pressures, Ppa: 26 and 34 mm Hg) during an hypoxic challenge at sea level.[204] After rapid ascent and exercise at high altitude (3,100 m), all subjects had pulmonary hypertension (mean Ppa: 39 mm Hg), which was much greater than that previously reported in normal subjects at higher altitude.[205] The pulmonary hypertension was moderately reduced by breathing 30% or 100% oxygen, indicating that hypoxic vasoconstriction could partially, but not entirely, account for the pathogenesis of HAPE.

The effect of vasodilators on systemic arterial oxygen tension illustrates another area where hypoxic pulmonary vasoconstriction is of clinical importance. Vasodilators have been shown to reduce pulmonary arterial pressure and systemic arterial oxygen tension in patients with chronic obstructive airways disease,[206,207] and with congestive heart failure,[208,209] who might be expected to have localized areas of hypoventilation. It is likely that the vasodilators inhibit the hypoxic vasoconstriction which both shunts blood away from poorly ventilated areas of atelectatic lung and gives rise to the recruitment of alveolar capillaries.[12,13] Consequently, if significant lung pathology is suspected, systemic arterial blood gases should be checked when vasodilator therapy is initiated.

CONCLUSION

An enormous amount of information has been obtained during the last 38 years about the characteristics of acute hypoxic pulmonary hypertension. We now appreciate the great range of species which demonstrate this phenomenon and the environmental and genetic factors that modify it. However, the mechanism which translates a reduction in oxygen tension into pulmonary vasoconstriction is still not certain. The current interest of the proponents of the mediator hypothesis is in leukotrienes. Several groups are studying the direct effects of changes in oxygen tension on the pulmonary vascular smooth muscle. An overall, but speculative, hypothesis which would bridge much of the available information is that a reduction in oxidative phosphorylation is associated with a decrease in NADPH, which in turn permits the oxidation of critical sulfhydryl groups, resulting in the influx of calcium across the cell membrane and the release of intracellular calcium.

Acknowledgments: I am most grateful to Miss Mary Bougetz and Mrs. Margaret Chelmo for their assistance in the preparation of this chapter. Supported by VA research funds and NHLBI Grant HL 23211.

REFERENCES

1. Acosta J: Excerpt from: The natural and moral history of the East and West Indies. 1604, London. In, West JB. *High Altitude Physiology.* Stroudsburg, Pennsylvania, Hutchinson Ross Publishing Co., 1981:9–15.
2. Euler von US, Liljestrand G: Observations on the pulmonary arterial blood pressure in the cat. *Acta Physiol Scand* 1946;12:301–320.
3. Assali MA, Kirschbaum TH, Dilts PV: Effects of hyperbaric oxygen on uteroplacental and fetal circulation. *Circ Res* 1968;22:573–588.

4. Cook CD, Drinker PA, Jacobson HN, Levinson H, Strang LB: Control of pulmonary blood flow in the foetal and newly born lamb. *J Physiol* 1963;169:10–29.
5. Cassin S, Dawes GS, Mott JC, Ross BB, Strang LB: The vascular resistance of the foetal and newly ventilated lung of the lamb. *J Physiol* 1964;171:61–79.
6. Marshall BE, Marshall C: Continuity of response to hypoxic pulmonary vasoconstriction. *J Appl Physiol* 1980;49:189–196.
7. Hiser W, Penman RW, Reeves JT: Preservation of hypoxic pulmonary pressor response in canine pneumococcal pneumonia. *Am Rev Resp Dis* 1975;112:817–822.
8. Goldzimer EK, Konopka RG, Moser KM: Reversal of the perfusion defect in experimental canine lobar pneumococcal pneumonia. *J Appl Physiol* 1978;37:85–91.
9. Colley PS, Cheney FW, Hlastala MP: Ventilation-perfusion and gas exchange effects of sodium nitroprusside in dogs with normal and edematous lungs. *Anesthesiology* 1979;50:489–495.
10. Colley PS, Cheney FW, Hlastala MP: Pulmonary gas exchange effects of nitroglycerin in canine edematous lungs. *Anesthesiology* 1981;55:114–119.
11. Dantzker DR, Bower JS: Pulmonary vascular tone improves VA/Q matching in obliterative pulmonary hypertension. *J Appl Physiol* 1981;51:607–613.
12. Wagner WW Jr, Latham LP, Capen RL: Capillary recruitment during airway hypoxia: Role of pulmonary artery pressure. *J Appl Physiol* 1979;47:383–387.
13. Capen RL, Wagner WW Jr: Intrapulmonary blood flow redistribution during hypoxia increases gas exchange surface area. *J Appl Physiol* 1982;52:1575–1581.
14. Heistad DD, Abboud FM: Circulatory adjustments to hypoxia. *Circulation* 1980;61:463–470.
15. Bohr DF: The pulmonary hypoxic response. *Chest* 1977;71:244–246.
16. Pittman RN: Influence of oxygen lack on vascular smooth muscle contraction. In: Vanhoutte PM, Leusen I, eds. *Vasodilatation.* New York: Raven Press, 1981:181–191.
17. Pittman RN, Quinn JV: A physicochemical model of adenosine's role in hypoxic relaxation of isolated vascular smooth muscle. *Microvasc Res* 1979;17:S37.
18. Scott JB, Chen WT, Swindall BT, Dabney JM, Haddy FJ: Evidence from bioassay studies indicating a role of adenosine in cardiac ischemic and hypoxic dilation in the dog. *Circ Res* 1979;45:451–459.
19. Mentzer RM Jr, Rubio R, Berne RM: Release of adenosine by hypoxic canine lung tissue and its possible role in pulmonary circulation. *Am J Physiol* 1975;229:1625–1631.
20. Satchell GH: Intrinsic vasomotion in the dogfish gill. *J Exp Biol* 1962;39:503–512.
21. Shelton G: The effect of lung ventilation on blood flow to the lungs and body of the amphibian, Xenopus laevis. *Respir Physiol* 1970;9:183–196.
22. Millard RW, Johansen K: Ventricular outflow dynamics in the lizard, Varanus niloticus: Responses to hypoxia, hypercarbia and diving. *J Exp Biol* 1974;60:871–880.

23. Cueva S, Sillau H, Valenzuela A, Ploog H: High altitude induced pulmonary hypertension and right heart failure in broiler chickens. *Res Vet Sci* 1974;16:370–374.
24. Kuida H, Brown AM, Thorne JL, Lange RL, Hecht HM: Pulmonary vascular response to acute hypoxia in normal, unanesthetized calves. *Am J Physiol* 1962;203:391–396.
25. Banchero N, Grover RF, Will JA; High altitude-induced pulmonary arterial hypertension in the llama (Lama glama). *Am J Physiol* 1971;220:422–427.
26. Grant BJB, Davies EE, Jones HA, Hughes JMB: Local regulation of pulmonary blood flow and ventilation-perfusion ratios in the coati mundi. *J Appl Physiol* 1976;40:216–228.
27. Parker HR, Purves MJ: Some effects of maternal hyperoxia and hypoxia on the blood gas tensions and vascular pressures in the foetal sheep. *Q J Exp Physiol* 1967;52:205–221.
28. Lewis AB, Heymann MA, Rudolph AM: Gestational changes in pulmonary vascular responses in fetal lambs in utero. *Circ Res* 1976;39:536–541.
29. Lock JE, Hamilton F, Olley PM, Coceani F: The effect of alveolar hypoxia on pulmonary vascular responsiveness in the conscious newborn lamb. *Can J Physiol Pharmacol* 1980;58:153–159.
30. Rendas A, Branthwaite M, Lennox S, Rein L: Response of the pulmonary circulation to acute hypoxia in the growing pig. *J Appl Physiol* 1982;52:811–814.
31. Kato M, Staub MC; Response of small pulmonary arteries to unilobar hypoxia and hypercapnia. *Circ Res* 1966;19:426–440.
32. Glazier JB, Murray JF: Sites of pulmonary vasomotor reactivity in the dog during alveolar hypoxia and serotonin, and histamine infusion. *J Clin Invest* 1971;50:2550–2580.
33. Quebbman EJ, Dawson CA: Influence of inflation and atelectasis on the hypoxic pressor response in isolated dog lung lobes. *Cardiovasc Res* 1976;10:672–677.
34. Malik AB, Kidd BSL: Pulmonary arterial wedge and left atrial pressures and the site of hypoxic pulmonary vasoconstriction. *Respiration* 1976;33:123–132.
35. Grimm DJ, Dawson CA, Hakin TS, Linehan JH: Pulmonary vasomotion and the distribution of vascular resistance in a dog lung lobe. *J Appl Physiol* 1978;45:545–550.
36. Bjertnaes LJ, Hauge A, Torgrinsen T: The pulmonary vasoconstrictor response to hypoxia. The hypoxia-sensitive site studied with a volatile inhibitor. *Acta Physiol Scand* 1980; 109:447–462.
37. Marshall C, Marshall BE: Influence of perfusate P_{O_2} on hypoxic pulmonary vasoconstriction in rats. *Circ Res* 1983;52:691–696.
38. Kapanci Y, Assimacopoulos A, Irle C, Zwahlen A, Gabbiani G: Contractile interstitial cells in pulmonary alveolar septa: A possible regulator of ventilation/perfusion ratio? *J Cell Biol* 1974;60:375–392.
39. Duane SF, Weir EK, Stewart RM, Niewoehner DE: Distal airway responses to changes in oxygen and carbon dioxide tensions. *Resp Physiol* 1979;38:303–311.
40. Stewart RM, Weir EK, Montgomery MR, Niewoehner DE: Hydrogen peroxide contracts airway smooth muscle: A possible endogenous mechanism. *Resp Physiol* 1981;45:333–342.

41. Sylvester JT, Mitzner W, Ngeow Y, Permutt S: Hypoxic constriction of alveolar and extra-alveolar vessels in isolated pig lungs. *J Appl Physiol* 1983;54:1660–1666.
42. Morgan B, Chruch S, Guntheroth W: Hypoxic constriction of pulmonary artery and vein in intact dogs. *J Appl Physiol* 1968;25:356–361.
43. Furnival CM, Linden RJ, Snow HM: The effect of hypoxia on the pulmonary veins. *J Physiol* 1970;210:43–44.
44. Nagasaka Y, Bhattacharya J, Cgopper MA, Staub NC: Micropuncture measurement of lung microvascular pressure profile during hypoxia in cats. *Fed Proc* 1983;42:595.
45. Koyama T, Horimoto M: Blood flow reduction in local pulmonary microvessels during acute hypoxic imposed on a small fraction of the lung. *Resp Physiol* 1983;52:181–189.
46. Benumof JL, Wahrenbrock EA: Dependency of hypoxic pulmonary vasoconstriction on temperature. *J Appl Physiol* 1977;42:56–58.
47. Daly J deB, Ramsey DJ, Waaler BA: Conditions governing the pulmonary vascular response to ventilation hypoxia in isolated perfused lungs of the dog. *J Physiol* 1962;163:46–47.
48. Nilsen H, Hauge A: Effects of temperature changes on the pressor response to acute alveolar hypoxia in isolated rat lungs. *Acta Physiol Scand* 1968;73:111–120.
49. Sylvester JT, Harabin AL, Peake MD, Frank RS: Vasodilator and constrictor responses to hypoxia in isolated pig lungs. *J Appl Physiol* 1980;45:820–825.
50. Tucker A, Reeves JT: Nonsustained pulmonary vasoconstriction during acute hypoxia in anesthetized dogs. *Am J Physiol* 1975;228:756–761.
51. Harabin AL, Peake MD, Sylvester JT: Effect of severe hypoxia on the pulmonary vascular response to vasoconstrictor agents. *J Appl Physiol* 1981;50:561–565.
52. Peake MD, Harabin AL, Brennan NJ, Sylvester JT: Steady-state vascular responses to graded hypoxia in isolated lungs of five species. *J Appl Physiol* 1981;51:1214–1219.
53. McMurtry IF, Hookway BW, Roos SD: Red blood cells but not platelets prolong vascular reactivity of isolated rat lungs. *Am J Physiol* 1978;234:H186–H191.
54. Hauge A, Melmon KL: Role of histamine in hypoxic pulmonary hypertension in the rat. II. *Circ. Res* 1968;22:385–392.
55. Weir EK, Seavy J, Mlczoch J, Genton E, Reeves JT: Platelets are not essential for the pulmonary vascular pressor response to hypoxia. *J Lab Clin Med* 1976;88:412–416.
56. McGrath RL, Weil JV: Adverse effects of normovolemic polycythemia and hypoxia on hemodynamics in the dog. *Circ Res* 1978;43:793–798.
57. Mlczoch J, Weir EK, Grover RF, Reeves JT: Pulmonary vascular effects of endotoxin in leukopenic dogs. *Am Rev Res Dis* 1976;118:1097–1099.
58. Gorsky BH, Lloyd TC: Effects of perfusate composition on hypoxic vasoconstriction in isolated lung lobes. *J Appl Physiol* 1967;23:683–686.
59. Lloyd TC Jr: Influence of blood pH on hypoxic pulmonary vasoconstriction. *J Appl Physiol* 1966;21:358–364.
60. Rudolph AM, Yuan S: Response of the pulmonary vasculature to hypoxia and H^+ ion concentration changes. *J Clin Invest* 1966;45:399–411.

61. Malik AB, Kidd BSL: Independent effects of changes in H^+ and CO_2 concentrations on hypoxic pulmonary vasoconstriction. *J Appl Physiol* 1973;34:318–324.
62. Silove ED, Inoue T, Grover RF: Comparison of hypoxia, pH, and sympathomimetic drugs on bovine pulmonary vasculature. *J Appl Physiol* 1968;24:355–365.
63. McMurtry IF, Morris KG, Petrun MD: Blunted hypoxic vasoconstriction in lungs from short-term high-altitude rats. *Am J Physiol* 1980; 238:H849–H857.
64. McMurtry IF, Petrun MD, Reeves JT: Lungs from chronically hypoxic rats have decreased pressor response to acute hypoxia. *Am J Physiol* 1978;235:H104–H109.
65. Newman JH, McMurtry IF, Reeves JT: Blunted pulmonary pressor responses to hypoxia in blood perfused, ventilated lungs isolated from oxygen toxic rats: Possible role of prostaglandins. *Prostaglandins* 1981; 22:11–18.
66. Weir EK, Tucker A, Reeves JT, Grover RF: Increased pulmonary vascular pressor response to hypoxia in highland dogs. *Proc Soc Exp Biol Med* 1977;154:112–115.
67. Weir EK, Will DH, Alexander AF, McMurtry IF, Looga R, Reeves JT, Grover RF: Vascular hypertrophy in cattle susceptible to hypoxic pulmonary hypertension. *J Appl Physiol* 1979;46: 517–521.
68. Moore LG, Reeves JT, Will DH, Grover RF: Pregnancy-induced pulmonary hypertension in cows susceptible to high mountain disease. *J Appl Physiol* 1979;46:184–188.
69. Moore LG, Reeves JT: Pregnancy blunts pulmonary vascular reactivity in dogs. *Am J Physiol* 1980;239:H297–301.
70. Fuchs KI, Moore LG, Rounds S: Pulmonary vascular reactivity is blunted in pregnant rats. *J Appl Physiol* 1982;53:703–707.
71. McMurtry IF, Davidson AB, Reeves JT, Grover RF: Inhibition of hypoxic pulmonary vasoconstriction by calcium antagonists in isolated rat lungs. *Circ Res* 1976;38:99–104.
72. Unger M, Atkins, M, Briscoe WA, King TKC: Potentiation of pulmonary vasoconstrictor response with repeated intermittent hypoxia. *J Appl Physiol* 1977;43:662–667.
73. Miller MA, Hales CA: Stability of alveolar hypoxic vasoconstriction with intermittent hypoxia. *J Appl Physiol* 1980;49:846–850.
74. Benumof JL, Wahrenbrock EA: Local effects of anesthetics on regional hypoxia pulmonary vasoconstriction. *Anesthesiology* 1975; 43:525–532.
75. Reeves JT, Grover RF: Blockade of acute hypoxic pulmonary hypertension by endotoxin. *J Appl Physiol* 1974;36:328–332.
76. Weir EK, Mlczoch J, Reeves J, Grover RF: Endotoxin and prevention of hypoxic pulmonary vasoconstriction. *J Lab Clin Med* 1976;88:975–983.
77. Tucker A, Reeves JT, Jackson DL, Grover RF: Decreased pulmonary vascular responses in dogs with increased pulmonary blood flow. *Can J Physiol Pharm* 1978;56:1011–1016.
78. Gregory TJ, Newell JC, Hakim TS, Levitzky MG, Sedransk N: Attenuation of hypoxic pulmonary vasoconstriction by pulsatile flow in dog lungs. *J Appl Physiol* 1982;53:1583–1588.
79. Campbell AGM, Dawes GS, Fishman AP, Hyman AI, Perks AM: The

release of a bradykinin-like vasodilator substance in foetal and new-born lambs. *J Physiol* 1968;195:83–96.
80. Barer GR: Reactivity of the vessels of collapsed and ventilated lungs to drugs and hypoxia. *Circ Res* 1966;18:366–378.
81. Hyman AL, Higashida RT, Spannhake EW, Kadowitz PJ: Pulmonary vasoconstrictor responses to graded decreases in precapillary blood PO_2 in intact-chest cat. *J Appl Physiol* 1981;51: 1009–1016.
82. Marshall C, Marshall BE: Effects of blood PO_2 on hypoxic pulmonary vasoconstriction. *Anesthesiology* 1982;57:A497.
83. Benumof JL, Pirlo AF, Johanson I, Trousdale FR: Interaction of Pv_{O_2} with Pa_{O_2} on hypoxic pulmonary vasoconstriction. *J Appl Physiol* 1981; 51:871–874.
84. Kennedy T, Summer W: Inhibition of hypoxic pulmonary vasoconstriction by nifedipine. *Am J Cardiol* 1982;50:864–868.
85. Tucker A, McMurtry IF, Grover RF, Reeves JT: Attenuation of hypoxic pulmonary vasoconstriction by verapamil in intact dogs. *Proc Soc Exp Biol Med* 1976;151:611–614.
86. Young TE, Lundquist LJ, Chesler E, Weir EK: Comparative effects of nifedipine, verapamil, and diltiazem on experimental pulmonary hypertension. *Am J Cardiol* 1983;51:195–200.
87. McMurtry IF, Reeves JT, Will DH, Grover RF: Reduction of bovine pulmonary hypertension by normoxia, verapamil and hexaprenaline. *Experientia* 1977;33:1191–1193.
88. Simonneau G, Escourrou P, Duroux P, Lockhart A: Inhibition of hypoxic pulmonary vasoconstriction by nifedipine. *N Engl J Med* 1981; 304:1582–1585.
89. Furchgott RF, Zawadzki JV: The obligatory role of endothelial cells in the relaxation of arterial smooth muscle by acetylcholine. *Nature* 1980; 288:373–376.
90. Cherry PD, Furchgott RF, Zawadzki JV, Jothianandan D. Role of endothelial cells in relaxation of isolated arteries by bradykinin. *Proc Natl Acad Sci* 1982;79:2106–2110.
91. Vanhoutte PM, DeMey J: Control of vascular smooth muscle function by the endothelial cells. *Gen Pharmacol* 1983;14:39–41.
92. Benumof JL, Mathers JM, Wahrenbrock EA: The pulmonary interstitial compartment and the mediator of hypoxic pulmonary vasoconstriction. *Microvasc Res* 1978;15:69–75.
93. Bergofsky EH: Active control of the normal pulmonary circulation. In: Moser KM, ed. *Pulmonary Vascular Diseases.* New York: Marcel Dekker, Inc., 1979:233–277.
94. Haas F, Bergofsky EH: Role of the mast cell in the pulmonary pressor response to hypoxia. *J Clin Invest* 1972;51:3154–3162.
95. Tucker A, Weir EK, Reeves JT, Grover RF: Histamine H_1- and H_2-receptors in the pulmonary and systemic vasculature of the dog. *Am J Physiol* 1975;229:1008–1013.
96. Hales CA, Kazemi H: Role of histamine in the hypoxic vascular response of the lung. *Resp Physiol* 1975;24:81–88.
97. Tucker A, Weir EK, Reeves JT, Grover RF: Failure of histamine antagonists to prevent hypoxic pulmonary vasoconstriction in dogs. *J Appl Physiol* 1976;40:496–500.

98. Stark RD, Joshi RC, Bishop JM: Failure of an antagonist of histamine—chlorpheniramine—to modify the pulmonary vascular response to hypoxia in chronic bronchitis. *Cardiovasc Res* 1977;11:219–222.
99. Rengo F, Trimarco B, Chiariello M, Ricciardelli B, Volpe M, Violini R, Rasetti G: Histamine and hypoxic pulmonary hypertension. A quantitative study. *Cardiovasc Res* 1978;12:752–757.
100. Rengo F, Trimarco B, Ricciardelli B, Volpe M, Violini R, Sacca L, Chiariello M: Effects of disodium cromoglycate on hypoxic pulmonary hypertension in dogs. *J Pharmacol Exp Ther* 1979;211: 686–689.
101. Mungall IPF: Hypoxia and lung mast cells; influence of disodium cromoglycate. *Thorax* 1976;31:94–100.
102. Tucker A, McMurtry IF, Alexander AF, Reeves JT, Grover RF: Lung mast cell density and distribution in chronically hypoxic animals. *J Appl Physiol* 1977;42:174–178.
103. Martin LF, Tucker A, Munroe ML, Reeves JT: Lung mast cells and hypoxic pulmonary vasoconstriction in cats. *Respiration* 1978; 36:73–77.
104. Zhu YJ, Kradin R, Brandstetter RD, Staton G, Moss J, Hales CA; Hypoxic pulmonary hypertension in the mast cell-deficient mouse. *J Appl Physiol* 1983;54:680–686.
105. Porcelli RJ, Viau A, Demeny M, Naftchi NE, Bergofsky EH: Relation between hypoxic pulmonary vasoconstriction, its humoral mediators and alpha-beta adrenergic receptors. *Chest* 1977;71: 249–251.
106. Porcelli RJ, Bergofsky EH: Adrenergic receptors in pulmonary vasoconstrictor responses to gaseous and humoral agents. *J Appl Physiol* 1973; 34:483–488.
107. Barer GR, McCurrie JR: Pulmonary vasomotor responses in the cat; the effects and inter-relationships of drugs, hypoxia and hypercapnia. *Q J Exp Physiol* 1969;54:156–172.
108. Barer GR, Emery CJ, Mohammed FH, Mungall IPF: H_1 and H_2 histamine actions on lung vessels; their relevance to hypoxic vasoconstriction. *Q J Exp Physiol* 1978;63:157–169.
109. Lloyd TC: Effect of alveolar hypoxia on pulmonary vascular resistance. *J Appl Physiol* 1964;19:1086–1094.
110. Silove ED, Grover RF: Effects of alpha adrenergic blockade and tissue catecholamine depletion on pulmonary vascular response to hypoxia. *J Clin Invest* 1968;47:274–285.
111. Malik AB, Kidd BSL: Adrenergic blockade and the pulmonary vascular response to hypoxia. *Res Physiol* 1973;19:96–106.
112. Daly I de B, Michel CC, Ramsay DJ, Waaler BA; Conditions governing the pulmonary vascular response to ventilation hypoxia and hypoxaemia in the dog. *J Physiol* 1968; 196:351–379.
113. Lewis AB, Heymann MA, Rudolph AM: Gestational changes in pulmonary vascular responses in fetal lambs in utero. *Circ Res* 1976;39: 536–541.
114. Lloyd TC: Role of nerve pathways in the hypoxic vasoconstriction of the lung. *J Appl Physiol* 1966;21:1351–1355.
115. Goldring RA, Turino GM, Cohen G, Jameson AG, Bass BG, Fishman AP: The catecholamines in the pulmonary arterial pressor response to acute hypoxia. *J Clin Invest* 1964;41: 1211–1220.
116. Berkov S: Hypoxic pulmonary vasoconstriction in the rat. *Circ Res* 1974; 35:256–261.

117. Hales CA, Rouse ET, Kazemi H: Failure of saralasin acetate, a competitive inhibitor of angiotensin II, to diminish alveolar hypoxic vasoconstriction in the dog. *Cardiovasc Res* 1977;11: 541–546.
118. Hyman A, Heyman MA, Levin DL, Rudolph AM: Angiotensin is not the mediator of hypoxia-induced pulmonary vasoconstriction in fetal lambs. *Circulation* 1975;52:II–132.
119. Prewitt RL, Leffler CW: Feline hypoxic pulmonary vasoconstriction is not blocked by the angiotensin I-converting enzyme inhibitor, captopril. *Cardiovasc Pharmacol* 1981;3:293–298.
120. Suggett AJ, Mohammed FH, Barer GR: Angiotensin, hypoxia, verapamil and pulmonary vessels. *Clin Exp Pharmacol Physiol* 1980;7:263–274.
121. Wanner A, Begin R, Cohn M, Sackner MA; Vascular volumes of the pulmonary circulation in intact dogs. *J Appl Physiol* 1978; 44:956–963.
122. Rickaby DA, Dawson CA, Maron MB: Pulmonary inactivation of serotonin and site of serotonin pulmonary vasoconstriction. *J Appl Physiol* 1980;48:606–612.
123. Harris P, Fritts HW Jr, Cournand A: Some circulatory effects of 5-hydroxytryptamine in man. *Circulation* 1969;21:1134–1139.
124. Boe J, Simonsson BG, Stahl E: Effect of histamine, 5-hydroxytryptamine and prostaglandins on isolated human pulmonary arteries. *Eur J Respir Dis* 1980;61:12–19.
125. Keith IM, Will JA: Hypoxia and the neonatal rabbit lung: Neuroendocrine cell numbers, 5-HT fluorescence intensity, and the relationship to arterial thickness. *Thorax* 1981;36:767–773.
126. Hakim TS, Michel RP, Minami H, Chang HK: Site of pulmonary hypoxic vasoconstriction studies with arterial and venous occlusion. *J Appl Physiol* 1983;54:1298–1302.
127. Said SI, Yoshida T, Kitamura S, Vriem C: Pulmonary alveolar hypoxia: Release of prostaglandins and other humoral mediators. *Science* 1974; 285:1181–1183.
128. Vaage J, Hauge A: Prostaglandins and the pulmonary vasoconstrictor response to alveolar hypoxia. *Science* 1975;189:899–900.
129. Weir EK, McMurtry IF, Tucker A, Reeves JT, Grover RF: Prostaglandin synthetase inhibitors do not decrease hypoxic pulmonary vasoconstriction. *J Appl Physiol* 1976;41:714–718.
130. Weir EK, Reeves JT, Grover RF: Meclofenamate and indomethacin augment the pulmonary pressor response to hypoxia and exogenous prostaglandin $F_2\alpha$ *Physiologist* 1974;17:355.
131. Afonso S, Bandow GT, Rowe GG: Indomethacin and the prostaglandin hypothesis of coronary blood flow regulation. *J Physiol* 1974;241: 299–308.
132. Vaage J, Bjertnaes L, Hauge A: The pulmonary vasoconstrictor response to hypoxia: Effects of inhibitors of prostaglandin biosynthesis. *Acta Physiol Scand* 1975;95:95–101.
133. Tyler TL, Wallis RG, Leffler CW, Cassin S: The effects of indomethacin on the pulmonary vascular response to hypoxia in the premature and mature newborn goat. *Proc Soc Exp Biol Med* 1975;150:695–698.
134. Weir EK, McMurtry IF, Tucker A, Reeves JT, Grover RF: Inhibition of prostaglandin synthesis or blockade of prostaglandin action increase the pulmonary pressor response to hypoxia. In: Samuelsson B, Paoletti R. eds. *Advances in Prostaglandin and Thromboxane Research*. Vol. 2. New York: Raven Press, 1976:914–915.

135. Hales CA, Rouse E, Buchwald IA, Kazemi H: Role of prostaglandins in alveolar hypoxic vasoconstriction. *Resp Physiol* 1977; 29:151–162.
136. Hanna CJ, Bach MK, Pare PD, Schellenberg RR: Slow-reacting substances (leukotrienes) contract human airway and pulmonary vascular smooth muscle in vitro. *Nature* 1981;290:343–344.
137. Piper PJ, Samborn MN: The mechanism of action of leukotrienes C_4 and D_4 in guinea pig isolated perfused lung and parenchymal strips of guinea pig, rabbit and cat. *Prostaglandins* 1981;21:793–803.
138. Gerber JG, Voelkel N, Nies AS, McMurtry IF, Reeves JT: Moderation of hypoxic vasoconstriction by infused arachidonic acid: Role of PGI_2. *J Appl Physiol* 1980;49:107–112.
139. Weir EK, Grover RF: The role of endogenous prostaglandins in the pulmonary circulation. *Anesthesiology* 1978;48:201–212.
140. Hamasaki Y, Tai HH, Said SI: Hypoxia stimulates prostacyclin generation by dog lung in vitro. *Prostaglandin Leuk Med* 1982;8: 311–316.
141. Hales CA, Rouse ET, Slate JL: Influence of aspirin and indomethacin on variability of alveolar hypoxic vasoconstriction. *J Appl Physiol* 1978; 45:33–39.
142. Ahmed T, Oliver W, Jr, Wanner A: Variability of hypoxic pulmonary vasoconstriction in sheep. *Am Rev Respir Dis* 1983;127: 59–62.
143. Ahmed T, Oliver W Jr: Does slow-reacting substance of anaphylaxis mediate hypoxic pulmonary vasoconstriction? *Am Rev Respir Dis* 1983; 127:566–571.
144. Morganroth ML, Murphy RC, Voelkel NF: Diethylcarbanazime (DEC), a leukotriene synthesis blocker, blocks hypoxic pulmonary vasoconstriction. *Fed Proc* 1983;42:303.
145. Sirois P, Brousseau Y: Leukotriene transformation by guinea-pig lungs. *Prostaglandins Leuk Med* 1983;10:133–143.
146. Ahmed T, Oliver W Jr, Frank BL, Robinson MJ, Wanner A: Hypoxic pulmonary vasoconstriction in conscious sheep. Role of mast cell degranulation. *Am Rev Respir Dis* 1982;126:291–297.
147. Porcelli RJ, Ventura DF, Mahoney WA, Bergofsky E: Role of histamine in regulating pulmonary vascular tone and reactivity. *J Appl Physiol* 1981; 51:1320–1325.
148. Mullane KM, Dusting GJ, Salmon JA, Moncada S, Vane J: Biotransformation and cardiovascular effects of arachidonic acid in the dog. *Eur J Pharmacol* 1979;54:217–228.
149. Spannhake EW, Hyman AL, Kadowitz PJ: Dependence of the airway and pulmonary vascular effects of arachidonic acid upon route and rate of administration. *J Pharmacol Exp Ther* 1980;212: 584–590.
150. Rounds S, McMurtry IF: Inhibitors of oxidative ATP production cause transient vasoconstriction and block subsquent pressor responses in rat lungs. *Circ Res* 1981;48:393–400.
151. McMurtry IF, Rounds S, Stanbrook HS: Studies of the mechanism of hypoxic pulmonary vasoconstriction. *Adv Shock Res* 1982; 8:21–33.
152. Rhoades RA, Shaw ME, Eskew ML: Influence of altered O_2 tension on substrate metabolism in perfused rat lung. *Am J Physiol* 1975;229: 1476–1479.
153. Longmore WJ, Mourning JT: Lactate production in isolated perfused rat lung. *Am J Physiol* 1976;231:351–354.
154. Tierney DF: Lactate metabolism in rat lung tissue. *Arch Intern Med* 1971; 127:858–860.

155. McDowall DG: Biochemistry of hypoxia: Current concepts. II: Biochemical derangements associated with hypoxia and their measurement. *Br J Anaesth* 1969;41:251–256.
156. Liang C-S: Metabolic control of circulation: Effects of iodoacetate and fluoroacetate. *J Clin Invest* 1977;60:61–69.
157. Stanbrook HS, McMurtry IF; Inhibition of glycolysis potentiates hypoxic vasoconstriction in rat lungs. *J Appl Physiol* 1983;55:1467–1473.
158. Lloyd TC: Pulmonary vasoconstriction during histotoxic hypoxia. *J Appl Physiol* 1965;20:488–490.
159. McMurtry IF, Stanbrook HS, Rounds S: The mechanism of hypoxic pulmonary vasoconstriction: A working hypothesis. In: Loeppky JA, Riedesel ML, eds. *Oxygen Transport to Human Tissues*. New York: Elsevier North Holland Inc.1982:77–89.
160. Kroeger E, Stephens NL: Effect of hypoxia on energy and calcium metabolism in airway smooth muscle. *Am J Physiol* 1971; 220:1199–1204.
161. Benumof JL, Fukunaga AF, Trousdale FR; ATP inhibits hypoxic pulmonary vasoconstriction. *Anesthesiology* 1982;57:A474.
162. Bassett DJP, Fisher AB: Metabolic response to carbon monoxide by isolated rat lungs. *Am J Physiol* 1976;230:658–663.
163. Sylvester JT, McGowen C: The effects of agents that bind to cytochrome P-450 on hypoxic pulmonary vasoconstriction. *Circ Res* 1978;43: 429–347.
164. Peres-Diaz J, Martin-Requero A, Parrilla R, Ayuso-Parrilla MS: Relationship between cellular energy production and rates of glucose utilization by lung cells. *Pflugers Arch* 1977;371:19–24.
165. Wilson DF, Erecinska M, Drown C, Silver IA: The oxygen dependence of cellular energy metabolism. *Arch Biochem Biophys* 1979;195:485–493.
166. Nuutinen EM, Nishiki K, Erecinska M, Wilson DF: Role of mitochondrial oxidative phosphorylation in regulation of coronary blood flow. *Am J Physiol* 1982;243:H159–H169.
167. Ebeigbe AB: Vascular smooth muscle responses to hypoxia and calcium withdrawal: Ultrastructural and mechanical observations. *IRCS Med Science* 1980;8:549.
168. Karki H, Suzuki T, Ozaki H, Urakawa N, Ishida Y: Dissociation of K^+-induced tension and cellular Ca^{2+} retension in vascular and intestinal smooth muscle in normoxia and hypoxia. *Pflugers Arch* 1982;394: 118–123.
169. Hurwitz L, Fitzpatrick DF, Debbas G, Landon EJ: Localization of calcium pump activity in smooth muscle. *Science* 1973;179:384.
170. Moore L, Hurwitz L, Davenport GR, Landon EJ: Energy-dependent calcium uptake activity of microsomes from the aorta of normal and hypertensive rats. *Biochem Biophys Acta* 1975;413: 432–443.
171. Weir EK, Tucker A, Reeves JT, Will DH, Grover RF: The genetic factor influencing pulmonary hypertension in cattle at high altitude. *Cardiovasc Res* 1974;6:745–749.
172. Vallieres J, Scarpa A, Somlyo AP: Subcellular fractions of smooth muscle: isolation, substrate utilization and Ca^{++} transport by main pulmonary artery and mesenteric vein mitochondria. *Arch Biochem Biophys* 1975;170:659–669.
173. Batra S: Some aspects of calcium uptake by human myometrial mitochondria and microsomes relevant to relaxation. *Acta Physiol Scand* 1982; 114:92–95.

174. Fitzpatrick DF, Landon EJ, Debbas G, Hurwitz L: A calcium pump in vascular smooth muscle. *Science* 1972;176:305–306.
175. Clyman RI, Manganiello VC, Vaughan M. Oxygen: Influence of cyclic nucleotides and calcium sequestration in the human umbilical artery. *Chest* 1977;71:247–249.
176. Greenberg S, Heitz DC, Brody MJ, Wilson WR, Diecke FPJ, Long JP: Differential effect of metabolic inhibitors on myogenic tone and contractility in isolated tibial arteries. *J Pharmacol Exp Ther* 1974;191:458–467.
177. Van Breeman C, Aaronson P, Loutzenhiser R, Meisheri K: Ca^{2+} movements in smooth mucle. *Chest* 1980;78:157–165.
178. Devine CE, Somlyo AV, Somlyo AP: Sarcoplasmic reticulum and excitation-contraction coupling in mammalian smooth muscles. *J Cell Biol* 1972;52:690–718.
179. Lehninger AL, Vercesi A, Bababunmi EA: Regulation of Ca^{2+} release from mitochondria by the oxidation-reduction state of pyridine nucleotides. *Proc Natl Acad Sci USA* 1978;75:1690–1694.
180. Lotscher HR, Winterhalter KH, Carafoli E, Richter C: Hydroperoxides can modulate the redox state of pyridine nucleotides and the calcium balance in rat liver mitochondria. *Proc Natl Acad Sci USA* 1979;76: 4340–4344.
181. Lotscher HR, Winterhalter KH, Carafoli E, Richter C: Hydroperoxide-induced loss of pyridine nucleotides and release of calcium from rat liver mitochondria. *J Biol Chem* 1980;255: 9325–9330.
182. Wolkowicz PE, McMillin-Wood J: Dissociation between mitochondrial calcium ion release and pyridine nucleotide oxidation. *J Biol Chem* 1980;255:10348–10353.
183. Beatrice MC, Palmer JW, Pfeiffer DR: The relationship between mitochondrial membrane permeability membrane potential, and the retention of Ca^{2+} by mitochondria. *J Biol Chem* 1980;255: 8663–8671.
184. Roth Z, Dikstein S. Inhibition of ruthenium red-insensitive mitochondrial Ca^{2+} release and its pyridine nucleotide specificity. *Biochem Biophys Res Comm* 1982;105:991–996.
185. Harris EJ, Al-Shaikhaly M, Baum H: Stimulation of mitochondrial calcium ion efflux by thiol-specific reagents and by thyroxine. *Biochem J* 1979;182:455–464.
186. Le-Quoc K, Le-Quoc D. Control of the mitochondrial inner membrane permeability by sulfhydryl groups. *Arch Biochem Biophys* 1982;216: 639–651.
187. Rydstrom J: Energy-linked nicotinamide nucleotide transhydrogenases. *Biochem Biophys Acta* 1977;463:155–184.
188. Lehninger AL, Reynafarje B, Vercesi A, Tew WP: Transport and accumulation of calcium in mitochondria. In, *Calcium Transport and Cell Function*. Scarpa A, Carafoli E, (Eds). Vol. 307, 1978; pp. 160–176.
189. Jewell SA, Bellomo G, Thor H, Orrenius S. Bleb formation in hepatocytes during drug metabolism is caused by disturbances in thiol and calcium ion homeostasis. *Science* 1982;217:1257–1259.
190. Boveris A: Mitochondrial production of superoxide radical and hydrogen peroxide. *Adv Exp Med Biol* 1977;78:67–82.
191. Freeman BA, Crapo JD: Hyperoxia increases oxygen radical production in rat lungs and lung mitochondria. *J Biol Chem* 1981;256: 10986–10992.

192. Freeman BA, Topolosky MK, Crapo JD: Hyperoxia increases oxygen radical production in rat lung homogenates. *Arch Biochem Biophys* 1982; 216:477–484.
193. Weir EK, Will JA. Oxidants: A new group of pulmonary vasodilators. *Bull Eur Physiopath Resp* 1982;18:81–95.
194. Weir EK, Will JA, Lundquist LJ, Eaton JW, Chesler E: Diamide inhibits pulmonary vasoconstriction induced by hypoxia or prostaglandin $F_2\alpha$. *Proc Soc Exp Biol Med* 1983;173:96–103.
195. Bellomo G, Jewell SA, Thor H, Orrenius S: Regulation of intracellular calcium compartmentation: Studies with isolated hepatocytes and t-butyl hydroperoxide. *Proc Natl Acad Sci USA* 1982;79: 6842–6846.
196. Scutari G, Ballestrin G, Covas AL: Divalent cation dependent ATPase activities of red blood cell membranes: Influence of the oxidation of membrane thiol groups close to each other. *J Supramol Struc* 1980;14: 1–11.
197. Gilbert HF: Biological disulfides: The third messenger? *J Biol Chem* 1982;257;12086–12091.
198. Hammarstrom S: Leukotrienes. *Ann Rev Biochem* 1983;52: 355–377.
199. Lebedev AV, Levitsky DO, Loginov VA, Smirnov VN: The effect of primary products of lipid peroxidation on the transmembrane transport of calcium ions. *J Mol Cell Card* 1982;14:99–103.
200. Levedev AV, Levitsky DO, Loginov VA: Oxygen as an inductor of divalent cation permeability through biological and lipid membranes. In: Chazov EI, Smirnov VN, Dhalla NS, Eds. *Advances in Myocardiology*, Vol. 3, New York: Plenum Publishing Corp., 1982:325–438.
201. Kappus H, Sies H: Toxic drug effects associated with oxygen metabolism: Redox cycling and lipid peroxidation. *Experientia* 1981;37: 1233–1241.
202. Knoblauch A, Sybert A, Brennan NJ, Sylvester JT, Gurtner GH: Effect of hypoxia and CO on a cytochrome P-450-mediated reaction in rabbit lungs. *J Appl Physiol* 1981, 51:1635–1642.
203. Fisher AB, Itakura N, Dodia C, Thurman RG: Relationship between alveolar PO_2 and the rate of p-nitroanisole O-demethylation by the cytochrome P-450 pathway in isolated rabbit lungs. *J Clin Invest* 1979; 64:770–774.
204. Hultgren HN, Grover RF, Hartley LH: Abnormal circulatory responses to high altitude in subjects with a previous history of high-altitude pulmonary edema. *Circulation* 1971;44:759–770.
205. Kronenberg RS, Safar P, Lee J, Wright F, Noble W, Wahrenbrock E, Hickey R, Nemoto E, Severinghaus JW: Pulmonary artery pressure and alveolar gas exchange in man during acclimatization to 12,400 feet. *J Clin Invest* 1971;50:827–844.
206. Chick TW, Kochukoshy KN, Matsumoto S, Leach JK: The effect of nitroglycerin on gas exchange, hemodynamics, and oxygen transport in patients with chronic obstructive pulmonary disease. *Am J Med Sci* 1978; 276:105–111.
207. Simonneau G, Escourrou P, Duroux P, Lockhart A: Inhibition of hypoxic pulmonary vasoconstriction by nifedipine. *N Engl J Med* 1981;304: 1582–1585.

208. Mookherjee S, Keighley JF, Warner RA, Bowser MA, Obeid AI: Hemodynamic, ventilatory and blood gas changes during infusion of sodium nitroferricyanide (Nitroprusside): Studies in patients with congestive heart failure. *Chest* 1977;72:273–278.
209. Pierpont GL, Hale KA, Franciosa JA, Cohn JN: Effects of vasodilators on pulmonary hemodynamics and gas exchange in left ventricular failure. *Am Heart J* 1980;99:208–216.

CHAPTER 7

PULMONARY HYPERTENSION SECONDARY TO LUNG DISEASE

Lewis J. Rubin

INTRODUCTION

The pulmonary vascular bed can be damaged by diseases which attack it primarily, such as idiopathic pulmonary hypertension, as well as by cardiac conditions which affect it secondarily, such as congenital or valvular heart disease. The intimate relationship between the pulmonary circulation and the lung parenchyma also renders the pulmonary vasculature vulnerable to disorders which interfere with the structure or function of the respiratory system. This chapter will address the effects of chronic respiratory diseases on the pulmonary circulation.

DEFINITION

The modern recognition of the effects of chronic respiratory diseases on the heart and pulmonary circulation dates back to 1931, when Dr. Paul Dudley White coined the term "cor pulmonale." The World Health Organization defines cor pulmonale as "hypertrophy of the right ventricle resulting from diseases affecting the function and/or structure of the lung, except when the pulmonary alterations are the result of diseases that primarily affect the left side of the heart or of congenital heart disease."[1] Although many clinicians equate cor pulmonale with overt right ventricular failure, it is worth emphasizing that right-sided failure is a late manifestation of pulmonary heart disease, and need not be present for the clinician to entertain the diagnosis of cor pulmonale. The classification of conditions causing cor pulmonale proposed by the World Health Organization provides a useful foundation for a discussion of this entity (Table 1).

EPIDEMIOLOGY

It is estimated that chronic lung diseases affect approximately 47 million people in this country and account for over 80,000 deaths per year. Equally sobering is the fact that chronic respiratory disease is the most rapidly increasing of the top 10 leading causes of death in the United States, rising at a rate of 1.4% per year.[2]

The prevalence of cor pulmonale among the population with chronic respiratory diseases is not known, but it has been estimated that between 16 and 38% of hospital admissions for congestive heart failure in this country are for exacerbations of chronic cor pulmonale.[3] Similar

TABLE 1
Conditions Associated with Cor Pulmonale

Diseases associated with hypoxic pulmonary vasoconstriction
- Chronic obstructive lung disease
- Bronchiectasis
- Chronic mountain sickness
- Cystic fibrosis
- Idiopathic alveolar hypoventilation
- Obesity hypoventilation syndrome
- Neuromuscular disease
- Kyphoscoliosis
- Pleuropulmonary fibrosis
- Upper airway obstruction

Diseases producing obstruction or obliteration of the pulmonary vasculature
- Pulmonary embolism
- Pulmonary fibrosis
- Pulmonary lymphangitic carcinomatosis
- Idiopathic pulmonary hypertension
- Progressive systemic sclerosis
- Sarcoidosis
- Intravenous drug use
- Pulmonary vasculitis
- Pulmonary venoocclusive disease

statistics have been generated from studies in large municipal hospitals in other industrialized countries where cigarette smoking, pollutants, and other environmental exposures undoubtedly contribute to the increasing incidence of chronic airways disease.[4-6] Next to hypertensive and atherosclerotic heart disease, cor pulmonale is the most common cardiac condition in patients beyond the fifth decade of life.

The importance of coexistent pulmonary hypertension in the setting of chronic respiratory disease lies not only with its contribution to the morbidity from lung disease but also to mortality. Burrows et al. reported that the presence and severity of pulmonary hypertension correlated more closely than any other variable with survival in a series of patients with chronic lung disease.[7] In their study, no patient with a pulmonary vascular resistance >550 dyne sec cm^{-5} survived 3 years, while 36% of patients with severe obstructive lung disease ($FEV_1 < 0.85$ litres) without pulmonary hypertension survived 3 years or longer. Similarly, Bishop studied a group of 128 patients with chronic bronchitis: 90% of patients with a normal pulmonary arterial pressure when first evaluated were alive 5 years later, and mortality rates in patients with elevated pulmonary arterial pressures increased progressively with increasing levels of pulmonary artery pressure[8] (Figure 1). Less than 10% of Bishop's patients who had a mean pulmonary artery pressure of 45 mm Hg or higher were alive at 5 years. Traver et al.[9] reported a mortality rate of 50% at 13.5 years in patients with high values for post-bronchodilator FEV_1 when there were no signs of cor pulmonale, and a 50% mortality rate at 7.0 years in the patients with comparable spirometric results in whom cor pulmonale was present.

PATHOGENESIS

The normal pulmonary circulation can accommodate a maximal right ventricular output with an increase in pressure of only several millimeters of mercury by one or both of two adaptive mechanisms—distension of existing vessels or recruitment of unused vessels. Patients with chronic lung diseases have larger than normal increases in pulmonary arterial pressure with maneuvers which increase pulmonary blood flow, such as exercise,[10-12] even at the stage when resting hemodynamics are normal, implying an inability to either further dilate the vasculature or recruit additional unused vasculature. Conditions such as emphysema and pulmonary fibrosis destroy large segments of lung parenchyma, but it is unlikely that loss of cross-sectional

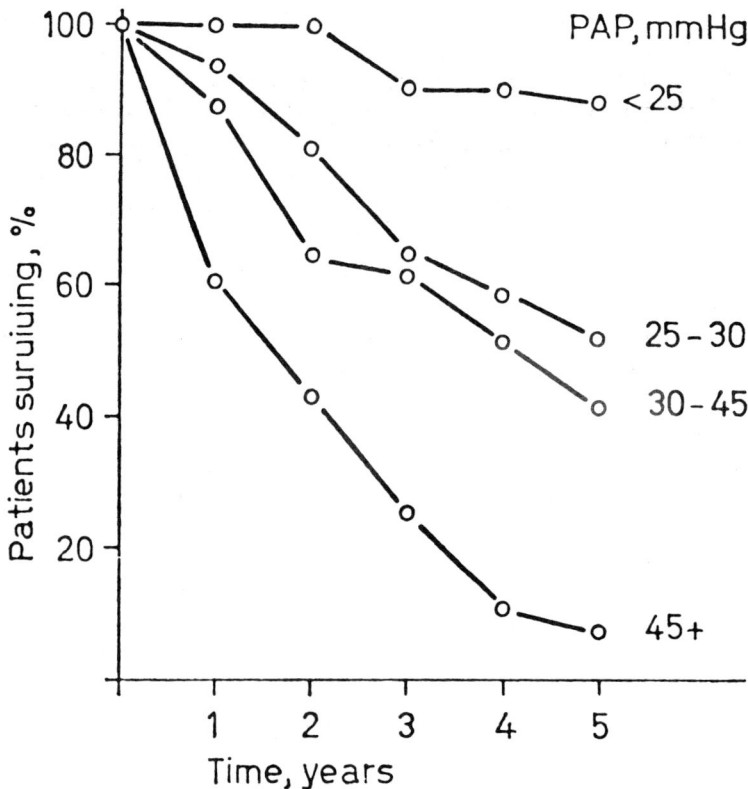

Figure 1. Correlation between mortality and mean pulmonary arterial pressure in patients with chronic bronchitis. (Reproduced with permission from Reference 8.)

surface area of the pulmonary vascular bed accounts for all the elevation in perfusion pressure because pulmonary hypertension is, at least in part, reversible in these conditions. In addition, experiments in dogs have shown that two-thirds of the lung parenchyma must be ablated before pulmonary arterial pressure increases appreciably.[13]

It is generally accepted that the derangements in intrapulmonary gas exchange which occur in chronic lung disease produce the major inciting factors of pulmonary hypertension. Alveolar hypoxia is a potent stimulus for constriction of precapillary pulmonary vessels,[14,15] and acidosis or hypercarbia potentiate this effect.[16,17] The pulmonary vasoconstrictor effects of alveolar hypoxia appear to be a locally mediated phenomenon, since an hypoxic pressor response can be elicited in denervated lungs in vivo and in isolated perfused lung systems.[18] These observations have prompted a search for chemical mediators which may be responsible for hypoxic pulmonary vasoconstriction. Although several candidates have been advocated, including histamine, serotonin, prostaglandins, and other products of the arachidonic acid cascade, there is to date no conclusive evidence supporting a role for any or all of these vasoactive substances as mediators of hypoxic pulmonary vasoconstriction.[19] (See Chapter 6.)

Factors other than alveolar hypoxia may play a role in the genesis and maintenance of pulmonary hypertension, since the use of continuous supplemental oxygen often has little effect on pulmonary artery pressure in lung disease, despite improving alveolar and arterial oxygenation. Harris et al.[20] have suggested that the increased airways resistance in patients with chronic obstructive lung disease may raise the transmural pulmonary vascular pressure and contribute to an increased pulmonary vascular resistance. Recent experiments in intact animals under conditions of controlled lobar flow have also suggested that the degree of mixed venous hypoxemia may be an additional stimulus for precapillary pulmonary vasoconstriction.[21,22] Secondary polycythemia might also contribute to the development of pulmonary hypertension in chronic hypoxia, presumably by increasing blood viscosity and raising both basal vascular resistance and the increase in vascular resistance produced by hypoxia.[23] It is also possible that other influences, such as extrapulmonary reflexes stimulated by systemic arterial hypoxemia or other as yet undefined stimuli unique to chronic lung disease, may contribute to the development of pulmonary vasoconstriction as well.

The sustained elevation in pulmonary vascular tone which results from active pulmonary vasoconstriction leads to an inexorable sequence of events (Figure 2): the increased right ventricular afterload causes pulmonary blood flow to decrease and eventually produces right ventricular failure. The decrease in systemic oxygen transport which results from the low cardiac output will produce tissue and mixed venous hypoxemia which, as mentioned previously, may provide a further stimulus for pulmonary vasoconstriction.

However, the incidence of heart failure seems disproportionately high considering the mild-to-moderate degree of pulmonary hypertension typically found in the hypoventilating pulmonary disease patients. This stands in contrast to the less frequent occurrence of heart failure in patients with primary pulmonary hypertension in whom the increase in pulmonary vascular resistance is often so severe as to have produced syncope due to inadequate cardiac output and cerebral

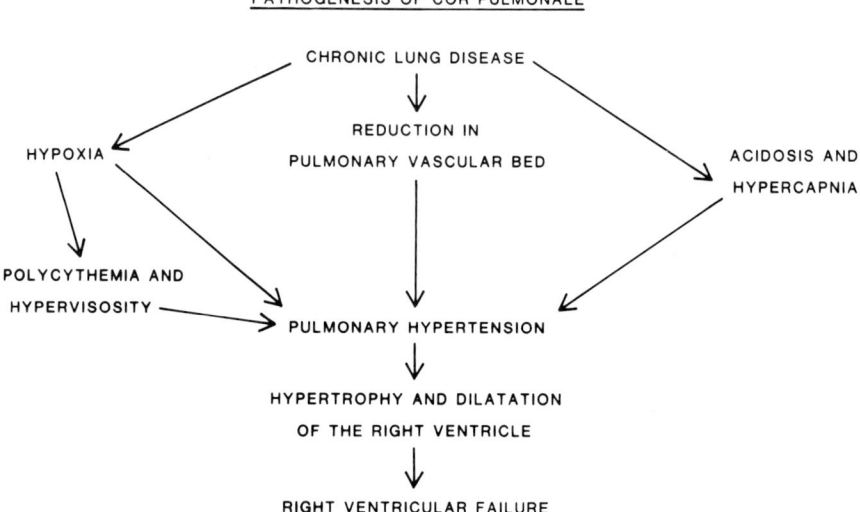

Figure 2. *Sequence of events contributing to the development and maintenance of cor pulmonale in chronic lung disease.*

blood flow, yet peripheral edema and other manifestations of heart failure are often absent (Chapter 4). Thus, in addition to pulmonary hypertension, other factors may be operating in hypoventilating pulmonary disease patients to promote the occurrence of heart failure in the face of pulmonary hypertension. Hypoxia could be such a factor but this seems unlikely, as increased right ventricular workloads seem to be well tolerated in cyanotic congenital heart disease (Chapter 3) and in subjects living at high altitude (Chapter 10). On the other hand, there does seem to be a close link between hypercapnia and the occurrence of heart failure at relatively low right ventricular workloads.[24,25] Perhaps hypercapnia in some way decreases the capacity of the myocardium to cope with increased afterload with resulting increases in right ventricular end diastolic pressure and systemic venous pressure, leading to the classic manifestations of right-sided heart failure. Another possible reason for the increased vulnerability of hypoventilating patients with lung disease to heart failure may be that intercurrent acute exacerbations of bronchitis lead to acute worsening of hypoventilation and hypertension. These abrupt changes may lead to heart failure, whereas more gradual increase in pulmonary vascular resistance seen in other disease states might be better tolerated.

The increased work of breathing common to many forms of chronic lung disease,[26] coupled with a diminishing oxygen delivery to the respiratory muscles, can precipitate or contribute further to respiratory failure, hypoxemia, and hypercapnia, and therefore produce an additional stimulus for pulmonary vasoconstriction. Additionally, repeated episodes of severe hypoxemia, which may occur during sleep in patients with sleep apnea syndromes or even in patients with chronic obstructive lung disease,[27] or during episodes of acute respiratory failure, may further contribute to the development of a chronic pulmonary hypertensive state—even if these episodes are interposed with prolonged periods of relative normoxia. (See Chapter 8.)

Left ventricular dysfunction can contribute to the pulmonary arterial hypertension of chronic lung disease, primarily by increasing pulmonary venous pressure and secondarily raising precapillary pressure. There has been considerable debate concerning the effects of chronic lung disease on ventricular function, and controversy exists as to the potential mechanisms responsible for left ventricular dysfunction in this setting.

Autopsy studies showing evidence of left ventricular hypertrophy in 10–90% of patients with chronic bronchitis[28-30] provided the earliest suggestion that the left ventricle may be affected by lung disease. Unfortunately, little clinical data concerning concomitant systemic conditions are provided in most of these reports, and the pathologic criteria used for left ventricular hypertrophy are not uniform. Baum et al.[31] reported 15 patients with chronic obstructive pulmonary disease who underwent complete hemodynamic studies; 10 of his 15 patients also underwent coronary angiography. Fourteen patients had abnormal left ventricular function curves, and 7 had elevations in left ventricular end diastolic pressure. Only 2 had significant coronary artery disease. They concluded that left ventricular dysfunction may be common in patients with chronic lung disease, even in the absence of coronary artery disease or systemic hypertension.

Several potential mechanisms for left ventricular hypertrophy or left ventricular dysfunction have been proposed, although conclusive evidence for any of these hypotheses is lacking:

- Severe systemic hypoxemia could decrease myocardial oxygen delivery and lead to left ventricular dysfunction. However, while hypoxemia is common in severe, stable lung disease, compensatory polycythemia frequently develops and maintains systemic oxygen transport at near normal levels. It is likely, however, that the left ventricular dysfunction which has been reported in patients with decompensated chronic lung disease and acute respiratory failure may be related to an acute deterioration in oxygen delivery to the myocardium.

- A high cardiac output, occasionally seen in the "blue bloater" with carbon dioxide retention, or left-to-right shunting through bronchopulmonary anastamoses,[32,33] could produce a high-output left ventricular failure. The cardiac output in stable chronic pulmonary disease, is usually normal,[34] and anastamoses, although present pathologically, do not appear to produce a significant left-to-right shunt. Additionally, increased flows, when seen, are usually modest and would not seem adequate, of themselves, to produce ventricular failure.

- Abnormal geometry of the left ventricle could impede left ventricular ejection. This hypothesis is based on echocardiographic and angiographic data which show that right ventricular pressure overload causes the interventricular septum to move paradoxically, and left ventricular filling and ejection may be limited by an alteration of the spatial geometry of the chamber.[31,35,36] Thus, left ventricular performance may be compromised by a distorted configuration of the left ventricle rather than by an intrinsic abnormality of the myocardium. In addition, the right ventricular muscle fibers are a syncitium which interlock with the left ventricular fibers. Each right ventricular contraction exerts some tension on the left ventricle. A hypertrophied, hypertensive right ventricle could thereby induce some hypertrophy of the left ventricle.

- Left ventricular dysfunction or hypertrophy could be secondary to other disease processes and thus merely coincidental. The bulk of reports in which careful selection of stable patients with lung disease were studied support this concept. Frank et al.[37] found that left ventricles of 11 patients with chronic cor pulmonale were normal with regard to contractile state, preload, afterload, and coronary blood flow. Davies and Overy[38] and Khaja and Parker[39] found no evidence of left ventricular dysfunction in their studies of carefully selected, stable patients with chronic lung disease and cor pulmonale. Similarly, Steele et al.[40] using radionuclide techniques, found that abnormalities in left ventricular ejection fraction in patients with chronic lung disese could be explained on the basis of coexistent coronary artery disease. Murphy et al.[41] found left ventricular hypertrophy in 20 of 72 patients (28%) with chronic bronchitis or emphysema: 10 had hypertensive and/or atherosclerotic heart disease, and 2 had aortic valve disease. Of the remaining 8 patients with left ventricular hypertrophy, the authors speculated that systemic hypertension may have been present but beyond the stringent criteria used for their study. It is thus likely that the presence of left ventricular hypertrophy or dysfunction results not from cor pulmonale, per se, but from coexistent cardiovascular disease. Although the spatial orientation of the left ventricle may be distorted in patients with cor pulmonale, it is unclear at this point whether this produces significant hemodynamic abnormalities in most cases.

Thromboembolic disease is an additional factor which can contribute to pulmonary hypertension in lung disease.[42] The true incidence is unknown, but patients with severe lung disease are particularly susceptible to pulmonary emboli or thrombosis, especially if heart failure is present. The diagnosis of pulmonary thromboembolism may be particularly elusive in patients with lung disease, since the signs and symptoms may be subtle and the usual preliminary diagnostic procedures such as arterial blood gases and perfusion lung scanning are not generally useful.[43] A high index of suspicion followed by pulmonary arteriography are necessary to make the diagnosis. (See Chapter 5.)

CLINICAL PICTURE

Symptoms

Most of the symptoms associated with cor pulmonale are attributable to the presence of underlying severe lung disease. Dyspnea and cough are common, and may be even more prominent during physical exertion. Precordial chest pain, thought by some to be right ventricular ischemia, is more common, in the author's experience, in other and more severe forms of pulmonary hypertension, such as idiopathic pulmonary hypertension or recurrent pulmonary thromboembolism. Epigastric pain and post-prandial nausea may be present, and are frequently due to hepatic congestion. These may be particularly bothersome when tricuspid insufficiency is present. Orthopnea is common and may be due to either the increased work of breathing in the supine position or the presence of coexistent left ventricular failure. Hemoptysis and syncope are rare, and should arouse suspicion either of other causes for pulmonary hypertension or of coexisting processes.

Signs

Tachycardia is common in stable chronic cor pulmonale, but significant systemic hypertension is reported to be unusual.[44,45] This may be due to the peripheral vasodilator effects of arterial hypoxemia, or to the decreased pulmonary activation of vasoactive substances such as angiotensin in the setting of alveolar hypoxia.[46] Cyanosis and clubbing are common, particularly in chronic bronchitis.

The neck veins are often distended, and a prominent "a" wave is frequently visualized. If tricuspid insufficiency is present, "cv" waves may also be seen. The cardiac impulse may be diffuse or a localized right ventricular impulse may be appreciated, particularly in the epigastric area, due to lung hyperinflation. Heart sounds are often distant and soft, particularly in the setting of severe obstructive airways disease. The pulmonic component of the second heart sound (P_2) may be increased on auscultation; I remember one asthenic patient with cor pulmonale in whom P_2 was not only palpable, but was clearly visible as well. A right-sided fourth heart sound is common; a third heart sound implies right ventricular failure.

Hepatic enlargement with pulsations suggests tricuspid regurgitation. Lower extremity edema is a frequent presenting sign, but it does not always imply that right ventricular failure is present, since it may be due to other conditions, such as chronic venous insufficiency.

Laboratory Studies

No single laboratory test is specific for, or diagnostic of, cor pulmonale. Polycythemia is common, and serves to facilitate tissue oxygen delivery in the setting of arterial hypoxemia. Serum electrolytes follow no specific pattern; elevation in the serum bicarbonate level generally reflects metabolic compensation for a chronic respiratory acidosis. Primary metabolic alkalosis and hypokalemia may be present when diuretics are used; the implications of these abnormalities will be discussed under *Therapy*.

A wealth of literature exists on the electrocardiographic features of cor pulmonale. Although several different criteria have been suggested for the ECG diagnosis of right ventricular hypertrophy, the electrocardiogram is not a sensitive tool for the diagnosis of cor pulmonale: Phillips[47] reported that only 30% of 18 cases with autopsy-proven cor pulmonale had electrocardiographic evidence of right ventricular hypertrophy, and Kilcoyne[48] found 28% of 81 living patients with cor pulmonale had right ventricular hypertrophy by elctrocardiogram criteria. Ferrer has suggested that the conventional electrocardiogram criteria for cor pulmonale are insensitive because they are based on the presence of right ventricular hypertrophy, which is a late manifestation of the disease.[49] Earlier changes on the electrocardiogram may suggest the presence of cor pulmonale (Table 2) and may be more useful diagnostically.

Vermeulen et al.[50] screened the records of 40,376 patients with silicosis and reported an incidence of 6% of chronic cor pulmonale based on the electrocardiogram. They suggested criteria for the electrocardiographic presence of cor pulmonale based on their study, although hemodynamic correlation is lacking. An example of right ventricular hypertrophy is seen in Figure 3.

Non-invasive techniques of evaluating left ventricular size and function have recently been applied to the evaluation of the right side of the heart. Wilson et al. evaluated 32 patients with chronic obstructive pulmonary disease with cardiac catheterization and with the vectorcardiogram.[51] No patient met electrocardiogram criteria for right ventricular hypertrophy, but there was a linear correlation between terminal rightward QRS forces and mean pulmonary arterial pressure during exercise in patients with posteriorly oriented horizontal loops on vectorcardiogram. Of 20 patients with hemodynamic abnormalities either at rest or during exercise, 85% had rightward terminal QRS forces of $\geq 5\%$ of the total loop area measured with a plastic grid. They concluded that the vectorcardiogram may be more useful than the electrocardiogram in identifying early hemodynamic abnormalities in the pulmonary circulation.

Nanda et al.[52] in 1974 suggested that the echocardiogram of the pulmonary valve was useful in evaluating the severity of pulmonary hypertension. His patient population, however, consisted of patients with postcapillary pulmonary hypertension and was devoid of cases of cor pulmonale. Acquatella et al.[53] studied 29 patients with congestive

TABLE 2
ECG Signs of Right Ventricular Hypertrophy

Early changes signaling right ventricular abnormality
- Shift of QRS axis $\geq 30°$ to the right
- Inverted, biphasic or flattened T waves in leads V1–V3
- ST segment depression in leads II, III, and aVF
- Right bundle branch block

Right ventricular hypertrophy
- Dominant R wave in aVR, V_1 or V_{4R}
- Dominant S wave in V_5 and V_6
- Frontal plane axis $> +90\%$
- P wave ≥ 2.5 mm

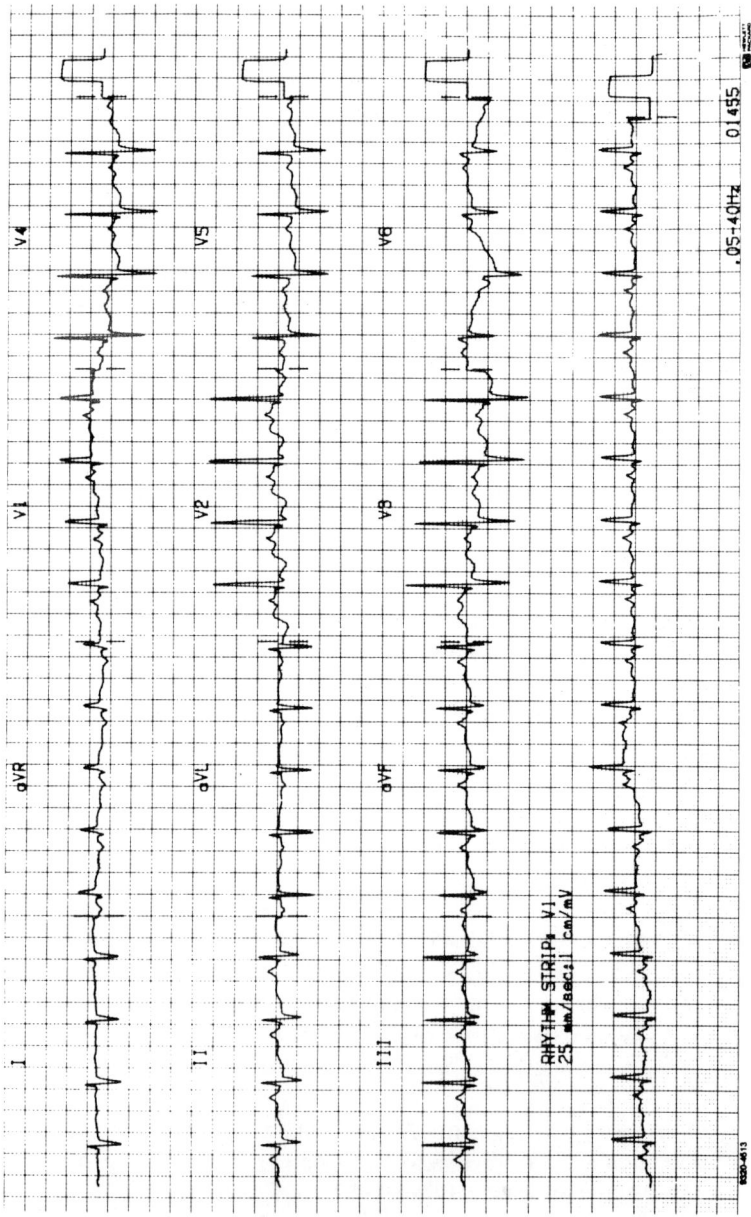

Figure 3. Electrocardiogram of a 50-year-old patient with severe interstitial lung disease and cor pulmonale.

heart failure (none with cor pulmonale) and were able to adequately visualize the pulmonic valve in 16. They found no correlation between hemodynamic measurements and any single abnormality of the pulmonary valve. Recently, Boyd et al.[54] studied 17 patients with chronic lung disease and found a close relationship between the pulmonary artery diastolic pressure and the time interval between tricuspid valve closure and pulmonary valve opening. The major limitation to the usefulness of echocardiography in cor pulmonale, however, has been that hyperinflation of the lungs often precludes adequate visualization of the cardiac chambers and valves, and may be accomplished in only 60% of patients with chronic obstructive pulmonary disease.[54] Nevertheless, if an adequate study can be performed, echocardiography may be useful not only in suggesting the presence of pulmonary hypertension but also in monitoring the effects of therapy (Figure 4).

Radionuclide angiocardiographic techniques have also been used to evaluate both right and left ventricular function in patients with pulmonary disease. Berger et al.[55] compared right ventricular function in patients with chronic obstructive pulmonary disease with normal patients and found a wide variability in right ventricular ejection fraction in chronic obstructive pulmonary disease patients, with a range of 19 to 71%. All 19 patients with right-sided heart failure, however, had a reduced right ventricular ejection fraction. Although it is often difficult to isolate and adequately quantify right ventricular function in patients who have large, dilated right ventricles, radionuclide techniques provide a promising tool for non-invasive evaluation of right ventricular function in cor pulmonale, and may be particularly useful in monitoring the effects of therapy.

Pulmonary function testing provides a qualitative and quantitative assessment of ventilatory defects. Abnormalities in pulmonary function may also suggest the likelihood that coexistent pulmonary hypertension is present, and can provide an indication of its magnitude. Enson[56] evaluated over 30 patients with interstitial lung disease and found that, when the vital capacity is between 50–80% of predicted the pulmonary vascular resistance is increased, but pulmonary arterial pressure may be increased only during exercise. When vital capacity is ≤ 50%, pulmonary arterial hypertension is usually present even at rest. Similarly, Timsit[57] and others have demonstrated a relationship between vital capacity or FEV_1 and the presence of pulmonary hypertension in obstructive airways disease. Ferrer and others have shown a close relationship between pulmonary arterial pressure and arterial hemoglobin saturation (Figure 5).

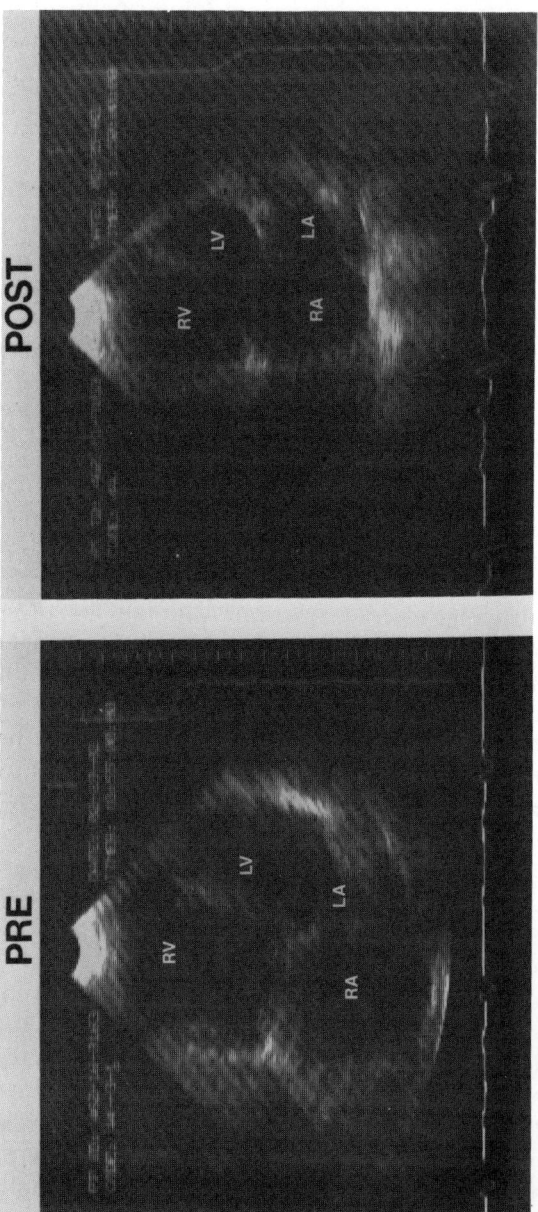

Figure 4. Two-dimensional echocardiogram of a patient with interstitial fibrosis and cor pulmonale before (pre) and 48 hours after (post) beginning vasodilator therapy with nifedipine 20 mg orally every 6 hours. LA, left atrium, LV, left ventricle, RA, right atrium, RV, right ventricle. Note the reduction in size of both right heart chambers after nifedipine.

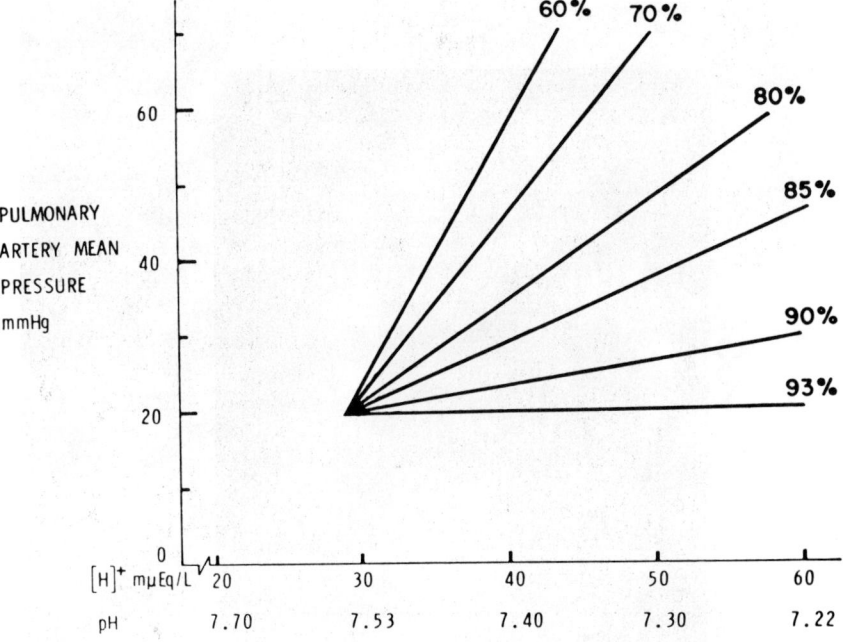

Figure 5. The relationship between pulmonary arterial pressure, arterial hemoglobin saturation, and blood hydrogen ion concentration in 43 patients with chronic obstructive lung disease. (Reproduced with permission from Bull NY Acad Med 1965;41:942.)

Chest radiography frequently demonstrates enlarged proximal pulmonary arteries (Figure 6), an enlarged right ventricle particularly in the lateral view, and azygos venous engorgement.

Therapy

The primary objective of therapy for cor pulmonale is to treat the underlying disease. Thus, the signs of cor pulmonale resulting from obstructive lung disease often improve with measures directed at improving air flow, such as bronchodilators, mucolytics, chest physiotherapy, and antibiotics. Theophylline compounds may improve hemodynamics in cor pulmonale secondary to chronic obstructive pulmonary disease in several ways: they may improve air flow and therefore provide more efficient alveolar gas exchange; they may reduce pulmonary transmural vascular resistance by producing bron-

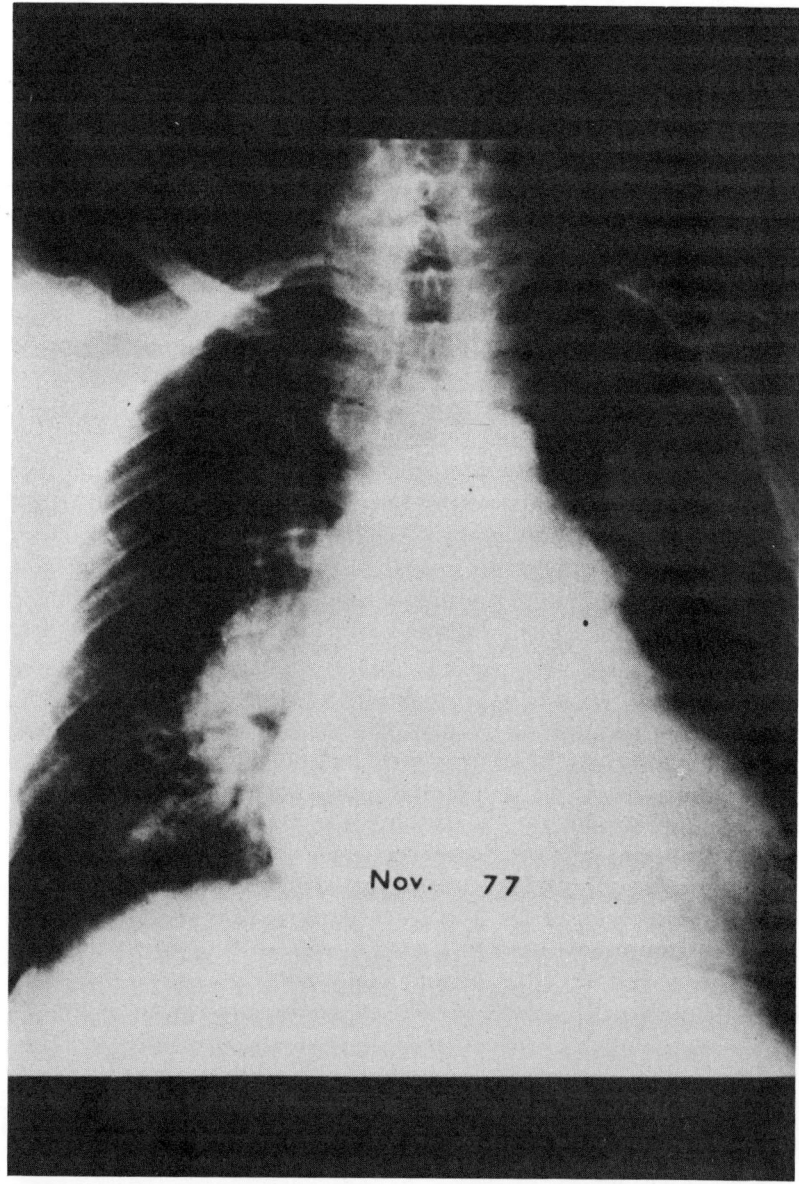

Figure 6. Posteroanterior (PA) chest radiograph of a 57-year-old man with severe pulmonary hypertension resulting from combined obstructive and restrictive ventilatory defects of undetermined etiology. Note the enlarged proximal pulmonary arteries and right ventricular configuration.

chodilation and decreasing intrathoracic pressure; and they may have a modest direct pulmonary vasodilating effect.[59,60]

As a result of chronic hypoxemia, polycythemia frequently develops in order to maintain systemic oxygen transport. Hyperviscosity resulting from polycythemia, however, can further increase pulmonary resistance and exacerbate or contribute to cor pulmonale. Weisse et al.[61] evaluated the hemodynamic effects of phlebotomy in 12 patients with cor pulmonale who had hematocrit levels above 55%. They found that reducing the hematocrit from a mean of 61 to 50% produced significant decreases in pulmonary arterial pressure and pulmonary vascular resistance, which was accompanied by improvement in exercise performance. No further benefit was obtained by reducing the hematocrit to a mean of 44%. Their study suggests that phlebotomy may be a useful therapeutic maneuver when severe polycythemia is present.

The goal of supplemental oxygen therapy is two-fold: to improve symptoms related to impaired systemic oxygen delivery, and to improve pulmonary hemodynamics. Several studies, using different approaches to supplemental oxygen therapy, have demonstrated both reductions in pulmonary vasomotor tone and prolonged survival in patients receiving supplemental oxygen. The British Medical Research Council study[62] demonstrated that patients with advanced chronic bronchitis who were treated with supplemental oxygen survived longer than patients not receiving oxygen. Exercise tolerance and quality of life were not critically evaluated in this study. The Nocturnal Oxygen Therapy Trial,[63] a cooperative study performed in the United States, compared physiologic, psychologic, and mortality parameters in two groups of patients—those receiving continuous oxygen therapy and those given only 12-hour nocturnal oxygen therapy. Mortality was nearly twice as high in the group receiving nocturnal oxygen alone. Although continuous oxygen therapy reduced pulmonary vascular resistance by 11%, the most striking beneficial effects on survival were seen in patients with small decreases in pulmonary vascular resistance, suggesting that the improved survival could not be directly attributed to the improved pulmonary hemodynamics in their patients.

Patients with severe arterial hypoxemia may, therefore, benefit from supplemental oxygen. The criteria used by the NOTT study[63] for inclusion are probably the most useful upon which to base the decision of which patients should receive supplemental oxygen: hypoxemia, i.e., $PaO_2 \leq 55$ mm Hg; edema; hematocrit $\geq 55\%$; and P pulmonale on ECG. The inspired concentration of oxygen and flow rate should be titrated to the level which produces an arterial pO_2 of 60 torr or greater without producing excessive carbon dioxide retention. It should be used for at least 16–18 hours per day, if possible, and most of this use should be at night, since nocturnal hypoxemia is common in chronic obstructive pulmonary disease[64,65] and may produce arrhythmias, sudden death, or contribute significantly to the development or maintenance of a pulmonary hypertensive state. The pulmonary vascular response to supplemental oxygen is slow, often taking weeks or months to produce its maximal vasodilation.[66] Frequently, oxygen has little effect on pulmonary vascular tone, and the pulmonary vascular responsiveness to supplemental oxygen may diminish with time.[67] Nevertheless, it may be worthwhile continuing supplemental oxygen therapy in such patients for its other important beneficial effects.[63,66]

The role of cardiac glycosides in therapy for cor pulmonale has been controversial for many years.[68] Ferrer showed a reduction in right ventricular end diastolic pressure after acute digitalization in a group of patients with cor pulmonale,[69] and a reduction in right ventricular and pulmonary arterial pressure at restudy after several weeks of chronic digitalis combined with intensive pulmonary toilet. In patients with cor pulmonale with normal right ventricular diastolic pressure and stable airways disease, however, Ferrer and others[70,71] have demonstrated that digitalis produces no hemodynamic changes. A recent study by Mathur et al.[72] using radionuclide techniques to quantitate right and left ventricular function demonstrated that digoxin improved right ventricular function only when concomitant left ventricular dysfunction was present. Additionally, several studies have demonstrated a high incidence of digitalis toxicity in patients with lung disease.[68] Thus, the risk of using cardiac glycosides, which are potentiated in cor pulmonale by hypoxemia, hypokalemia if diuretics are used, and impaired drug excretion if renal function is abnormal, probably outweigh the potential benefits in most patients without left ventricular failure. Digoxin may, however, be useful in the management of supraventricular arrhythmias, which are common in patients with lung disease, but they should be used only when reversible causes of these arrhythmias, such as hypoxemia, sympathomimetic, or other bronchodilator-induced cardiac irritability or metabolic derangements have been excluded.

Diuretics have been advocated in the management of cor pulmonale both because they can reduce salt and water retention and because they may have independent effects on alveolar ventilation and pulmonary vascular tone.[73–75] Potent diuretics, such as furosemide, can cause hypokalemia and, by enhancing the reabsorbtion of bicarbonate in the kidney, produce a metabolic alkalosis which is poorly tolerated by the chronic obstructive pulmonary disease patient with chronic hypercapnia. In addition, a decreased intravascular volume as the result of aggressive diuresis can reduce right ventricular preload and further decrease cardiac output.[75] Thus, diuretics should be used sparingly, and potassium supplements should be given as needed.

The concept of vasodilator therapy for left ventricular failure has recently been applied to conditions which exclusively affect the right side of the heart and pulmonary circulation. The rationale for vasodilator therapy for cor pulmonale is based on the demonstration that right ventricular failure is the result of an increased right ventricular afterload and that active pulmonary vasoconstriction constitutes a significant component of the elevation in vascular resistance. A vasodilator which reduces pulmonary vasomotor tone would produce a reduction in right ventricular afterload and an increase in cardiac output. Systemic vascular resistance is reduced as well by vasodilators, but if cardiac output is significantly increased, blood pressure may fall slightly or remain unchanged. Although no specific or even preferential pulmonary vasodilators are available, several potent systemic vasodilators have been reported to exert beneficial hemodynamic effects in patients with cor pulmonale.

Williams et al.[76] and Lockhart et al.[77] both demonstrated an increase in cardiac output and a reduction in pulmonary vascular resistance in response to intravenous isoproterenol in patients with chronic obstructive pulmonary disease and pulmonary hypertension. It is unclear whether the improved hemodynamic state was the result of a direct vasodilatory effect of isoproterenol, or whether an increase in air flow from the known bronchodilatory effects of isoproterenol improved gas exchange and indirectly led to a reduction in pulmonary tone.

Phentolamine, an alpha-adrenergic antagonist which has been used to treat patients with persistent fetal circulation and pulmonary hypertension resulting from congenital intracardiac shunts, has also been reported to produce reductions in pulmonary arterial pressure and pulmonary vascular resistance in patients with cor pulmonale without affecting ventilatory parameters or air flow rates.[78,79]

Recently, Rubin and Peter reported the beneficial hemodynamic effects of oral hydralazine in 12 patients with cor pulmonale resulting from obstructive or restrictive ventilatory defects[80] (Figures 7–9). All of the patients had persistent pulmonary hypertension despite being treated with a conventional medical regimen for at least 6 months. After 48 hours of therapy with hydralazine 50 mg orally every 6 hours, there were significant decreases in mean pulmonary arterial pressure and pulmonary vascular resistance and increases in cardiac output,

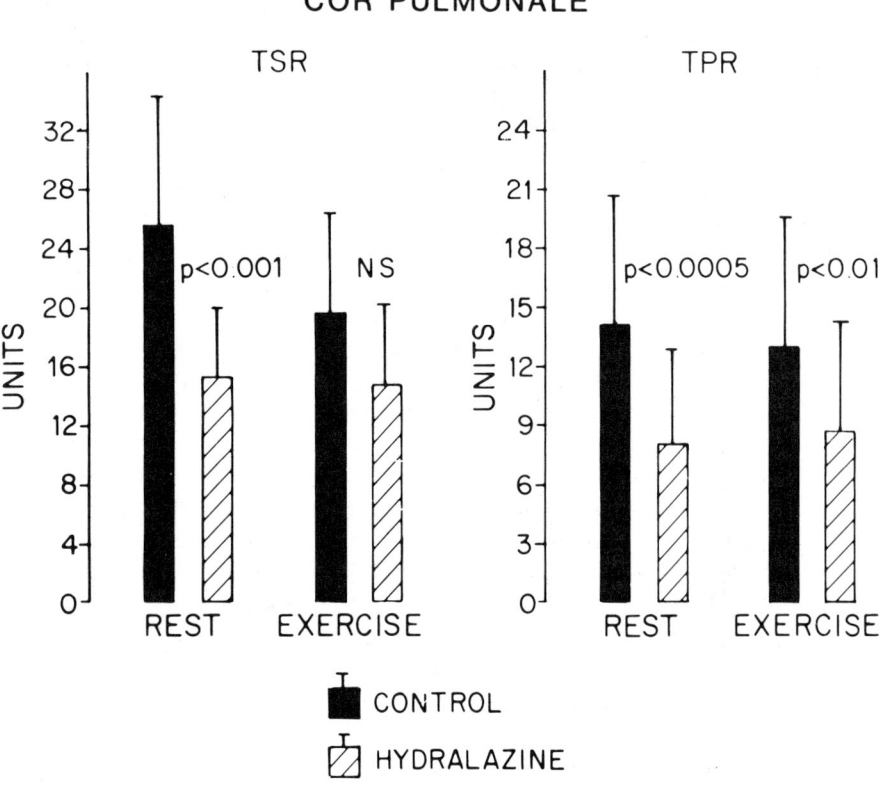

Figure 7. The effects of oral hydralazine on total systemic (TSR) and total pulmonary (TPR) resistances in 12 patients studied at rest and during submaximal sitting bicycle exercise. (Reproduced with permission of the authors and the American Heart Association from Reference 80.)

both at rest and during submaximal exercise. Rubin et al. have also demonstrated a reduction in right ventricular end diastolic pressure in patients with pulmonary hypertension and right ventricular failure who were treated with hydralazine, suggesting that right ventricular function improves with afterload reduction therapy[81] (Figure 10). Similarly, Brent et al.[82] demonstrated a significant improvement in right ventricular ejection fraction after administration of hydralazine in 6 patients with cor pulmonale studied by radionuclide angiocardiography. The recent demonstration by Simmonneau et al. that nifedipine, a cal-

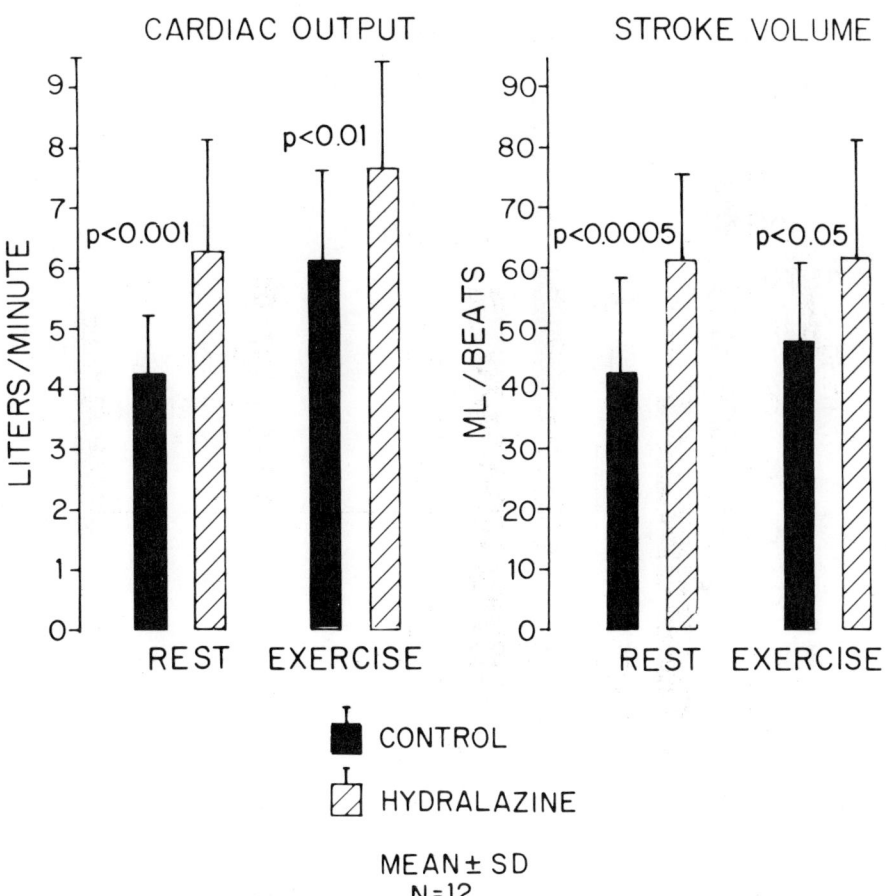

Figure 8. *The effects of hydralazine on cardiac output and stroke volume in cor pulmonale.*

cium channel blocker, inhibited hypoxic pulmonary vasoconstriction in 13 patients with acute respiratory failure[83] suggests that this drug might also be useful in the management of chronic cor pulmonale.

The two major potential adverse effects of vasodilator administration to patients with cor pulmonale are systemic hypotension and worsening hypoxemia. The risk of developing systemic hypotension can be minimized if intravascular volume is replete and small doses of a vasodilator are administered initially. Since not all patients have a

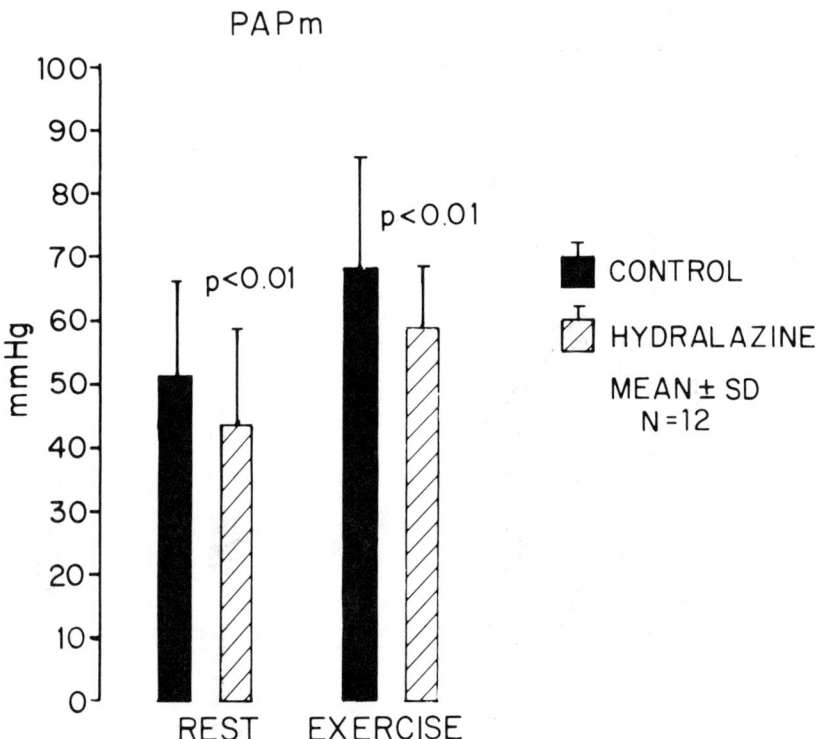

Figure 9. The effects of hydralazine on mean pulmonary arterial pressure (PAPm) in cor pulmonale.

beneficial response to vasodilators, hemodynamic monitoring during a trial of vasodilator therapy is crucial.

Vasodilators can worsen hypoxemia either by increasing perfusion to poorly ventilated units or by recruitment of shunt vessels. In our experience, vasodilators do not generally worsen arterial oxygenation, possibly because the worsening VA/Q relationship is offset by an increase in mixed venous oxygen content which results from the improved cardiac output.

There may be marked swings in pulmonary arterial pressure in the resting state especially during exercise, owing to the wide respiratory fluctuations in intrathoracic pressure occurring in patients with obstructive airways disease (Figure 11). These must be taken into account

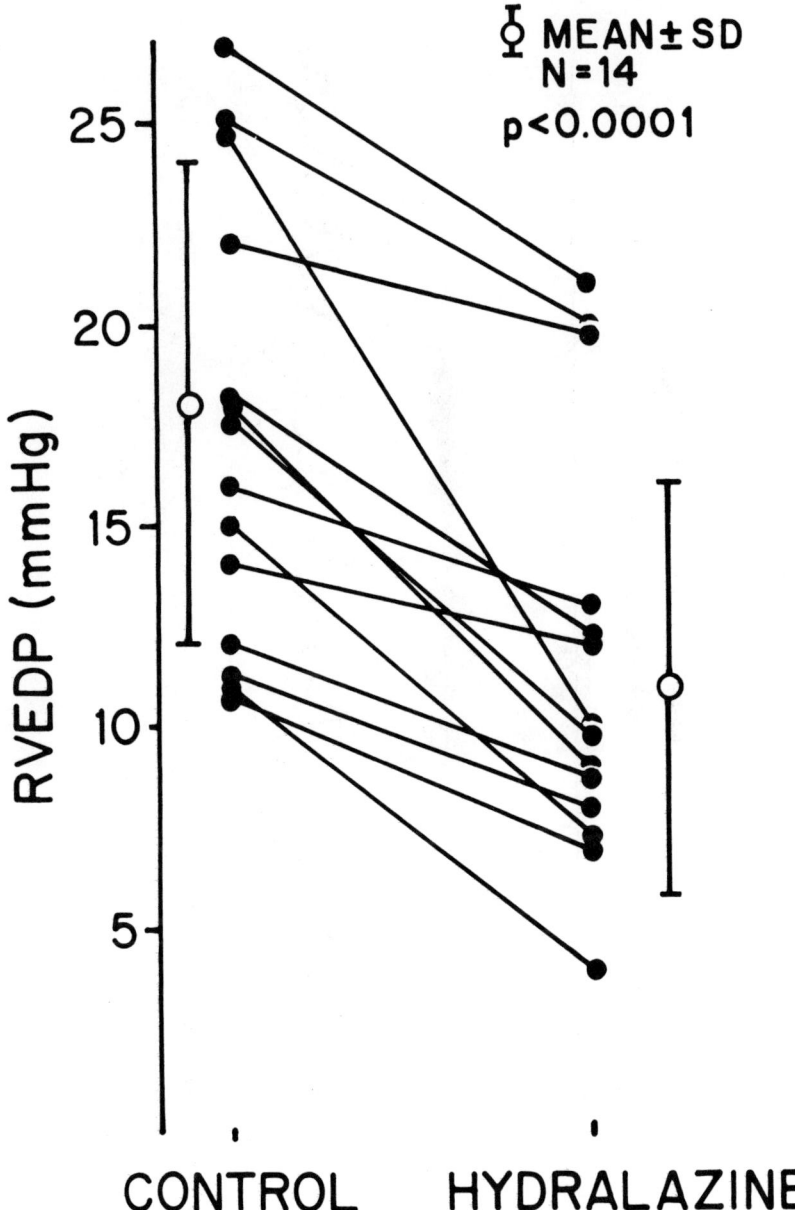

Figure 10. The effects of hydralazine on right ventricular end diastolic pressure (RVEDP) in 14 patients with right ventricular failure. (Reproduced with permission from Reference 81.)

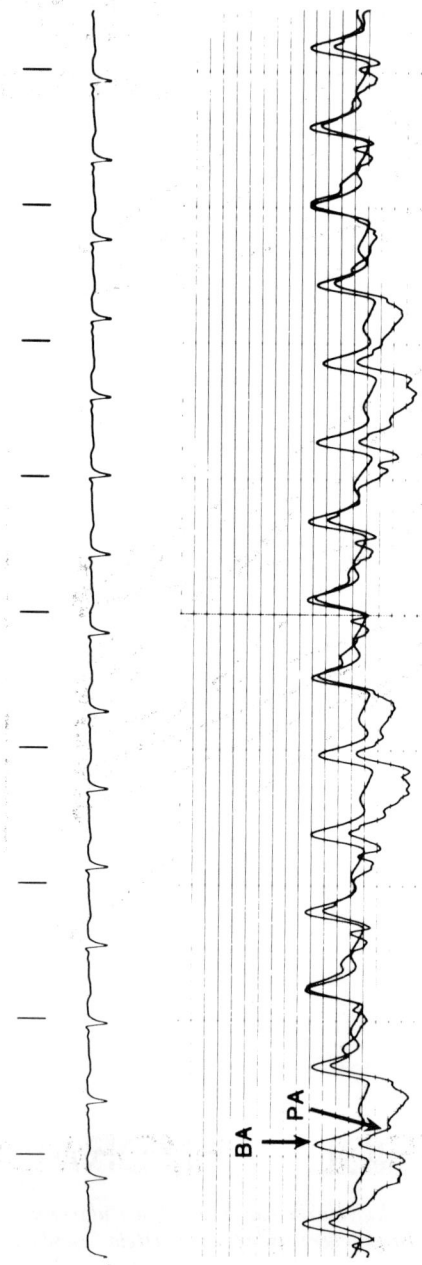

Figure 11. Simultaneous tracing of brachial arterial (BA) and pulmonary arterial (PA) pressures in a patient with severe obstructive airways disease and pulmonary hypertension. There are marked swings in PA pressure during respiration.

when evaluating the response to vasodilator agents. The approach in our laboratory is to take the mean of pulmonary arterial pressure measurements over three respiratory cycles as representative values.

The role of vasodilator therapy for cor pulmonale is uncertain: while vasodilators may improve hemodynamics, the long-term effects of these agents on right ventricular function have not yet been addressed. In addition, whether vasodilators improve exercise tolerance or alter survival rates is unknown. Vasodilators should be reserved for patients who, despite an aggressive approach with conventional therapy, have signs of pulmonary hypertension or right ventricular failure. The institution of vasodilator therapy should be done cautiously and under hemodynamic or non-invasive monitoring.

SUMMARY

Despite advances in our understanding and treatment of pulmonary diseases, cor pulmonale remains a frequent and serious complication of chronic lung disease. The development and application of newer diagnostic techniques may enable the clinician to identify the presence of pulmonary hypertension in patients with lung disease at an earlier and, therefore, a more reversible stage. Therapy should be individualized for each patient based on the underlying disease and both objective and subjective responses.

Acknowledgments: I am indebted to Ms. Becky Rendon and Mr. Walter Craig for their assistance in the preparation of this manuscript.

REFERENCES

1. World Health Organization: Chronic cor pulmonale. A report of the expert committee. *Circulation* 1963;27:594–615.
2. U.S. Department of Health and Human Services, National Heart, Lung and Blood Institute: *Division of Lung Disease Program Report*, 1980, p. 121.
3. Intersociety Commission for Heart Disease Resources: Primary prevention of pulmonary heart disease. *Circulation* 1970;41:A-17.
4. Flint FJ: Cor pulmonale, incidence and etiology in an industrial city. *Lancet* 1954;2:51–58.
5. Stuart-Harris CH, Twidle RSH, Clifton M: A hospital study of congestive heart failure with special reference to cor pulmonale. *Br Med J* 1959; 2:201–208.

6. Slavkovic J, Konecni J, Kovacevic M, Djuric D: Anoxic cor pulmonale. *Serb Arch Med* 1959;83:36–40.
7. Burrows B, Kettel LJ, Niden AH, Rabinowitz M, Diener CF: Patterns of cardiovascular dysfunction in chronic obstructive lung disease. *N Engl J Med* 1972;286:912–917.
8. Bishop JM: Hypoxia and pulmonary hypertension in chronic bronchitis. *Prog Resp Res* 1975;9:10–16.
9. Traver GA, Cline MG, Burrows B: Predictors of mortality in chronic obstructive pulmonary disease. *Am Rev Respir Dis* 1979;119:895–902.
10. Riley RL, Himmelstein A, Motley HL, Weiner HM, Cournand A: Studies of the pulmonary circulation at rest and during exercise in normal individuals and in patients with chronic pulmonary disease. *Am J Physiol* 1948;152:372–382.
11. Mohsenifar Z, Tashkin DP, Levy SE, Bjerke RD, Clements PJ, Furst D: Lack of sensitivity of measurements of VD/VT at rest and during exercise in detection of hemodynamically significant pulmonary vascular abnormalities in collagen vascular disease. *Am Rev Resp Dis* 1981;123:508–572.
12. Widimsky J, Riedel M, Stanek V: Central hemodynamics during exercise in patients with restrictive pulmonary disease. *Bull Eur Physiopath Resp* 1977;13:369–379.
13. Fishman AP: Dynamics of the pulmonary circulation. In: Hamilton, WF, Dow P., eds. *Handbook of Physiology*, Sec. Z, Circulation, Vol. II, Washington, D. C., American Physiology Society, 1963:1667.
14. Von Euler US, Liljestrand G: Observations on the pulmonary arterial blood pressure in the cat. *Acta Physiol Scand* 1946;12:301–320.
15. Barer GR, Howard P, Shaw JW: Stimulus-response curves for the pulmonary vascular bed to hypoxia and hypercapnia. *J Physiol* 1970;211:139–155.
16. Barer GR, McCurrie JR, Shaw JW: Effect of changes in blood pH on the vascular resistance of normal and hypoxic cat lung. *Cardiovas Res* 1971;5:490–497.
17. Harvey RM, Enson Y, Betti R, Lewis ML, Rochester DF, Ferrer MI: The influence of hydrogen ion concentration and hypoxia on the pulmonary circulation. *J Clin Invest* 1964;43:1146–1162.
18. Fishman AP: Respiratory gases in the regulation of the pulmonary circulation. *Physiol Rev* 1961;41:214–280.
19. Fishman AP: Hypoxia on the pulmonary circulation. *Circ Res* 1975;38:221–231.
20. Harris P, Segal N, Green I, Housley E: The influence of the airways resistance and alveolar pressure on the pulmonary vascular resistance in chronic bronchitis. *Cardiovasc Res* 1968;2:84–92.
21. Hyman AL, Higashida RT, Spannhake EW, Kadowitz PJ: Pulmonary vasoconstrictor responses to graded decreases in precapillary blood pO_2 in intact-chest cat. *J Appl Physiol* 1981;51:1009–1016.
22. Benumof JL, Pirlo AF, Johanson I, Trousdale FR: Interaction of PVO_2 with PAO_2 on hypoxic pulmonary vasoconstriction. *J Appl Physiol* 1981;51:871–874.
23. McGrath RL, Weil JV: Adverse effects of normovolemic polycythemia and hypoxia on hemodynamics in the dog. *Circ Res* 1978;43:793–798.

24. Campbell EJM, Short DS: The cause of oedema in "cor pulmonale." *Lancet* 1960;1:1184–1186.
25. Platts MM, Greaves MS: Arterial blood gas measurements in the management of patients with chronic bronchitis and emphysema. *Thorax* 1957;12:236–240.
26. Field S, Kelly SM, Macklem PT: The oxygen cost of breathing in patients with cardiorespiratory disease. *Am Rev Respir Dis* 1982;126:9–13.
27. Wynne JW, Block AJ, Hemenway J, Hunt LA, Flick MR: Disordered breathing and oxygen desaturation during sleep in patients with chronic obstructive lung disease (COLD). *Am J Med* 1979;66:573–579.
28. Scott RW, Garvin CF: Cor pulmonale: Observations in fifty autopsy cases. *Am Heart J* 1941;22:56–63.
29. Michelson N: Bilateral ventricular hypertrophy due to chronic pulmonary disease. *Dis Chest* 1960;38:435–446.
30. Fluck DC, Chandrasekar RG, Gardner RV: Left ventricular hypertrophy in chronic bronchitis. *Br Heart J* 1966;28:92–97.
31. Baum GL, Schwartz A, Llamas R, Castillo C: Left ventricular function in chronic obstructive lung disease. *N Engl J Med* 1971;285:361–365.
32. Cudkowicz L, Armstrong JB: The bronchial arteries in pulmonary emphysema. *Thorax* 1953;8:46–58.
33. Roosenberg JG, Deenstra H: Bronchial-pulmonary vascular shunts in chronic pulmonary infections. *Dis Chest* 1954;26:664–671.
34. Shaw DB, Grover RF, Reeves JT, Blount SG Jr: Pulmonary circulation in chronic bronchitis and emphysema. *Br Heart J* 1965;27:674–683.
35. Weber KT, Janicki JS, Shroff S, Fishman AP: Contractile mechanics and interaction of the right and left ventricles. *Am J Cardiol* 1981;47:686–695.
36. Summer WR, Permutt S, Sagawa K, Shoukas AA, Bromberger-Barnea B: Effects of spontaneous respiration on canine left ventricular function. *Circ Res* 1979;45:719–728.
37. Frank MJ, Weisse AB, Moschos CB, Levinson GE: Left ventricular function, metabolism and blood flow in chronic cor pulmonale. *Circulation* 1973;47:798–806.
38. Davies H, Overy HR: Left ventricular function in cor pulmonale. *Chest* 1970;58:8–14.
39. Khaja F, Parker JO: Right and left ventricular performance in chronic obstructive lung disease. *Am Heart J* 1971;82:319–327.
40. Steele P, Ellis JH, Van Dyke D, Sutton F, Creagh E, Davies H: Left ventricular fraction in severe chronic obstructive airways disease. *Am J Med* 1975;59:21–28.
41. Murphy ML, Adamson J, Hutcheson F: Left ventricular hypertrophy in patients with chronic bronchitis and emphysema. *Ann Intern Med* 1974;81:307–313.
42. Fanta CH, Wright TC, McFadden ER: Differentiation of recurrent pulmonary emboli from chronic obstructive lung disease as a cause of cor pulmonale. *Chest* 1981;79:92–95.
43. Sharma GVRK, Sasahara AA: Diagnosis of pulmonary embolism in patients with chronic obstructive pulmonary disease. *J Chron Dis* 1975;28:253–257.
44. Anderson AE, Bedrossian CWM, Foraker AG: Systemic blood pressure in subjects with and without emphysema. *Am Rev Respir Dis* 1971;576–578.

45. Schrijen F, Uffholtz H, Polu JM, Poincelot F: Pulmonary and systemic hemodynamic evolution in chronic bronchitis. *Am Rev Respir Dis* 1978; 117:25–31.
46. Szidon P, Bairey N, Oparil S: Effect of acute hypoxia on the pulmonary conversion of angiotensin I to angiotensin II in dogs. *Circ Res* 1980; 45:221–226.
47. Phillips RW: The electrocardiogram in cor pulmonale secondary to pulmonary emphysema: A study of 18 cases proved by autopsy. *Am Heart J* 1958;56:352–371.
48. Kilcoyne MM, Davis AL, Ferrer MI: A dynamic electrocardiographic concept useful in the diagnosis of cor pulmonale. *Circulation* 1970;42:903–924.
49. Ferrer MI: Clinical and electrocardiographic correlations in pulmonary heart disease (cor pulmonale). *Cardiovasc Clin* 1977;8:215–224.
50. Vermeulen R, Kenis J, Groetenbriel C, Lahaye D: Electrocardiographic signs of chronic cor pulmonale in 40,376 patients with silicosis. *Acta Cardiologica* 1978;33:263–278.
51. Wilson JR, Mason UG, Bahler RC, Chester EH, Picken JJ, Baum GL: Vectorcardiographic detection of early hemodynamic abnormalities in chronic obstructive pulmonary disease. *Chest* 1979;76:160–165.
52. Nanda NC, Gramiak R, Robinson TI, Shah PM: Echocardiographic evaluation of pulmonary hypertension. *Circulation* 1974;50:575–581.
53. Acquatella H, Schiller NB, Sharpe DN, Chatterjee K: Lack of correlation between echocardiographic pulmonary valve morphology and simultaneous pulmonary arterial pressure. *Am J Cardiol* 1979;43:946–950.
54. Boyd MJ, Williams IP, Turton CWG, Brooks N, Leech G, Millard FJC: Echocardiographic method for the estimation of pulmonary artery pressure in chronic lung disease. *Thorax* 1980;35:914–919.
55. Berger HJ, Matthay RA, Loke J, Marshall RC, Gottschalk A, Zaret B: Assessment of cardiac performance with quantitative radionuclide angiocardiography: Right ventricular ejection fraction with reference to findings in chronic obstructive pulmonary disease. *Am J Cardiol* 1978;41:897–905.
56. Enson Y: Pulmonary heart disease: Relation of pulmonary hypertension to abnormal lung structure and function. *Bull NY Acad Med* 1977;53:551–566.
57. Timsit G, Neukirch F, du Perron MC, Verdier F, Drutel P, Legrand M, Botto MJ, Lesorbe R: Statistical correlation between PAP, spirographic data and arterial and mixed venous blood gases in 22 subjects with chronic obstructive lung disease. *Prog Resp Res* 1975;9:105–111.
58. Ferrer MI: Disturbances in the circulation in patients with cor pulmonale. *Bull NY Acad Med* 1965;41:942–958.
59. Parker JO, Kelkar K, West RO: Hemodynamic effects of aminophylline in cor pulmonale. *Circulation* 1966;33:17–25.
60. Barer GR, Gunning AJ; Action of a sympathomimetic drug and of theophylline ethylene diamine on the pulmonary circulation. *Circ Res* 1979; 7:383–389.
61. Weisse AB, Moschos CB, Frank MJ, Levinson GE, Canilla JE, Regan TJ: Hemodynamic effects of staged hematocrit reduction in patients with stable cor pulmonale and severely elevated hematocrit levels. *Am J Med* 1975;58:92–98.

62. British Medical Research Council Working Party: Long term domiciliary oxygen therapy in chronic hypoxic cor pulmonale complicating chronic bronchitis and emphysema. *Lancet* 1981;1:681–685.
63. Nocturnal Oxygen Therapy Trial Group: Continuous or nocturnal oxygen therapy in hypoxemic chronic obstructive lung disease. *Ann Intern Med* 1980;93:391–398.
64. Boysen PG, Block AJ, Wynne JW, Hunt LA, Flick MR: Nocturnal pulmonary hypertension in patients with chronic obstructive pulmonary disease. *Chest* 1979;76:536–542.
65. DeMarco FJ, Wynne JW, Block AJ, Boysen PG, Taasan VC: Oxygen desaturation during sleep as a determinant of the "blue and bloated" syndrome. *Chest* 1981;79:621–625.
66. Bishop JM: Hypoxia and pulmonary hypertension in chronic bronchitis. *Prog Resp Res* 1975;9:10–16.
67. Anderson PB, Campbell RHA, Brennan SR, Howard P: The problem of pulmonary hypertension in chronic cor pulmonale. *Prog Resp Res* 1975; 9:37–40.
68. Green LH, Smith TW: The use of digitalis in patients with pulmonary disease. *Ann Intern Med* 1977;87:459–465.
69. Ferrer MI, Harvey RM, Cathcart RT, Webster CA, Richards DW, Cournand A: Some effects of digoxin upon the heart and circulation in man: Digoxin in chronic cor pulmonale. *Circulation* 1950;1:161–186.
70. Howarth S, McMichael J, Sharpey-Schafer EP: Effects of oxygen, venesection and digitalis in chronic heart failure from disease of the lungs. *Clin Sci* 1948;6:187–196.
71. Jezek V, Schrijen F: Hemodynamic effect of deslanoside at rest and during exercise in patients with chronic bronchitis. *Br Heart J* 1973; 35:2–8.
72. Mathur PN, Powles P, Pugsley SO, McEwan MP, Campbell EJM: Effect of digoxin on right ventricular function in severe chronic airflow obstruction. *Ann Intern Med* 1981;95:283–288.
73. Noble NIM, Trenchard D, Guz A: The value of diuretics in respiratory failure. *Lancet* 1966;2:257–260.
74. Whitman V, Stern RC, Bellet P, Doershuk CF, Liebman J, Boat TF, Borkat G, Matthews LW: Studies on cor pulmonale in cystic fibrosis. I. Effects of diuresis. *Pediatrics* 1975;55:83–85.
75. Heinemann HO: Right-sided heart failure and the use of diuretics. *Am J Med* 1978;64:367–370.
76. Williams JF, White DH, Behnka RH: Changes in pulmonary hemodynamics produced by isoproterenol infusion in emphysematous patients. *Circulation* 1963;28;396–403.
77. Lockhart A, Lissac J, Salmon D, Zappacosta C, Benismail M: Effects of isoproterenol on the pulmonary circulation in obstructive airways disease. *Clin Sci* 1967;32:177–187.
78. Van Mieghem W, de Bakcer G, de Wispehere B, Biliet L, Cosemans J: Phentolamine infusion in cor pulmonale due to chronic obstructive pulmonary disease. *Acta Cardiologica* 1978;4:253–262.
79. Gould L, DeMartino A, Gomprecht RF, Umali F, Michael A: Hemodynamic effects of phentolamine in cor pulmonale. *J Clin Pharm* 1972;12: 153–157.

80. Rubin LJ, Peter RH: Hemodynamics at rest and during exercise after oral hydralazine in patients with cor pulmonale. *Am J Cardiol* 1981;47:116–122.
81. Rubin LJ, Handel F, Peter RH: The effects of oral hydralazine in right ventricular end-diastolic pressure in patients with right ventricular failure. *Circulation* 1982;65:1369–1373.
82. Brent B, Berger H, Mahler D, Matthay R, Zaret B: Acute effects of hydralazine on the pulmonary circulation and right ventricular function in chronic lung disease and pulmonary hypertension. *Clin Res* 1982;30:4A (Abstract).
83. Simmoneau G, Escourrou P, Duroux P, Lockhart A: Inhibition of hypoxic pulmonary vasoconstricton by nifedipine. *N Engl J Med* 1981;304:1582–1585.

CHAPTER 8

PULMONARY HYPERTENSION AND COR PULMONALE IN HYPOVENTILATING PATIENTS

John V. Weil

Hypoventilation is now a widely recognized cause of pulmonary hypertension, with congestive heart failure or cor pulmonale. This association accounts for much of the pulmonary hypertension and right-sided heart failure seen in patients with chronic obstructive lung disease, mechanical dysfunction of the thorax as in kyphoscoliosis, or weakness of respiratory muscles as in neuromuscular diseases. In such patients hypoventilation is usually attributed to obvious disease-imposed mechanical or anatomic limitation of the patient's ability to breathe, as outlined in the preceding chapter. This chapter deals with those patients in whom hypoventilation, pulmonary hypertension, and right-sided congestive failure occur in a setting where strict structural or functional limitation on the ability to breathe is not obvious. The evidence will be reviewed that in such individuals decreased ventilatory drive plays a prominent role in the pathogenesis of hypoventilation and its sequelae.

VENTILATORY DRIVE—ITS VARIABILITY AND IMPLICATIONS

A critical step in understanding the origin of these syndromes has been the recognition that ventilatory drives are not constant, but instead are variable both between and within individuals (Figure 1). This was initially appreciated in studies of persons residing at high altitude

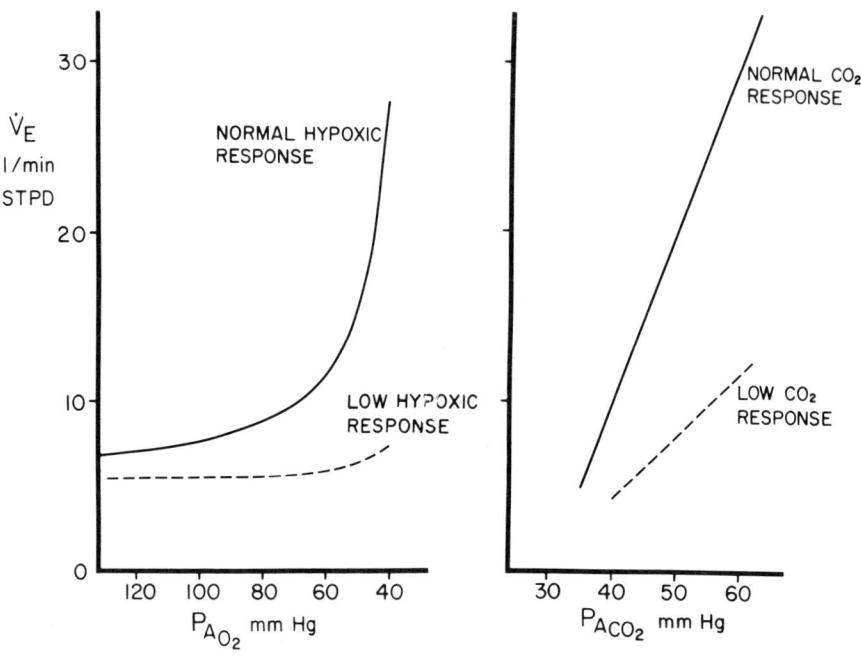

Figure 1. *Ventilatory responses to hypoxia (left) and hypercapnia (right) depicting examples of low and high responses. There is considerable variability in both hypoxic and hypercapnic responses which are largely attributable to differences between individuals.*

where there is considerable variation in oxygenation and ventilation among subjects living at the same altitude.[1] Search for the source of this variation led to the discovery that ventilatory drives, in particular the ventilatory response to hypoxia, span a considerable range. Blunted ventilatory drives are especially common in native or very long-term residents of high altitude, while brisk responses are more frequent in newcomers[2] (Figure 2). This suggested that long-term hypoxia leads to blunting of ventilatory drives. Although the mechanism of this effect is unknown, it may have implications for hypoxic disease at low altitude. For example, ventilatory drives are typically strikingly blunted in persons with long-standing severe hypoxemia, as in cyanotic congenital heart disease, and may remain so for many years after surgical correction of the cardiac defect.[3] A low ventilatory drive may predispose some individuals to hypoventilation, which may become apparent under special circumstances, such as during recovery from general anesthesia. A low drive may also be a factor in the pathogenesis of hypoventilation in patients with antecedent long-standing hypoxia due

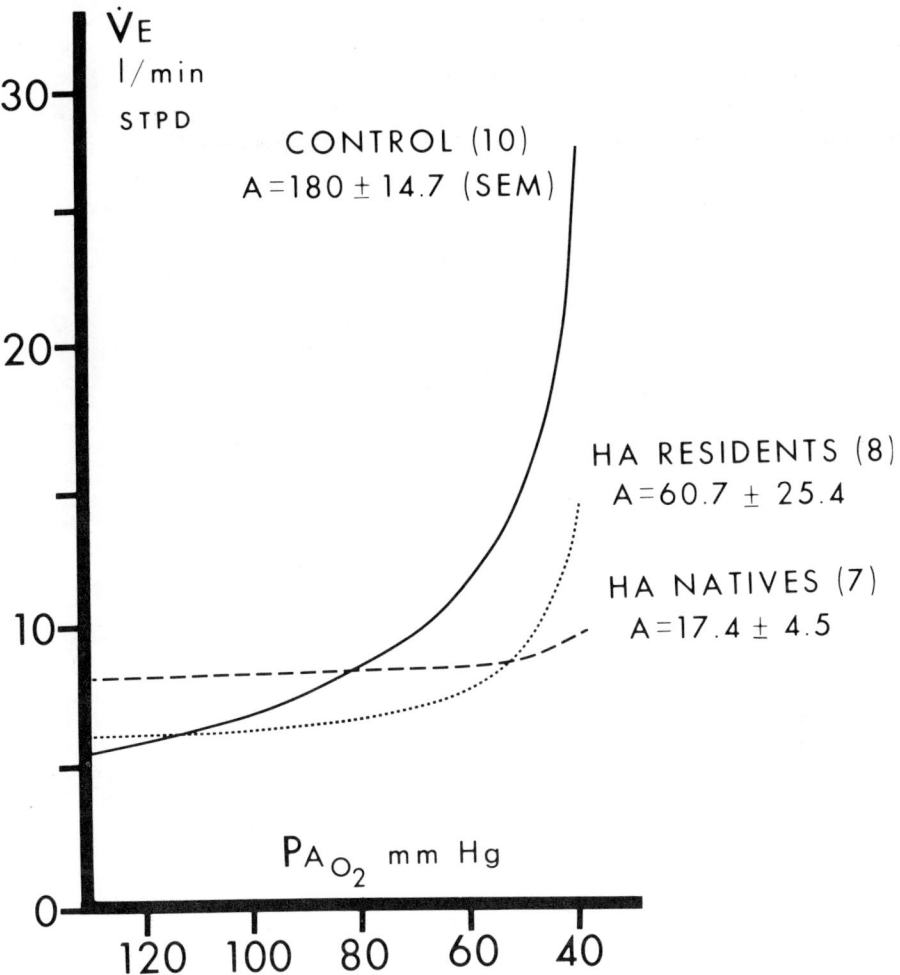

Figure 2. Decreased hypoxic ventilatory drive in high altitude residents and natives. Hypoxic ventilatory responses were uniformly and markedly decreased in natives of Leadville, Colorado (elevation 3,100 M). Non-native residents at that altitude showed an intermediate degree or depression of hypoxic response which is proportional to their length of residence at high altitude. (Reproduced with permission from Reference 2.)

to lung disease, although as we shall see this phenomenon probably has another explanation.

Subsequent studies revealed that there is also considerable variation in ventilatory drives among individuals at low altitude[4] (Figure 3). This

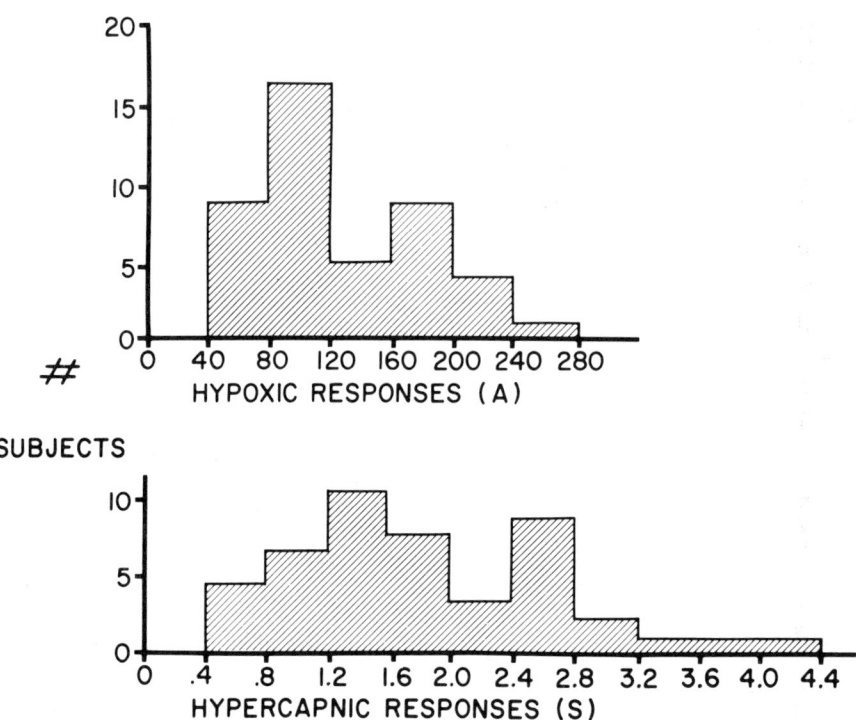

Figure 3. Distribution of ventilatory responses to hypoxia (above) and to hypercapnia (below) in 44 normal subjects at low altitude. Note the broad flat distribution of responses indicating that within the normal population high, low, and mid range responses exist in roughly comparable proportions. (Figure drawn from data in Reference 4.)

led to studies which indicated that patterns of high or low ventilatory drive tend to run in families[5] and that there is greater concordance for ventilatory drive among identical than fraternal twins.[6] Thus, much of the variation in ventilatory drive at low altitude seems to reflect the influence of familiar or genetic factors (Figure 4). This broad range of ventilatory drives in the normal population may be an important antecedent determinant of ventilation in the setting of subsequent disease-induced mechanical or functional impediment to breathing. When ventilatory drives are low, this may predispose to hypoventilation with even mild respiratory disability, whereas the same disability associated with high ventilatory drives may not lead to hypoventilation. Thus, in the face of respiratory disease a patient's ventilatory status may depend upon the balance of the positive effects of ventilatory drive, tending to preserve ventilation, and the negative influence of diseases of the lung, skeletal thorax, and respiratory muscles which act

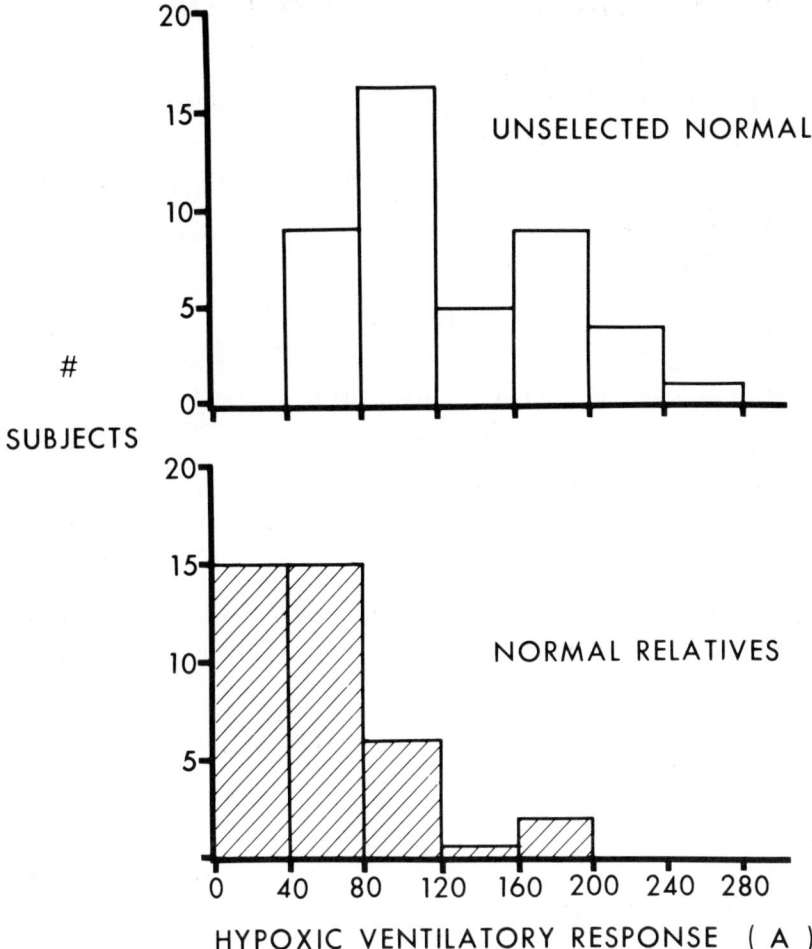

Figure 4. Familial aggregation of decreased ventilatory drives. Distribution of hypoxic responses in an unselected normal population are shown in the top panel, while the bottom panel shows the distribution of responses in another group of normal subjects of comparable age and sex distribution, but selected because they were immediate relatives (parents or siblings) of individuals in whom a low hypoxic ventilatory response had been measured. Thus, a low hypoxic response in one family member was predictive of low responses in other healthy family members.

to reduce ventilation (Figure 5). This is illustrated by the finding that hypoventilating chronic obstructive pulmonary disease patients have decreased ventilatory drives[7,8] compared to those measured in patients who maintain normal ventilation despite comparable severity of airways' obstruction. Similar patterns have been described in the families

FUNDAMENTAL CAUSES OF HYPOVENTILATION

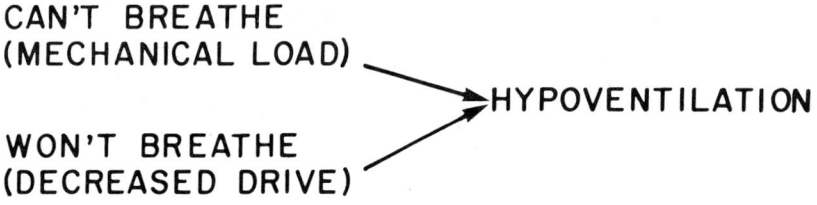

Figure 5.

of such patients, i.e., ventilatory drives are decreased in the families of hypoventilating patients with obstructive lung disease[9,10] (figure 6).

In addition to chronic hypoxia, and familial or genetic influences, other factors may also operate to depress ventilatory drives. These include respiratory depressant drugs such as the barbiturates and opiates. Decreased metabolic rate can also depress ventilatory drive and is probably responsible for the hypoventilation seen in myxedema. However, these are uncommon or short-lived causes of hypoventilation which usually do not lead to pulmonary hypertension or cor pulmonale. Sleep also decreases ventilatory drives, and as we shall see, this may be an important cause of hypoventilation, and because it exerts its influence over a considerable portion of each day can lead to pulmonary hypertension and cor pulmonale.

Because clinical hypoventilation most commonly reflects a combination of an impediment to breathe and a deficit in ventilatory drives, variation in the relative roles played by these factors is responsible for a broad spectrum of patients presenting with hypoventilation. Thus, there are hypoventilating patients with little or no dysfunction of the respiratory apparatus, but major deficits in ventilatory drive, as seen in primary hypoventilation or mild neuromuscular disease where hypoventilation may be a presenting feature but conventional tests of pulmonary function show normal or near-normal results. There are other patients who have diseases associated with impediment to breathing which, however, seem too mild to explain hypoventilation. This is seen in the obesity hypoventilation syndrome[11] and in mild neuromuscular disease, especially myotonic dystrophy,[12] where hypoventilation is often disproportionate to the nearly normal performance on pulmonary function testing. Finally, there are patients in whom hypoventilation is associated with severe anatomical or functional derangement of respiratory apparatus, yet as discussed, even in such patients hypoventilation is typically associated with decreased ventilatory drives.

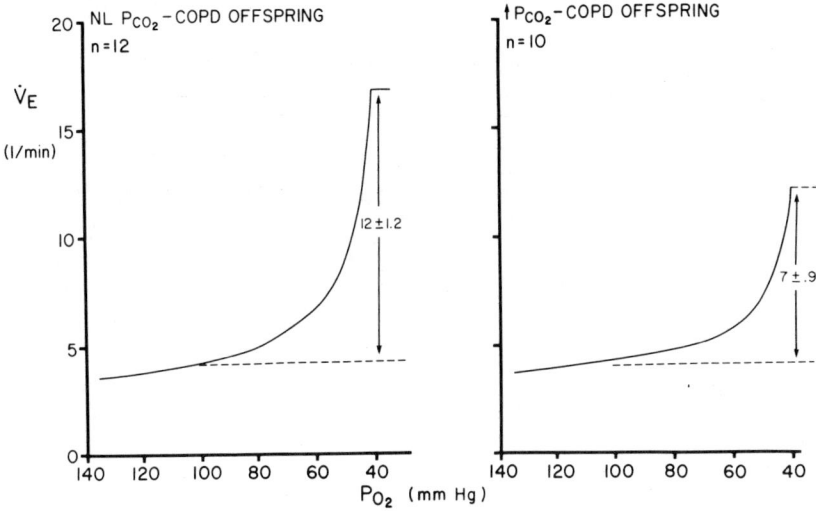

Figure 6. Hypoxic responses in the normal adult offspring of patients with severe chronic obstructive pulmonary disease. Normal offspring of hypoventilating chronic obstructive pulmonary disease patients had decreased hypoxic ventilatory (right panel) responses in comparison with those measured in normal offspring of patients with equally severe airways obstruction who maintained normal ventilation (left panel). The results suggest that hypoventilation in chronic obstructive pulmonary disease is associated with familial decreases in ventilatory drive. (Figure drawn from data in Reference 9.)

RESPIRATORY DISORDERS OF SLEEP

It is now broadly recognized that hypoventilation out of proportion to coexistent respiratory apparatus dysfunction is especially common and may be very severe during sleep.[13] This discovery largely arose from studies aimed at determining the cause of the marked sleepiness observed in hypoventilating, obese subjects with the obesity hypoventilation of Pickwickian syndrome, named after the obese, plethoric, somnolent boy described by Charles Dickens. Gastaut[14] and others in the mid-60's investigated the sleep of such patients using a novel approach which employed conventional electroencephalographic techniques for sleep staging combined with measures of air flow, intrapleural pressure, diaphragmatic electromyogram, and ear oximetery. They found that these patients had frequent and prolonged respiratory pauses, apneas, as often as hundreds of times each night and single apneas occasionally lasted as long as 3 minutes (Figure 7). Analysis of an entire night's sleep revealed that in some individuals more than half

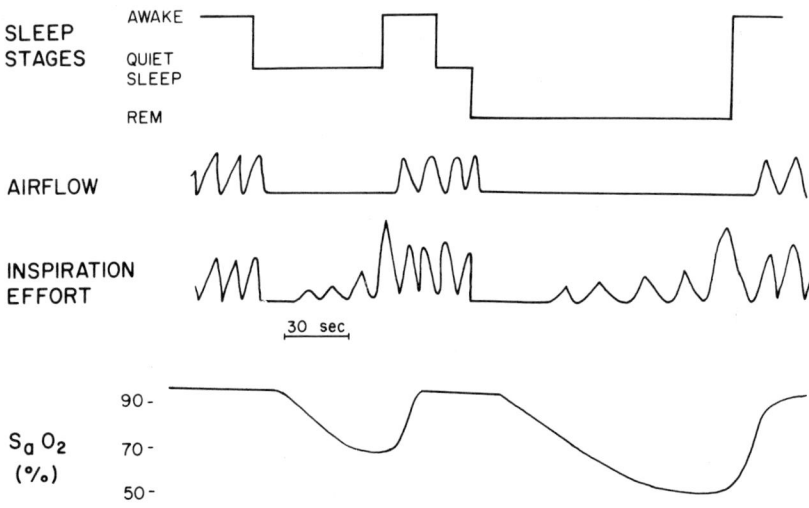

Figure 7. Schematic illustration of interrelationships between sleep stage, air flow, inspiratory effort, and arterial oxygen saturation in a patient with obstructive apnea. During sleep there is a cessation of air flow, apnea, which may last from 10 sec to a few minutes. While there is often a brief decrease or cessation of inspiratory effort, measured as diaphragmatic EMG or intrapleural pressure, effort is eventually resumed, yet there is no air flow. Hence the designation of such an apnea as obstructive. There are associated decreases in arterial oxygen saturation. Following termination of the apnea there is commonly a brief arousal of which there may be hundreds in each night. REM sleep is often associated with the most prolonged apneas and severe hypoxemia.

of the total sleep period was spent in an apneic state. Some apneas were due to a primary cessation of inspiratory activity (central apneas). However, the majority of the more severe and prolonged episodes were clearly related to repetitive upper airway obstruction manifested as cessation of air flow despite continued inspiratory rhythmic activity evidenced by continued cycling of diaphragmatic EMG or intrapleural pressure. Not surprisingly, apneas are associated with phasic hypoxemia and hypercapnia, and the hypoxemia can be very severe with arterial oxygen saturation below 50% and oxygen tensions as low as 20–25 mm Hg. This in turn can lead to pulmonary hypertension presumably through mechanisms identical to those outlined in the preceding chapters. Indeed, it can be shown that with each apneic episode, pulmonary arterial pressure rises coincident with hypoxia and hypercapnia and resolves, albeit only partially, at the end of each apnea with improvement in blood gases[15,16] (Figure 8). The consequence of this partial resolution is that the baseline pulmonary arterial pressure seems to gradually drift higher throughout the night's sleep so that

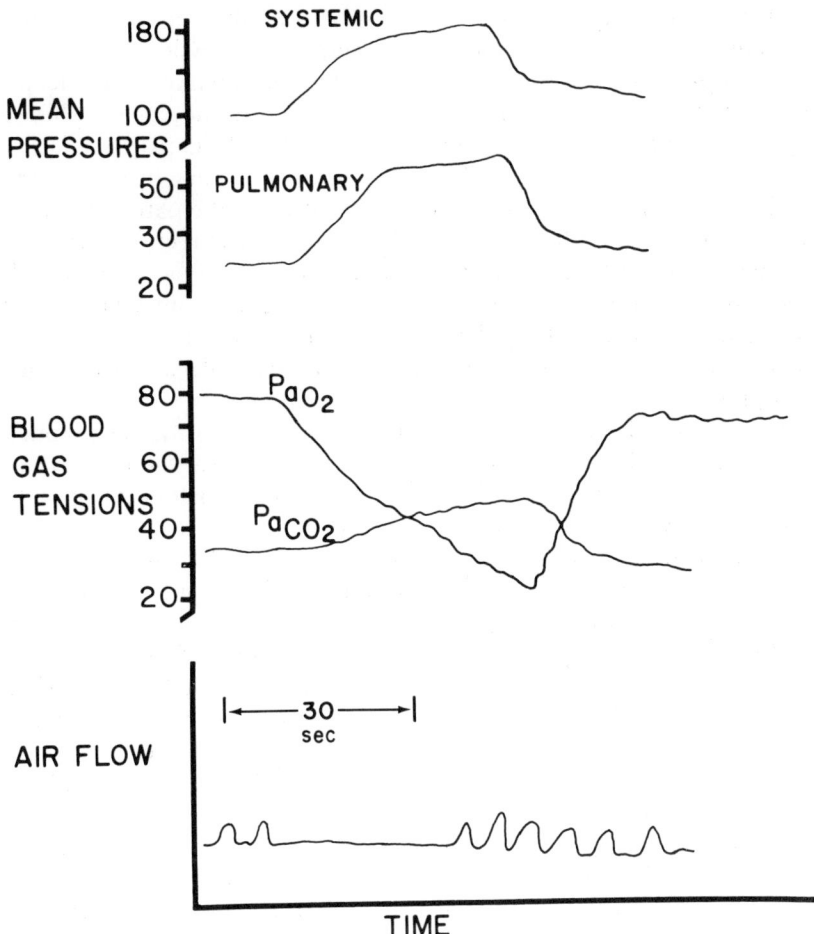

Figure 8. Schematic respresentation of hemodynamic and blood gas events during an apnea. Respiratory pauses are associated with a fall in PaO_2 that generally exceeds the rise in $PaCO_2$ which may reflect the relatively small body store of oxygen compared to CO_2. The combined hypoxia and hypercapnia are probably responsible for the rise in pulmonary arterial pressure which occurs with each apnea. Note that baseline pulmonary arterial pressure is slightly higher following each apnea. (Figure drawn from data in Reference 15.)

pulmonary hypertension is most severe in the morning, resolves gradually during the daytime, only to rise progressively with the apneic episodes during the next night's sleep. Pulmonary hypertension arising from phasic asphyxia with each apnea can lead to residual chronic pulmonary hypertension and cor pulmonale. Similarly, the hypoxemia of the apneic episodes can eventually lead to erythrocytosis.

Apneas are frequently terminated by brief awakenings of which the patient remains unaware, but it is thought that they lead to chronic sleep deprivation or fragmentation resulting in the irresistible sleepiness which is such a striking feature of patients with the classical obesity hypoventilation syndrome. Long-term sequelae of sleep apnea, in addition to severe, irresistible sleepiness and pulmonary hypertension, include an increase in systemic arterial pressure,[16] the pathogenesis of which is not well understood, and the common occurrence of cardiac arrhythmias. Although a variety of arrhythmias have been described, the most common are bradyarrhythmias ranging from severe sinus bradycardia to asystole and occasionally heart block. They appear to be cholinergically mediated as they are typically abolished with atropine.[17]

Collectively these disorders are now referred to as the sleep apnea syndromes, and a number of interesting facts have emerged regarding the setting in which they occur. While these disorders, as already mentioned, were initially described in the rare patients with the classic obesity hypoventilation syndrome, it is now clear that they are more common than was once thought. Pronounced sleep apnea seems especially frequent in middle-aged or older men and is often associated with obesity and a history of heavy snoring. Some degree of sleep apnea is common in otherwise healthy middle-aged men[18] as is snoring, which probably represents a mild form of upper airway obstruction. Indeed, there does not appear to be a clear dividing line between the normal sleep apnea of middle-aged snoring men and the pathological sleep apnea seen in symptomatic patients. Remarkably, premenopausal women are commonly regular breathers with little or no apnea but following the menopause, erratic breathing and apneas emerge, resembling that seen in men.[18] This suggests that hormonal factors are somehow involved in the maintenance of respiratory rhythm and upper airway patency during sleep. Hypoventilation and hypoxemia also occur during sleep in the absence of clear cut apneas, and this is seen in normal subjects,[18] in asthma,[19] and in patients with the "blue bloater" type of chronic obstructive pulmonary disease in whom sleep hypoxemia may be quite severe especially during REM sleep[20] (Figure 9).

It is not entirely clear why hypoventilation and apnea should be so frequent during sleep, but a number of important factors bearing on this issue are now apparent. First, decreased ventilatory drives may be important in either producing or permitting hypoventilation or apnea in sleep. In many cases of sleep apnea or hypoxemia, as in patients with the obesity hypoventilation syndrome or the "blue bloater" variety of

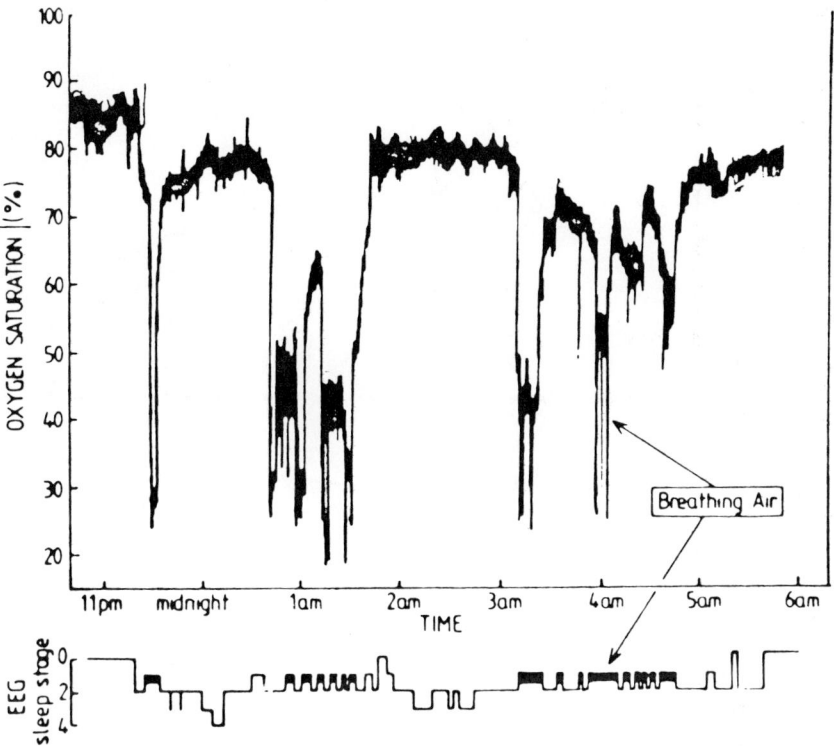

Figure 9. Severe, episodic hypoxemia during sleep in a patient with the "blue bloater" type of chronic obstructive pulmonary disease. Most of the severe hypoxic episodes occur during REM sleep. (Reproduced with permission from Reference 20.)

chronic obstructive pulmonary disease, ventilatory drives measured during wakefulness are decreased.[7,8,21] Further, it is now clear that even in normal subjects sleep itself leads to marked attenuation of ventilatory drives[22–25] (Figure 10). This effect is especially pronounced in dreaming or rapid eye movement (REM) sleep where hypoventilation and apnea are often most frequent and severe. Thus, ventilatory drives which may be reduced during wakefulness may be further and markedly depressed during sleep and might explain or contribute to occurrence of hypoventilation or apneas resulting from a primary decrease or cessation of ventilatory effort. Although these decreases in ventilatory drive might explain hypoventilation, the reasons for upper airway obstruction and obstructive apnea during sleep are less apparent. Curiosity about the pathogenesis of obstructive apneas stimulated research into mechanisms involved in the normal maintenance of

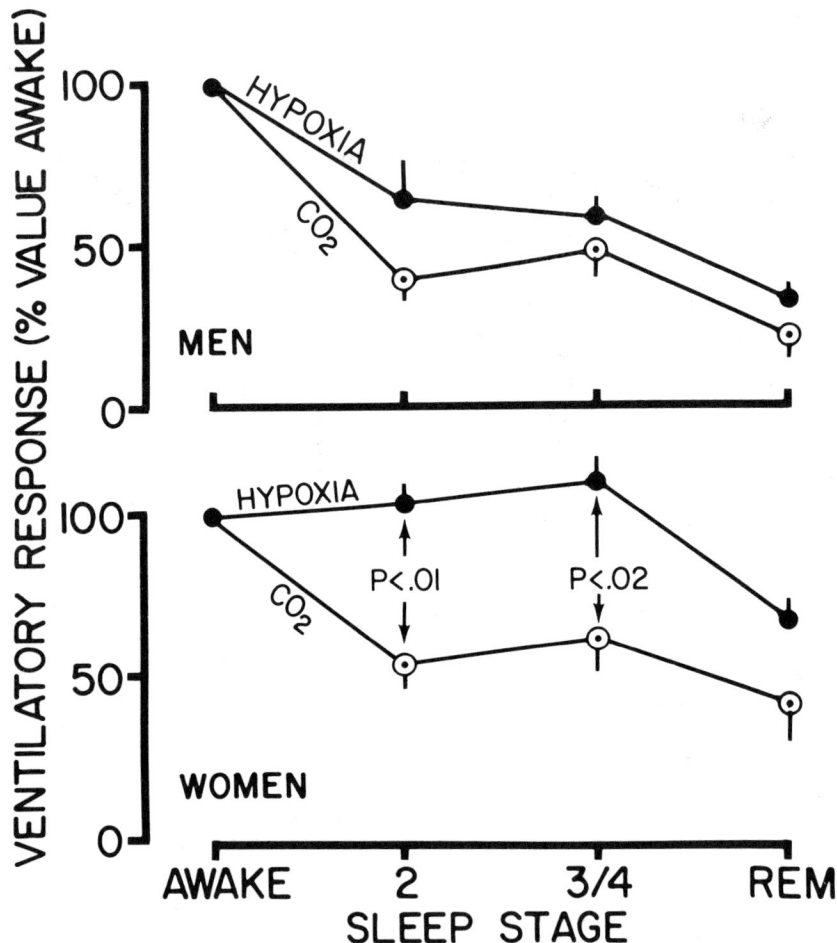

Figure 10. Ventilatory responses to hypoxia and CO_2 are depressed in sleep. Hypercapnic responses are depressed in both men and women, reaching their lowest values in REM sleep. Hypoxic response shows a similar pattern in men, but in women there is better preservation of this response in sleep. (Reproduced with permission from Reference 23.)

Figure 11. Upper airway muscle activity in sleep. This figure illustrates the activity of the genioglossus muscle which acts to pull the base of the tongue forward opening the upper airway. This muscle has clear-cut EMG bursts synchronous with inspiration (left panel). In the supine position, when upper airway patency is threatened there is an associated increase in the inspiratory bursts as well as increased tonic activity (middle panel). In patients with obstructive sleep apnea genioglossal EMG activity is greatly attenuated (right panel). This loss of upper airway muscle activity combined with anatomic encroachment probably represents an important contributor to the pathogenesis of upper airway obstruction in sleep. (Reproduced with permission from Reference 26.)

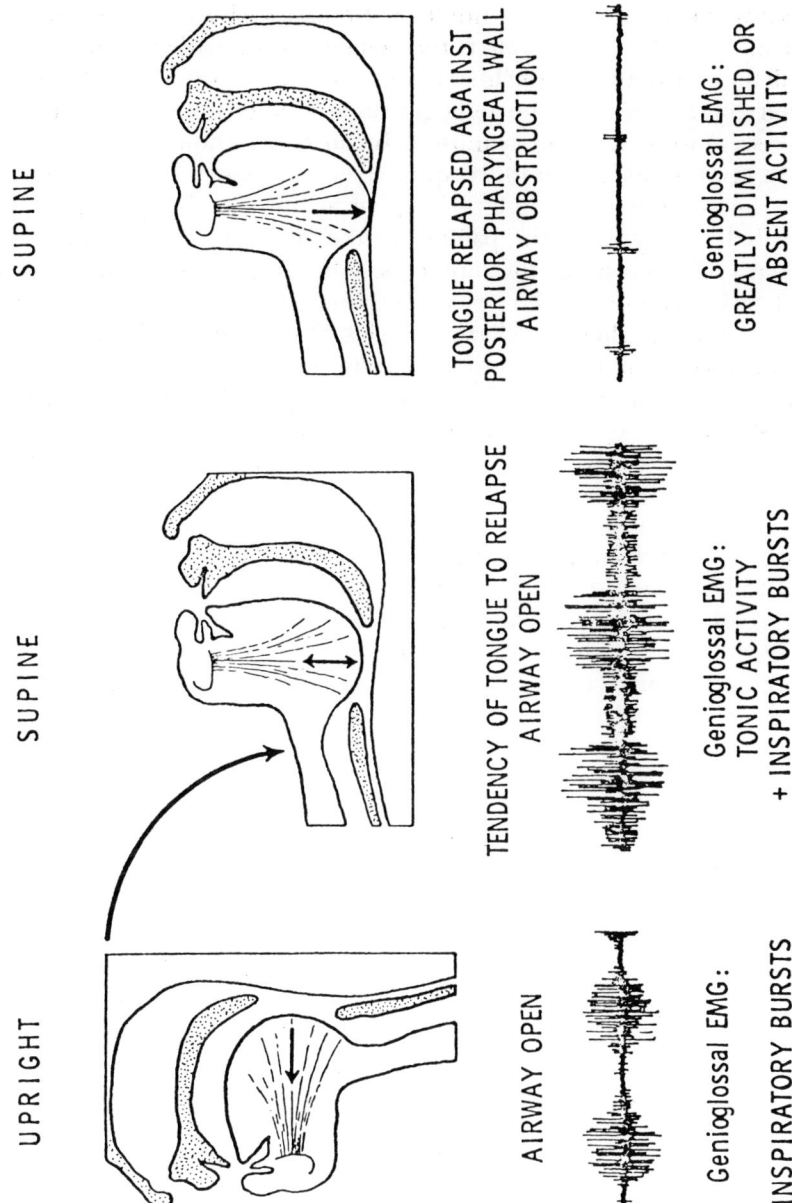

upper airway patency. It now seems likely that the upper airway remains patent in part because of its anatomic structure but also in part because of the activity of a number of muscles which act to keep the airway open.[13] An example is the genioglossus muscle which acts to pull the base of the tongue forward away from the posterior wall of the pharynx (Figure 11). The genioglossus and other upper airway muscles seem to be respiratory muscles because they show phasic activity with inspiration, and in this respect resemble classic inspiratory muscles such as the diaphragm.[25,26] Upper airway muscles also show increased activity when the patency of the airway is compromised, as when a subject assumes the supine position which causes the tongue to fall back and obstruct the airway. It is also apparent that these upper airway muscles, like the classic muscles of inspiration, are linked to ventilatory drives in that most of the classic ventilatory stimuli, such as hypercapnia and hypoxia, lead to increased activity of these muscles. This would act to insure upper airway patency at times when blood gases are in jeopardy and there is a need for increased ventilation. This link between ventilatory drives and upper airway muscles may explain the association of upper airway obstruction and obstructive apneas with depressed ventilatory drives during sleep.

In addition to the failure of active muscular mechanisms for maintenance of upper airway patency, it is clear that anatomical factors also contribute to upper airway obstruction. In some cases obvious and specific anatomic encroachment on the upper airway is apparent, as in children with enlarged tonsils and adenoids, or in adults with congenital skeletal deformities such as micrognathia, or tumors of the larynx and pharynx. The most common anatomic contribution to upper airway obstruction is obesity where pharyngeal CAT scans show marked narrowing of the upper airway presumably due to encroachment by cervical adipose tissue.[27] Present evidence suggests that the patient most likely to develop obstruction is an individual with an anatomically narrowed upper airway and a loss of synchronous inspiratory upper airway muscle activity due perhaps in part to depressed ventilatory drives.

Diagnosis of these disorders can be difficult because the most striking abnormalities occur in sleep and because the daytime manifestations of the disorder can be subtle, nonspecific, and protean. Indeed, there is an impressive array of presenting manifestations including somnolence, hypoventilation, obesity, hypertension, congestive heart failure, or polycythemia. The somnolence arising from sleep fragmentation can be mistaken for a primary disorder, such as narcolepsy, or may be attributed to CO_2 narcosis due to lung disease, such as chronic obstructive pulmonary disease, until spirometry reveals normal or near normal lung function and blood gas measurements show only mild elevations in $PaCO_2$. Polycythemia is often attributed to primary erythrocytosis because only red cells are increased. Absence of leukocytosis, thrombocytosis, and splenomegaly help in ruling out polycythemia vera. However, the near-normal blood gases during wakefulness may misleadingly suggest that the problem is not secondary to hypoxemia.

The key to diagnosis of respiratory disorders of sleep is frequently a high index of suspicion and a careful history taken from both the patient and other individuals sharing the same household. Patients with severe apnea are often middle-aged males or post-menopausal females, and loud snoring, a common feature of the history, is often sufficiently severe to necessitate separate bedrooms for spouses. Family members often comment on the restless nature of the patient's sleep. Patients often complain of awakening in the morning feeling fatigued, and occasionally a morning headache may reflect the cerebral vasodilator effects of hypercapnia during sleep. The patient, and quite often his associates, describe excessive, sometimes irresistible, daytime somnolence with dozing at inappropriate times and there are often personality changes and loss of intellectual function.

Features of the physical examination are variable, the patient is commonly middle-aged and obese, as already mentioned, and may have a sleepy or lethargic demeanor. Systemic hypertension is often present, and there may be any or all of the stigmata of pulmonary hypertension and right-sided congestive heart failure outlined in the preceding chapter with the exception that evidence of obvious disease of the lungs, chest wall, or respiratory muscles is typically absent. Laboratory data may reveal an elevated hematocrit, and arterial blood gases may show mild hypercapnia and hypoxemia.

Patients in whom the history and laboratory features suggest the possibility of a respiratory disorder of sleep should undergo studies during sleep. The simplest of these is the monitoring of arterial oxygenation with an ear oximeter in sleep to determine whether frequent and severe episodes of hypoxemia occur. The advantages of the test are that it requires only an ear oximeter, which is becoming a widely available instrument. The disadvantages are that it is often uncertain whether the patient slept during the study, and such a study does not exclude the possibility that frequent apneas might have occurred but were insufficient in duration to lead to significant desaturation. Still, the majority of patients with serious respiratory disorders of sleep will probably be detected during such a test. A more sophisticated approach is the combination of ear oximetery, electroencephalography,

EKG monitoring, and measures of respiratory air flow. Such a test will document that sleep occurred, detect apneas, demonstrate their type, and document the extent of cardiac arrthymias and the severity of hypoxemia. This test is commonly conducted throughout a full night's sleep, but good information can also be obtained during a daytime nap.

Therapy of respiratory disorders of sleep remains controversial and largely unsettled. The most definitive remedy for severe obstructive apneas is tracheostomy[13,15,16] but this is an invasive procedure with a number of problems, and is being used with decreasing frequency as alternative approaches evolve. In obese patients weight loss, while difficult to achieve, is commonly effective. It is typically not necessary for the patient to shed large amounts of weight, regaining a normal habitus, but often reduction of 20 to 30 pounds can lead to substantial improvement.[11] The problem is that such weight loss, even if achieved, can be difficult to sustain, and surgical procedures such as intestinal bypass and gastric fundal plication have been used.[28] Intestinal bypass has largely been abandoned because of a number of late and serious complications, and gastric plication has only a partial success rate. Some patients, particularly those with obesity and daytime hypoventilation corresponding to the classic Pickwickian picture may benefit from the administration of progestational agents[29] which seem to act as stimulants of ventilatory drive. Other patients with sleep apnea have shown improvement when treated with protriptyline,[30] a nonsedating tricyclic antidepressant. Nocturnal oxygen administration has had variable results leading to prolonged apneas in some patients and to resolution of apnea in others.[31,32] Finally, preliminary reports suggest impressive resolution of obstructive sleep apnea with the application of continuous positive airway pressure applied to the upper airway during sleep with a tightly fitting nose mask.[33] Presumably this positive pressure acts to maintain the patency of the upper airway and thereby prevents obstructive apnea. As more practical techniques are developed for the application of such nasal positive pressure, this may become an increasingly popular form of therapy.

SUMMARY

Ventilation is largely a balance of the positive contributions of ventilatory drive and the negative effects of dysfunction of the respiratory apparatus leading to mechanical or physiological impediment to breathing or gas exchange. Thus, hypoventilation and its sequelae, pulmonary hypertension, and cor pulmonale can occur in individuals with little respiratory dysfunction but with major defects in ventilatory drive. This combination occurs fairly often because ventilatory drives are highly variable. There are numerous instances of low ventilatory drives in the normal population, due occasionally to exposure to chronic hypoxia, but more often due to spontaneous variation or the operation of familial–genetic effects. While such low drives in themselves seem to do no harm, when this is combined with even small degrees of respiratory dysfunction, it contributes to the development of clinically significant hypoventilation. Ventilatory drives are particularly likely to be depressed during sleep, and this together with factors which narrow the upper airway, such as obesity, may explain the development of severe sleep apnea leading to hypoxia, hypercapnia, pulmonary hypertension, and cor pulmonale. In other disease states, such as chronic airways obstruction, decreased ventilatory drive may worsen hypoventilation and hypoxemia leading to increased pulmonary hypertension and heart failure. Thus, in addition to the extent of disease of the lungs, chest wall, or respiratory muscles, the status of ventilatory drives should be considered as important determinants of ventilation and events in the pulmonary circulation.

REFERENCES

1. Severinghaus JW. Hypoxic respiratory drive and its loss during chronic hypoxia. *Clin Physiol* 1971;2:57–79.
2. Weil JV, Byrne-Quinn E, Sodal IE, Filley GF, Grover RF: Acquired attenuation of chemoreceptor function in chronically hypoxic man at high altitude. *J Clin Invest* 1971;50:186–195.
3. Sorenson SC, Severinghaus JW: Respiratory insensitivity to acute hypoxia persisting after correction of tetralogy of Fallot. *J Appl Physiol* 1968;25:221–223.
4. Hirshman CA, McCullough RE, Weil JV: Normal values for hypoxic and hypercapnic ventilatory drives in man. *J Appl Physiol* 1975;38:1095–1098.
5. Moore GC, Zwillich CW, Battaglia JD, Cotton EK, Weil JV: Respiratory failure associated with familial depression of ventilatory response to hypoxia and hypercapnia. *N Engl J Med* 1976;295:861–865.
6. Collins DD, Scoggin CH, Zwillich CW, Weil JV: Hereditary aspects of decreased hypoxic response. *J Clin Invest* 1978;62:105–110.
7. Matthews AW, Howell JBL: Assessment of responsiveness to carbon dioxide in patients with chronic airways obstruction by rate of isometric inspiratory pressure development. *Clin Sci Molec Med* 1976;50:199–205.
8. Bradley CA, Fleetham JA, Anthonisen NR: Ventilatory control in patients with hypoxemia due to obstructive lung disease. *Am Rev Resp Dis* 1979;120:21–31.

9. Mountain R, Zwillich C, Weil J: Hypoventilation in obstructive lung disease: The role of familial factors. *N Eng J Med* 1978;298:521–525.
10. Kawakami Y, Irie T, Shida A, Yoshikawa T: Familial factors affecting arterial blood gas values and respiratory chemosensitivity in chronic obstructive pulmonary disease. *Am Rev Resp Dis* 1982;125:420–425.
11. Rochester DF, Enson Y: Current concepts in the pathogenesis of the obesity hypoventilation syndrome. *Am J Med* 1974;57:402–420.
12. Carroll JE, Zwillich CW, Weil JV: Ventilatory response in myotonic dystrophy. *Neurology* 1977;27:1125–1128.
13. Guilleminault C, Dement WC: *Sleep Apnea Syndromes*. New York: Alan R. Liss, Inc., 1978.
14. Gastaut H, Tassinari CA, Duron B: Polygraphic study of the episodic diurnal and nocturnal (hypnic and respiratory) manifestations of the pickwick syndrome. *Brain Res* 1966;2:167–186.
15. Guilleminault C, Tilkian A, Dement WC: The sleep apnea syndromes. *Ann Rev Med* 1976;27:465–484.
16. Motta J, Guilleminault C, Schroeder JS, Dement WC: Tracheostomy and hemodynamic changes in sleep-induced apnea. *Ann Intern Med* 1978;89:454–458.
17. Tilkian AG, Motta J, Guilleminault C: Cadiac arrhythmias in sleep apnea. In, *Sleep Apnea Syndromes*. Guilleminault C, Dement W. (Eds.) New York, Alan R. Liss, Inc., 1978; pp. 197–210.
18. Block AJ, Boysen PG, Wynne JW, Hunt IA: Sleep apnea, hypopnea and oxygen desaturation in normal subjects. *N Engl J Med* 1979;300:513–517.
19. Catterall JR, Calverley PMA, Brezinova V, Douglas NJ, Brash HM, Shapiro CM, Flenley DC: Irregular breathing and hypoxaemia during sleep in chronic stable asthma. *Lancet* 1982;1:301–304.
20. Douglas NJ, Leggett RJE, Calverley PMA, Brash HM: Transient hypoxaemia during sleep in chronic bronchitis and emphysema. *Lancet* 1979;1:1–4.
21. Zillich CW, Sutton FD, Pierson DJ, Creagh EM, Weil JV: Decreased hypoxic ventilatory drive in the obesity-hypoventilation syndrome. *Am J Med* 1975;59:343–348.
22. Bulow K: Respiration and wakefulness in man. *Acta Physiol Scand* 1963;209:10–110.
23. Douglas NJ, White DP, Weil JV, Pickett CK, Zwillich CW: Hypercapnic ventilatory response in sleeping adults. *Am Rev Respir Dis* 1982;126:758–762.
24. White DP, Douglas NJ, Pickett CK, Weil JV, Zwillich CW: Hypoxic ventilatory response during sleep in normal premenopausal women. *Am Rev Resp Dis* 1982;126:530–533.
25. Douglas NJ, White DP, Weil JV, Pickett CK, Martin RJ, Hudgel DW, Zwillich CW: Hypoxic ventilatory response decreases during sleep in normal man. *Am Rev Resp Dis* 1982;125:266–269.
26. Harper RM, Sauerland EK: The role of the tongue in sleep apnea. *Sleep Apnea Syndrome*. New York: Alan R. Liss, Inc., 1978:219–234.
27. Haponik EF, Bohlman M, Smith PL, Allen R, Goldman S, Bleecker ER: CT scanning in obstructive sleep apnea: Correlation of structure with airway physiology during sleep and wakefulness. *Am Rev Resp Dis* 1982;125:107 (Abstract).

28. Pochi PE: Surgical therapy for obesity. (Editorial) *N Engl J Med* 1983: 308:1026–1027.
29. Strohl KP, Hensley MJ, Saunders NJ, Scharf SM, Brown R, Ingram RN: Progesterone administration and progressive sleep apneas. *J Am Med Assn* 1981;245:1230–1232.
30. Brownell LG, West P, Sweatman P, Acres JC, Kryger MH: Protriptyline in obstructive sleep apnea. *N Eng J Med* 1982;307:1037–1042.
31. Motta J, Guilleminault C: Effects of oxygen administration in sleep-induced apneas. In, Guilleminault C, Dement WC eds. *Sleep Apnea Syndromes*. New York: Alan R. Liss, Inc., 1978:137–144.
32. McNicholas WT, Carter JL, Rutherford R, Zamel N, Phillipson EA: Beneficial effect of oxygen in primary alveolar hypoventilation with central sleep apnea. *Am Rev Resp Dis* 1982;125:773–775.
33. Sullivan CE, Berthon-Jones M, Issa FG, Eves L: Reversal of obstructive sleep apnoea by continuous positive airway pressure applied through the nares. *Lancet* 1981;1:862–865.

CHAPTER 9

DRUG AND DIETARY INDUCED PULMONARY HYPERTENSION

Johannes Mlczoch

INTRODUCTION

Twenty-five years ago the possibility that drugs or diet might induce or contribute to pulmonary hypertension was not considered. Today, the proven facts are still few, because we do not know the mechanism by which a suspected substance can induce pulmonary hypertension.

How might an ingested substance work?
- It could be toxic or have toxic metabolites which may affect the pulmonary vasculature either directly, or through an action on circulating cells.
- It could disturb liver function, thus allowing the circulation of vasoactive substances which are normally inactivated in the liver.
- It may act only in certain persons in whom hormonal balance, neural activity, or immune status allow the substance to be toxic.

The interest in this problem increased dramatically when an epidemic of pulmonary hypertension occurred in Europe between 1966 and 1969 following the introduction of anorectic drugs such as Aminorex.[1-5] This epidemic was the first indication of a link between drugs and the development of pulmonary hypertension in man. The epidemic in man was reminiscent of the 1961 discovery that crotaline alkaloids, when fed to rats, caused pulmonary hypertension. Although we are not certain that it is possible to induce pulmonary hypertension in man by drug administration or dietary measures, the following discussion summarizes our present knowledge.

DRUGS

Amorexigens

Aminorex

Aminorex fumarate (menocil) became available in November 1965 in Switzerland, in April 1966 in Germany, and in August 1966 in Austria. By acting directly on the central nervous system the substance not only depressed appetite but also had an euphoric effect. Aminorex was soon the most common anorectic drug used in these countries, with more than 1 million tablets sold in 1967 in Switzerland alone.[6] Aminorex is a sympathicomimetic drug and its chemical structure (2-amino-5-phenyl-2-oxazoline) resembles amphetamine, norepinephrine, and ephedrine. Even aminorex intoxication[7,8] or intravenous infusion of aminorex in patients with normal pulmonary arterial pressure[9] did not result in an increase in pulmonary pressure. Before a connection with pulmonary hypertension was suspected, only one case of pulmonary hypertension was identified in several clinical trials involving the administration of aminorex to a total of 4,400 subjects.[10] Only nonspecific cardiovascular side effects were reported in other subjects.[10-12] For these reasons and because symptoms did not develop until 4 to 11 months after beginning aminorex,[13] it has been difficult to demonstrate a connection between aminorex and the increased incidence of pulmonary hypertension. However, there have been some patients who developed dyspnea and syncope after aminorex intake, which disappeared after withdrawal and reappeared when the drug was used again.[14,15]

Epidemology

The strongest point in favor of aminorex as an etiologic factor in the development of pulmonary hypertension is the epidemiology.[1,16,17] The sudden increase in the incidence in pulmonary hypertension in Switzerland, Germany, and Austria cannot be attributed to improved clinical or hemodynamic methods of investigation. This increase was first noted in Switzerland[4,5]; the initial detailed report was made by Gurtner in 1968.[3] As a result, an International Symposium was held in Vienna in November of that year,[18] after which aminorex was withdrawn from the market by the company. The number of patients diagnosed as having pulmonary hypertension peaked in 1968 with an approximately 20-fold increase (Figure 1). In a cooperative study of the German Society of Cardiology, with centers in Switzerland and Austria, 582 patients were identified after 1966 as new cases of pulmonary hypertension of unknown origin.[1,17] Sixty-one percent gave a history of taking aminorex, either alone, or in combination with another anorectic drug. Other anorectic drugs without aminorex were taken by 6.4%, in 5.5% a history of drug intake was not available, and in 27.1% the patients gave a history of no anorectic drug intake.[17] This relatively high percentage of patients without anorectic drug intake suggested that the epidemic outbreak of pulmonary hypertension might be unrelated to anorectic drugs. However, in that case, it would still be unclear why the outbreak of pulmonary hypertension was only seen in these 3 countries where aminorex was on the market, and disappeared after withdrawal of the drug. Furthermore, several clinicians reported that even patients with definitive proof of aminorex intake denied the use of this drug for unknown reasons.[13,19]

Gurtner, in Switzerland, found no definite relationship between the risk of developing pulmonary hypertension and the individual dose of

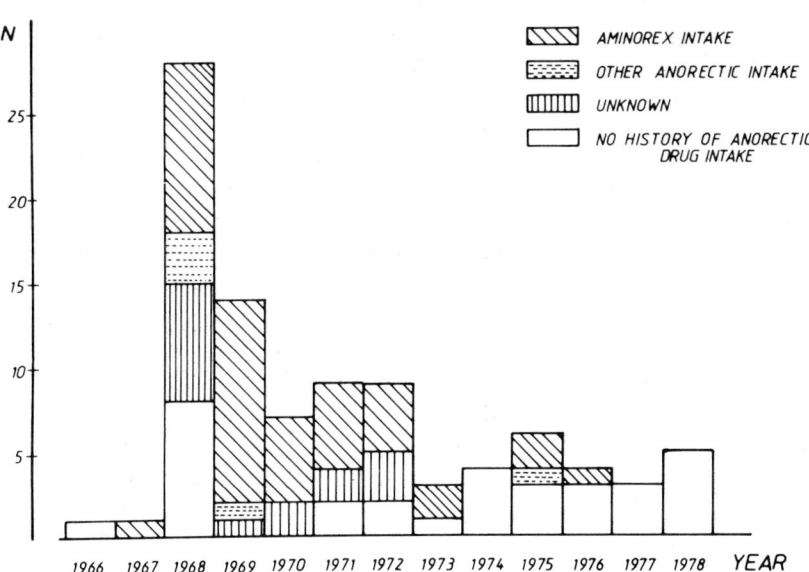

Figure 1. Increase in incidence of pulmonary hypertension of unknown origin in Vienna 1968.

aminorex,[13] but in a report from Hannover, the risk of developing pulmonary hypertension was about 0.5% after 40 tablets (14 mg per tablet) of aminorex and increased to up to 10% in patients with 320 or more tablets of aminorex.[17] The overall incidence of developing pulmonary hypertension in those who took aminorex was about 1–2%,[13] but the risk of developing pulmonary hypertension in this group was 52:1 compared to patients without aminorex intake.[17] Although aminorex is an anorectic agent, obesity was not an important etiological factor. Among the first 31 patients described by Gurtner,[3] only 10 patients were definitely overweight.

Clinical Data

The clinical features of the patients with aminorex-related pulmonary hypertension are not different from the patients without anorectic drug intake.[13,18,20] The early symptoms are palpitations, tachycardia, and hyperventilation, which were at first misinterpreted as a "neurovegetative disorder."[4] Later on, the principal symptom in all patients is dyspnea,[19] initially occurring only on exertion and later at rest. Then, in the course of the disease the following signs and symptoms occur in decreasing frequency: edema, hepatomegaly, angina, cough, syncope, and hemoptysis.[21] The auscultation of an accentuated second pulmonic sound is the main finding at physical examination.[16,19]

The ECG usually shows right axis deviation and an incomplete right bundle branch block. The majority of patients have additional signs of severe right ventricular hypertrophy such as those described in Chapter 1. The chest x-ray is typical for pulmonary hypertension, with prominence of the main pulmonary artery segment, widening of the diameter of the central pulmonary arteries, and narrowing of the peripheral vessels.[22] Hemodynamic measurements show marked precapillary pulmonary hypertension with a mean pulmonary arteriolar resistance of about 10 units[14,15] and a range of 2 to 37.5 units (mm Hg/L/min). Pulmonary angiograms were performed at the beginning of the epidemic in most patients and showed widening of the pulmonary trunk, followed by sudden narrowing of the pulmonary arteries, almost no capillary phase, and rapid opacification of the pulmonary veins.[22] Pulmonary function studies have been essentially normal and a reduction in PaO_2 is only observed occasionally.[16,23] Marked hyperventilation at rest has been reported in several studies.[23] Pulmonary perfusion scintigrams have usually been normal.[24]

Histologic Data

The histology of the pulmonary vasculature was of great interest in these patients, in the hope that it might define a possible—so far undetected—reason for the pulmonary hypertension. In lung biopsies taken in 1968 from 8 patients with Aminorex-related pulmonary hypertension, the main findings were concentric fibrous thickening and edema of the intima, with extensive proliferation of the endothelial cells (Figure 2).[25,26] The lumina of the vessels were nearly obstructed by the proliferating endothelial cells, and there were only capillary-like slits in between (Figure 3). In some areas intravascular fibrin deposition was observed.[25,26] The biopsies did not show the medial hypertrophy and inflammatory vessel wall changes seen in primary pulmonary hypertension as discussed in detail in Chapter 11. Skin biopsies were performed in some patients who developed cyanotic areas on the cheeks and at the extremities. The histologic changes in the small arteries were essentially the same as those found in the lung biopsies[27] (Figure 4). The capillaries and non-muscular arterioles showed dilata-

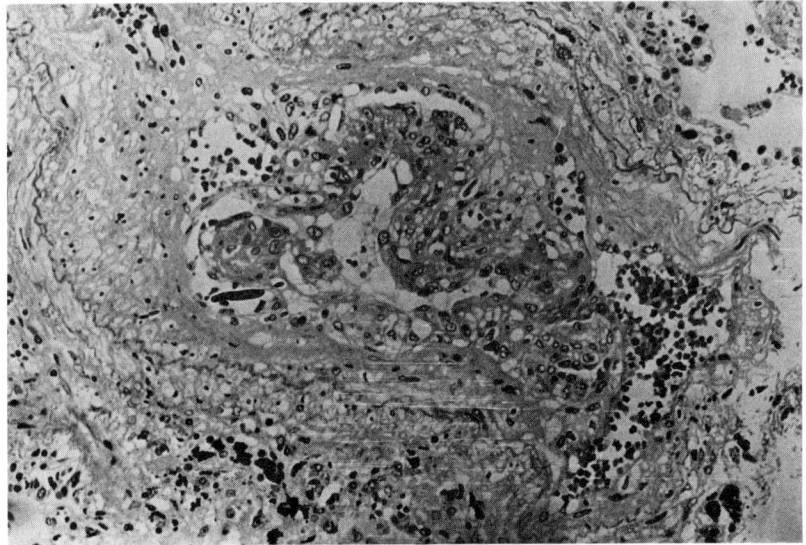

Figure 2. Lung biopsy: muscular pulmonary artery with enlarged endothelial cells and irregular endothelial cell proliferation into the lumen (toluidin-blue). (Unpublished figure courtesy of Prof. Dr. I. Mayer-Obiditsch.)

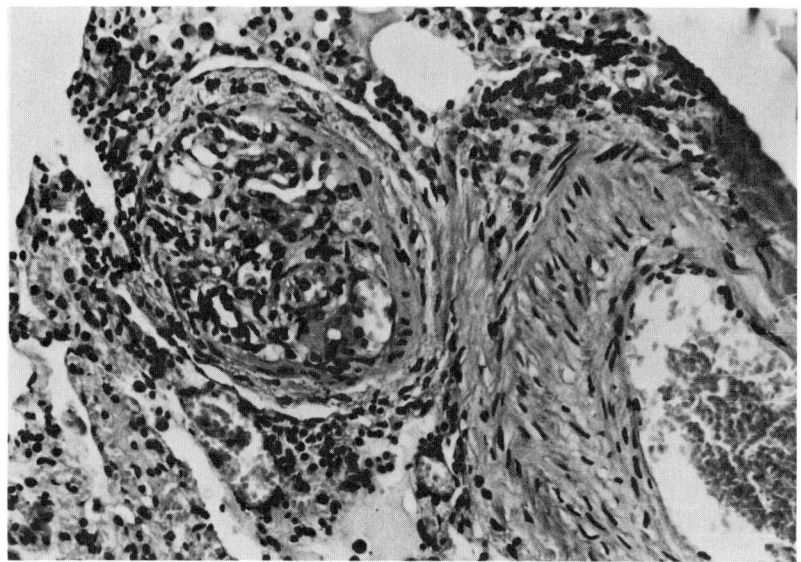

Figure 3. Lung biopsy: muscular pulmonary artery with cell-rich intima proliferation with slit-like perforation (haematoxylin-eosin). (Unpublished figure courtesy of Prof. Dr. I. Mayer-Obiditsch.)

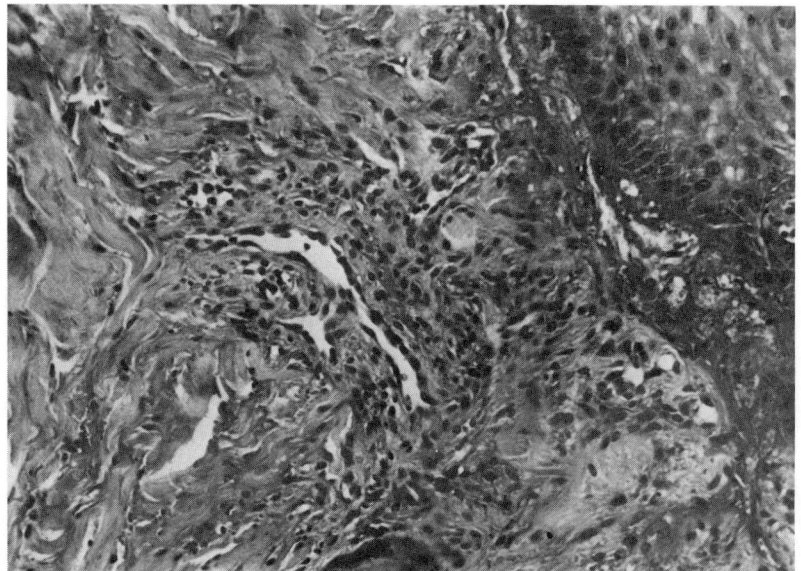

Figure 4. Skin biopsy showing arteriole with increase in endothelial cells and enlargement of nuclei (haematoxylin-osin). (Unpublished figure courtesy of Prof. Dr. I. Mayer-Obiditsch.)

tion and endothelial proliferation. However, more extensive morphologic studies in autopsies of patients with a history of Aminorex intake showed that the lesions of the muscular pulmonary arteries are in fact comparable to those described in primary pulmonary hypertension and no specific changes could be discerned[28,29] (Figure 5). The ultrastructure of intimal hyperplasia consists of myointimal cells and smooth muscle cells.[28] Widgren summarized the histology as a vicious cycle consisting of "morphologic healing" (fibrosis and dilatation), "histologic activity" (intimal proliferation and plexiform lesions), "functional activity" (muscular spasm and muscularization of the intima), and "functional inactivity" (angiomatoid lesions).[28]

Follow-up Data

At first, there was a general impression that most of the patients had a rapidly deteriorating course. The mortality rate was initially reported to be about 44%[23] and in another report 20%.[13] However, a follow-up study on more than 200 patients after 2 years, revealed a mortality of approximately 10%, with a time interval of about 1½ years between the onset of symptoms and death.[13] Survival rate at 5 years is about 75% and at 10 years 44%.[21] Some authors felt that patients with anorectic drug intake had a better prognosis than those with primary pulmonary

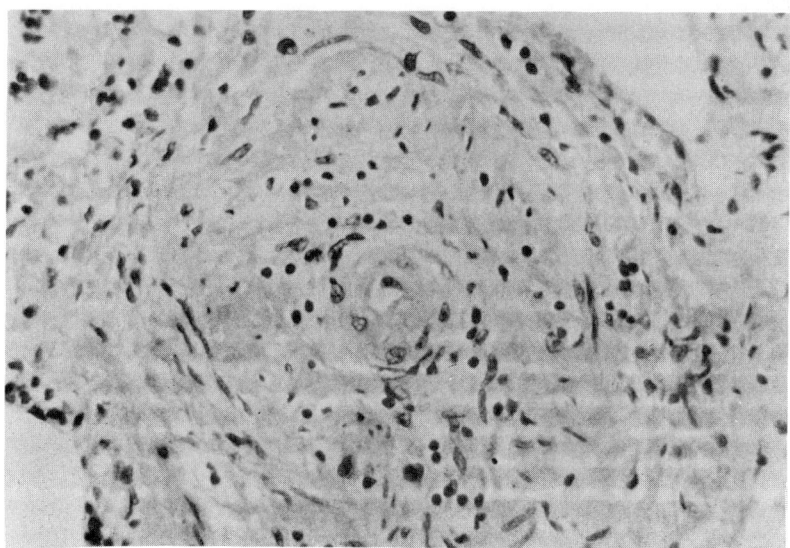

Figure 5. Muscular pulmonary artery with medial hypertrophy and intimal proliferation at autopsy (haematoxylin-eosin). (Unpublished figure courtesy of Prof. Dr. I. Mayer-Obiditsch.)

hypertension; however, this is not supported by the survival rates.[21,30]

Recent follow-up has revealed that long-term survival is possible, even for patients with very high pulmonary arterial pressures at diagnosis.[21] Hemodynamic improvements have been found (Figure 6), especially in patients who had only modest increases in pulmonary pressures initially. Cases have been reported with normalization of the pulmonary arterial pressure, at least at rest.[31,32] It may be that the pulmonary hypertension is reversible if the condition is recognized early and the stimulus withdrawn. Pulmonary function tests continue to be almost normal in patients with long-standing disease. The hypocapnia seen early in the course of the disease is no longer present and the arterial oxygen levels are normal.[33]

Other Anorexigens

Other anorectic drugs have also been noted in the history of patients with pulmonary hypertension. The development of pulmonary hypertension has been attributed to chlorphentermine and phenmetrazin.[1]

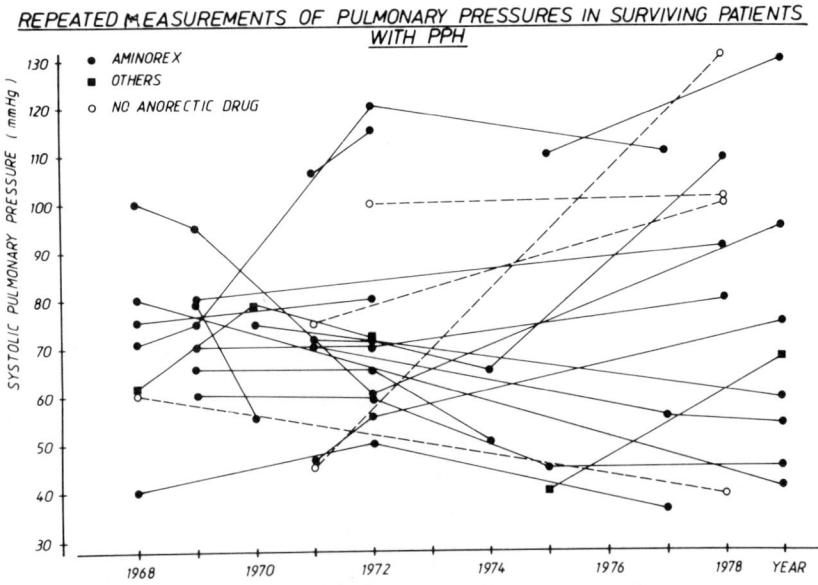

Figure 6. Long-term changes in systolic pulmonary pressures in surviving patients with pulmonary hypertension.

About 20% of the patients collected by the German Society of Cardiology took another anorectic drug, either alone (6.4%) or in addition to aminorex (13.4%).[17] The other anorectic substances did not attain the publicity, or suffer the fate, of aminorex and both are still available on the market. Since then however, no more cases related to the intake of these agents have been reported, at least to my knowledge.

Recently, fenfluramine, another anorectic substance, with a different mode of action, was associated with pulmonary hypertension.[34] Two patients were described who showed coincidental intake of fenfluramine and pulmonary hypertension, with reversion of the pulmonary hypertension after withdrawal of fenfluramine. One of the patients again developed breathlessness on exertion 6 weeks after fenfluramine was restarted, and these symptoms disappeared 2 days after the drug was stopped. A third patient with pulmonary hypertension gave a history of fenfluramine intake as the only striking point.[35] Again, this coincidence might be without relevance. Interference with serotonin metabolism was discussed as a possible mechanism.

Animal Experiments

After the first report of aminorex-related pulmonary hypertension in man, numerous studies were conducted in other species and under different conditions (for example, in obese and non-obese animals). However, none of these studies induced either significant chronic pulmonary hypertension or histologic pulmonary vascular changes comparable to those observed in man. Some increase in pulmonary vascular resistance and pressure was demonstrated in dogs after acute and chronic administration of aminorex.[36-38] Pulmonary hypertension could not be elicited in rats,[39] monkeys,[40] cattle,[41] or pigs,[42] even after making the pulmonary circulation susceptible by high altitude exposure[41] or ligation of one pulmonary artery.[42] However, the increase in pulmonary perfusion pressure caused by experimental microemboli has been reported to be accentuated by the injection of aminorex or amphetamine.[10]

In rat experiments, an increase in the number of circulating platelets has been demonstrated after aminorex treatment.[43] After chronic treatment of rats with aminorex the content of serotonin in the lungs has been found to be significantly increased. Similar changes have been produced by chlorphentermin and phenmetrazin. This increase in serotonin may have resulted from an inhibition of monoamine oxidase by these substances.[44]

Management of Patients

Different therapeutic interventions have been described. However, even in patients with either subjective or hemodynamic improvement, no single effective therapeutic measure could be identified. Since no specific treatment is available, most patients have been treated symptomatically for right heart failure. No data are available on the possible effects of long-term vasodilator therapy, although treatment with nitroglycerin was instituted in some patients.[14,32] Long-term anticoagulants were also used but have not been shown to influence the course of the disease.[30]

Summary

Summarizing the available information on the connection between anorexigens and the development of pulmonary hypertension, it can be said that the clinical facts, together with the epidemiologic aspects, are the strongest arguments for a cause–effect relationship.[1,20,45] However, a clear-cut proof has not been possible, whether clinically or in numerous animal studies. Without knowing what factor or factors might render the pulmonary vasculature susceptible, it is probably impossible to detect or to prove this relationship. Pulmonary hypertension was only recognized in 1 to 2% of those who took aminorex, and this incidence is too low to allow evaluation by the usual methods. So far, the question of the missing link remains open. The aminorex-related epidemic of pulmonary hypertension also provides important information for the overall approach to the management of pulmonary hypertension of unknown etiology. After discontinuing the use of aminorex, about 30% of the patients noted, on long-term follow-up, an increase in exercise capacity[21] and hemodynamic improvement occurred in some, as mentioned earlier. It may be that if primary pulmonary hypertension could be detected and treated early, or if an etiologic factor could be identified and removed, then the prognosis could be improved.

Other Drugs

The interest in drugs affecting the pulmonary vasculature has been focused mainly on substances which dilate an acutely or chronically constricted pulmonary vascular bed, rather than on searching for substances constricting the pulmonary arterial vessels. There are many difficulties in assessing the specificity of a drug action on the pulmonary vasculature, and a complete hemodynamic study with almost simulataneous measurements of pulmonary artery pressure, pulmonary capillary wedge pressure, cardiac output, and systemic pressures is necessary. In addition, pulmonary blood volume and lung compliance may be of importance. Because of species differences, animal experiments are not necessarily representative of changes in the pulmonary circulation in man. Some of the substances which may increase pulmonary vascular resistance are discussed below.

Alpha-sympathicomimetics

Administraton of an alpha-agonist has been reported to induce pulmonary vasoconstriction through stimulation of alpha receptors, but this has not been a consistent finding.[46] Chronic inhalation or abuse of oximetazolin, a nasal mucous membrane shrinking substance, has been reported as a possible reason for the pulmonary hypertension found in one patient.[47]

Histamine

Infusion of histamine in man causes a decrease in pulmonary vascular resistance,[46] while isolated human pulmonary arteries contract in response to histamine.[48] The finding of two separate histamine receptors,[49] one with vasodilator and the other with vasoconstrictor effects, together with the possibility of selective blockade, has increased our understanding, but again we do not know if these receptors play a pathophysiological role.

Serotonin

In some species serotonin is a potent pulmonary vasoconstrictor.[46] In man infusion of serotonin does not change pulmonary vascular resistance, but isolated pulmonary vessels vasoconstrict.[48] It may be that serotonin receptors with opposite actions, similar to the histamine-2 receptors, are present and therefore mask the action of serotonin.

Prostaglandins

An increase in pulmonary arterial pressure and pulmonary vascular resistance is seen in women with prostaglandin F2 alpha-induced abortion.[50] Prostaglandin F2 alpha is a potent pulmonary vasoconstrictor in animals. The possible pathophysiologic role of other prostaglandin-like substances such as thromboxanes in the human pulmonary vasculature remains to be determined.[51]

Oral Contraceptives

Shortly after the introduction of oral contraceptive substances, there were reports of cardiovascular complications induced by these drugs.[52] Venous thromboembolic disease in particular has been under discussion since then. In a recent review it was concluded that oral contraceptives increase the risk of both occult and overt venous thromboembolic disease, "primarily by increase in the size of the intravenous clots formed in response to endothelial injury or other stimuli that lead to thrombin formation."[53] However, it remains uncertain whether oral contraceptives might affect the pulmonary vasculature directly, or only indirectly by pulmonary embolization. A rapid increase in pulmonary pressure was reported in some patients using oral contraceptives, with potential predisposing causes for severe pulmonary hypertension, such as increased pulmonary flow, already elevated pulmonary vascular resistance, and pulmonary vascular disease.[52] In these patients no evidence of thrombosis or thromboembolic disease could be found. Several years later a similar report was published including patients without any apparent predisposing factors.[54]

Phenformin

Biguanides have been widely used in the treatment of diabetes mellitus. There have been reports of some patients developing pulmonary hypertension during phenformin treatment. After withdrawal an improvement gradually occurred. At necropsy "non-specific" signs of pulmonary hypertension were found.[55] One serious side effect of the biguanides is the incidental induction of severe lactic acidosis, and for that reason phenformin is no longer on the market in some countries. The metabolic effect might be of pathogenic importance, because in animal experiments pulmonary vasoconstriction can be induced by infusion of lactic acid.

DIET

A dietary origin of pulmonary hypertension in animals has been clearly demonstrated and the best example is the pulmonary vascular change induced by crotaline alkaloids in rats.

Herbal Toxins

Crotalaria Spectabilis

Monocrotaline, a pyrrolizidine alkaloid, occurs in the stems, foliage, and seeds of different crotalaria species. Crotalaria spectabilis is found in tropical and subtropical regions of the world, crotalaria retusa in West Australia, crotalaria crispata in West Australia, and crotalaria dura in South Africa.[56] In early reports on the toxicity of monocrotaline and similar pyrrolizidine alkaloids toxic to farm and experimental animals, pulmonary vascular changes were not even mentioned. The most prominent lesions were described in the liver. In 1961 Lalich and Merkow[57] found predominant changes in the pulmonary vasculature of rats fed with the ground-up seeds of crotalaria spectabilis. Since then monocrotaline-induced pulmonary hypertension has been studied extensively in rats, as described in detail in Chapter 10. Monocrotaline has not been reported to cause pulmonary hypertension in man.

Crotalaria Fulvia

Crotalaria fulvia is a plant used in Jamaica to prepare "bush tea." Fulvine, another pyrrolizidine alkaloid, has a similar structural formula to monocrotaline and is more hepatotoxic. It is now thought to cause veno-occlusive disease of the liver, but so far no changes in the lungs have been observed in adults or children.[58] In rats a single dose can lead to death with hepatic necrosis, but the surviving animals develop the same pulmonary vascular and parenchymal changes as those seen with monocrotaline.[58]

Crotalaria Laburnoides

Crotalaria laburnoides is a leguminous plant occurring in East Africa and the alkaloid has not yet been isolated or identified. Powdered seeds of this plant fed to rats have been found to induce pulmonary vascular changes, including medial hypertrophy and muscularization of the pulmonary arterioles, but not necrotizing arteritis. In Tanzania, Heath was shown necropsy material from a 19-year-old boy who had died of unexplained pulmonary hypertension, possibly related to ingestion of crotalaria laburnoides' seeds.[59] Histology showed hypertensive pulmonary vascular disease with angiomatoid lesions. However, angiomatoid lesions have never been reported in animals given pyrrolizidine alkaloids.

Senecio Jacobaea

This is a plant commonly seen in England which contains several pyrrolizidine alkaloids. When powdered senecia was fed to rats, all developed right ventricular hypertrophy and hypertensive pulmonary vascular disease.[60] Again, it has not been recognized to cause pulmonary hypertension in man.

Diet Composition

It is not known whether changes in diet can directly modify pulmonary vascular reactivity. However, recently there have been reports that dietary changes can influence platelet aggregability,[61] thromboxane formation,[61] and the induction of endothelial damage.[62] Thus the pulmonary vasculature might be affected indirectly, as suggested by the following studies. Greenland Eskimos have a high intake of monounsaturated and polyunsaturated fatty acids, which may be one of the reasons why they have a low incidence of cardiovascular disorders. The effect of a mackerel diet has been studied in healthy men and a decrease in platelet aggregation and thromboxane formation was demonstrated.[61] This suggests that a change in fatty acid consumption can alter platelet properties, which may be of importance in their activation.[62,63] Several studies had shown that in hyperlipidemic patients platelets are hyperresponsive and might be involved in atherogenesis.[64] High fat diets lead to endothelial changes in mice, with holes and crater-like lesions. Fibrin and platelets are commonly found in and around the crater-like defects.[62] Endothelial cells appear to be able to recognize the presence of certain vasoactive agents and to generate signals that alter the contractile behavior of the smooth muscle cells of the media.[65] Although the cited studies did not look for pulmonary vascular changes and such changes have not been reported by others, it is tempting to speculate that dietary or drug-induced interference in platelet-endothelium interaction might be of importance in pulmonary vascular pathophysiology.

PATHOPHYSIOLOGIC PATHWAYS

The pathways by which drugs or diet might initiate pulmonary hypertension are not known. In a proposed scheme for the pathogenesis of primary pulmonary hypertension, Voelkel and Reeves[66] suggested that any of several stimuli may induce vasoconstriction as the starting point for subsequent pulmonary vascular changes. The same initial mechanism might apply for drug and dietary-induced pulmonary hypertension, either alone, or in combination with one or more predisposing factors. According to this hypothesis, vasoconstriction would come first and lead to intimal endothelial cell lesions, together with medial hypertrophy.[66]

Another possibility might be that the pulmonary endothelium is the primary target. Following endothelial damage and increased capillary permeability, circulating cells could be activated with subsequent release of chemical or vasoactive factors.[67] Indeed, a trigger mechanism, followed by the subsequent development of autonomous pulmonary hypertension, would explain why patients with only minor aminorex intake sometimes develop pulmonary hypertension. The histologic appearance on lung biopsy of some aminorex patients favors the possibility that the endothelium is affected first.[25,26] In these patients, concentric fibrous thickening and edema of the intima, with extensive proliferation of the endothelial cells, are the main findings. In some cases fibrin deposition has been described and the plexiform lesion may be a fibrin-induced hyperplasia of the endothelium.[26,68] Recently, symptoms of acute pulmonary distress were described after ingestion of a toxic cooking oil.[69] Pulmonary hypertension was found in some of these patients and lung biopsies in 2 patients showed intimal proliferation with subtotal occlusion of the capillary bed. It may be that this is another example of diet-induced pulmonary hypertension involving the endothelium.

So the question remains, what might cause the endothelial damage? In the last few years our knowledge of prostaglandins in relation to the lung has increased tremendously, and the balance between thromboxane in platelets and prostacyclin in the endothelial cell has been recognized as an important factor.[51] Teleologically, this system is considered to react to endothelial injury by the adherence of activated platelets on the injured areas. On the other hand, platelet activation can lead to endothelial injury. The fact that diet can alter platelet function and dietary components can induce endothelial damage, opens new possibilities in the speculative pathways of drug or diet-induced pulmonary hypertension.

Many questions remain to be resolved: if a platelet endothelial interaction is the starting process, why is it restricted to the pulmonary vasculature? Is the lung more susceptible? Is the predisposing factor—which is at least necessary for the aminorex-related cases—restricted to the lung? The skin biopsy findings would be in favor of a more general vascular process. In the majority of patients with aminorex-related pulmonary hypertension, no increase in fibrinolytic activity could be detected by the euglobulin lysis test after stimulation by venous occlusion.[70] The lack of stimulation of fibrinolytic activity might also point to a generalized defect of endothelial cell function. The uncertainty about mechanisms, the probability that more than one drug may precipitate pulmonary hypertension, and the possibility that these studies may throw light on the etiology of primary pulmonary hypertension, encourage further research.

REFERENCES

1. Backmann R, Dengler H, Gahl K, et al.: Primaere pulmonale hypertonie. *Verh Dtsch Ges f Kreislaufforschung* 1972;38:134–141.
2. Blankart R: Epidemiologische untersuchungen zur haeufung der pulmonalen hypertonie in den jahren 1967–1969. In: Blankart R, ed.: *Symposium on Obesity, Circulation and Anorexigens.* Bern: Huber, 1974:187.
3. Gurtner HP, Gertsch M, Salzmann C, et al: Haeufen sich die primaer vasculaeren formen des chronischen cor pulmonale? *Schweiz Med Wschr* 1968;98:1579–1581 and 1695–1707.
4. Kraehenbuehl B, Laperrouza C, Moret P: L'hypertension pulmonaire "essentielle" ou "thrombo-embolique." *Schweiz Med Wschr* 1968;98:1311–1320.
5. Sangra R, Tsicotis A, Reymond C, et al.: L'hemodynamique de l'hypertension arterielle pulmonaire d'origine vasculaire. *Schweiz Med Wschr* 1968;98:1252–1255.
6. Rivier JL: Hypertension arterielle pulmonaire primitive. *Schweiz Med Wschr* 1970;100:143.
7. Borbely F, Pasi A, Velvart J: Die akute perorale vergiftung durch 2-amino-5-phenyl-oxazolin-fumarat beim menschen anhand von 30 beobachtungsfaellen. *Arch Toxikol* 1970;26:117–124.
8. Schuster HP, Lang K, Baum P: Akute intoxikation mit aminorex-fumarat bericht ueber den verlauf eines falles mit schwerer suizidaler vergiftung ohne anzeichen einer pulmonalen hypertonie. *Med Welt* 1969;40:2212–2215.
9. Steim H: Zur aetiologie der primaeren pulmonalhypertension. *Wein Z inn Med* 1969;50:497–499.
10. Peters L, Gourzis JT: Pharmacological, toxicological and clinical observations with Aminorex in the United States. In: Blankart R ed.: *Symposium on Obesity, Circulation and Anorexigens.* Bern: Huber, 1974.
11. Hadler AJ: Studies of aminorex, a new anorexigenic agent. *J Clin Pharmacol* 1967;7:296–302.
12. Hadler AJ: Further studies on aminorex, a new anorexigenic agent. *Curr Ther Res* 1970;12:639–644.
13. Gurnter HP: Pulmonary hypertension, "plexogenic pulmonary arteriopathy" and the appetite depressant drug aminorex: Post or propter? *Bull Eur Physiopath Res* 1979;15:897–923.

14. Follath F, Burkart F, Schweizer W: Drug-induced pulmonary hypertension. *Br Med J* 1971;1:265–266.
15. Lang E, Haupt E, Koehler JA, et al.: Cor pulmonale durch Appetitzuegler. *Muench Med Wschr* 1969; 111:405–412.
16. Gahl K, Fabel H, Greiser E, et al.: Primaer vaskulaere pulmonale hypertonie. *Ztschr f Kreislaufforschung* 1970;59:868–883.
17. Greiser E: Epidemiologische untersuchungen zum zusammenhang zwischen appetitzueglere innahme und primaer vasculaer pulmonaler hypertonie. *Internist* 1973;14:437–442.
18. Kaindl F: Primaere pulmonale hypertension. *Wien Z Inn Med* 1969;50: 449–511.
19. Kaindl F: Medikamentoes bedingte pulmonale Hypertonie. *Wien Klin Wochenschr* 1971;21:373–375.
20. Loogen F, Both A: Primaere pulmonale hypertonie. *Zeitschr f kardiologie* 1976;65:1–16.
21. Mlczoch J, Probst P, Szeless S, et al.: Primary pulmonary hypertension: Follow up of patients with and without anorectic drug intake. *Cor et Vasa* 1980;22:;251–257.
22. Kotscher E, Lobenwein E: Radiologischer beitrag zur primaeren pulmonalen hypertension nach appetitzueglern. *Fortschr Roentgenstr* 1973; 119: 141–146.
23. Voss H, Gadermann E, Hauch HJ: Die primaere vasculaere pulmonale hypertonie. *Internist* 1973;14:463–469.
24. Luther M, Czempiel H: Das lungenszintigramm bei primaer vasculaerem cor pulmonale chronicum. *Z Kreislaufforsch* 1970;59:1061–1073.
25. Obiditsch-Mayer I: Lingulabiopsien bei patienten mit primaerer pulmonaler hypertonie. *Wien Z Inn Med* 1969;50:486–489.
26. Obiditsch-Mayer I, Kletter G: Morphologische untersuchungen am bioptischen und sektionmaterial bei pulmonaler hypertonie nach "menocil"-medikation. *Verh Dtsch Ges Pathol* 1972;56:509–512.
27. Tappeiner J, Mannheimer E, Pfleger L: Angiopathia cutanea bei medikamentoes induzierter primaer vasculaerer pulmonaler hypertension. *Wien Med Wschr* 1975;125:52–56.
28. Widgren S: Pulmonary hypertension related to aminorex intake. *Curr Topics Pathol* 1977;64:1–64.
29. Widgren S, Kapanci Y: Menocilbedingte pulmonale hypertonie. *Z Kreislaufforch* 1970;59:924–930.
30. Turina J, Wirz P, Krayenbuehl HP: Verlauf und prognose der primaeren pulmonalen hypertonie. *Schweiz Med Wschr* 1977;107:1825–1828.
31. Gertsch M, Stucki P: Weitgehend reversible primaer vaskulaere pulmonale hypertonie bei einem patienten mit menocil-einnahme. *Zeitschr f Kreislaufforschung* 1970;59:902–908.
32. Simon H, Felix R: Reversible pulmonalarterielle hypertension nach einnahme von menocil. *Med Klin* 1977;72:1685–1688.
33. Mlczoch J, Kaindl F: Pulmonary hemodynamics and lung function in long standing primary pulmonary hypertension. VII. *Eur Congress Cardiol Abstract book* 1980;59, Paris.
34. Douglas JG, Munro JF, Kitchin AH, et al.: Pulmonary hypertension and fenfluramine. *Br Med J* 1981;283:881–883.
35. Gaul G: A case of chronic pulmonary hypertension after fenfluramine intake. *Clin Resp Physiol* 1982;18:89P (Abstract).

36. Kraupp D, Stuehlinger W, Raberger G, et al.: Die wirkung von aminorex (menocil) auf die haemodynamik des kleinen und grossen kreislaufs bei i.v. darreichung am hund. *Naunyn/Schmiedebergs Arch Pharmak* 1969;264: 389–405.
37. Stuehlinger W, Turnheim K, Kraupp D: Vergleichende untersuchungen ueber die wirkung von aminorex; noradrenalin, amphetamin und ephedrin auf die haemodynamik des grossen und kleinen kreislaufs an hunden. *Z Kreislaufforschung* 1971;60:73–82.
38. Stepanek J, Zak F: Zweijaehrige perorale applikation von aminorex am hund. *Zeitschr f Kardiologie* 1975;64:749–781.
39. Kay JM, Smith P, Heath D: Aminorex and the pulmonary circulation. *Thorax* 1971;26:262–270.
40. Smith P, Heath D, Kay JM, et al.: Pulmonary artery pressure and structure in the patas monkey after prolonged administration of aminorex fumarate. *Cardiovasc Res* 1973;7:30–36.
41. Byrne-Quinn E, Grover RF: Aminorex (menocil) and amphetamine: Acute and chronic effects on pulmonary and systemic haemodynamics in the calf. In: Blankart R ed: *Symposium on Obesity, Circulation and Anorexigens*. Bern: Huber, 1974;154.
42. Mlczoch J, Weir EK, Reeves JT, et al.: Long term effects of the anorectic agent fenfluramine alone and in combination with aminorex on pulmonary and systemic circulation in the pig. *Basic Res Cardiol* 1979;74: 313–320.
43. Credner C: Einfluss von chronisch hypoxischer pulmonaler hypertonie auf die wirkung von aminorex am kleinen kreislauf. *Verh Dtsch Ges Inn Med* 1977;47:1700–1702.
44. Mielke H, Seiler KU, Stumpf U, et al.: Ueber eine bexiehung zwischen dem serotoninstoffwechsel und der pulmonalen hypertonie bei ratten nach gabe verschiedener anorektika. *Zeitschr f Kardiologie* 1973;62: 1090–1097.
45. Hatano S, Strasser T: Primary pulmonary hypertension. Report on a WHO-meeting. Geneva, Oct., 1973. WHO 1973.
46. Harris P, Heath D: Pharmacology of the pulmonary circulation. In: *The Human Pulmonary Circulation* Edinburgh-London-New York: Churchill Livingstone 1977:182–210.
47. Schnabel KH, Schuly V, Busch S: Medikamenteninduzierte primaer vasculaere pulmonalhypertonien. *Med Welt* 1976;27:1300–1303.
48. Boe J, Simonsson BG, Stahl E: Effect of histamine, 5-hydroxy-tryptamine and prostaglandins on isolated human pulmonary arteries. *Eur J Respir Dis* 1980;61:12–19.
49. Tucker A, Weir EK, Reeves JT, et al.: Histamine H1 and H2 receptors in the pulmonary and systemic vasculature in the dog. *Am J Physiol* 1975;229:1008–1113.
50. Weir EK, Greer BE, Smith SC, et al.: Bronchoconstriction and pulmonary hypertension during abortion induced by 15-methyl-prostaglandin F2 alpha. *Am J Med* 1976;60:556.
51. Hyman AL, Mathe AA, Lippton HL: Prostaglandins and the lung. *Med Clin N Am* 1981;65:789–808.
52. Dakley C, Somerville J: Oral contraceptives and progressive pulmonary vascular disease. *Lancet* 1968;I:890.

53. Stadel BV: Oral contraceptives and cardiovascular disease. *N Engl J Med* 1981;305:612–618.
54. Kleiger RE, Boxer M, Ingham RE, et al.: Pulmonary hypertension in patients using oral contraceptives. A report of six cases. *Chest* 1976; 69:143–147.
55. Fahlen M, Bergman H, Helder G, et al.: Phenformin and pulmonary hypertension. *Br Heart J* 1973;35:824–828.
56. Kay JM, Heath D: Crotalaria spectabilis. The pulmonary hypertension plant. Springfield, Thomas, 1969.
57. Lalich J, Merkow L: Pulmonary arteritis produced in rats by feeding crotalaria spectabilis. *Lab Invest* 1961;10:744.
58. Kay JM, Heath D, Smith P, et al.: Fulvine and the pulmonary circulation. *Thorax* 1971;26:249–256.
59. Heath D: A pulmonary hypertension producing plant from Tanzania. *Thorax* 1975;30:389.
60. Burns J: The heart and pulmonary arteries in rats fed on senecio jacobaea. *J Pathol* 1972;106:187.
61. Siess W, Scherer B, Boehlig B, et al.: Platelet-membrane fatty acids, platelet aggregation and thromboxane formation during a mackerel diet. *Lancet* 1980;1:441–444.
62. Davenport WD, Ball CR: Diet induced arterial endothelial damage. A Scanning Electron-microscope Study. *Atherosclerosis* 1981;40:145–152.
63. Hammerschmidt DE: Platelets and the environment. *JAMA* 1982;15: 345–350.
64. Harker LA, Hazzard W: Platelet kinetic studies in patients with hyper-.lipoproteinemia: Effects of clofibrate therapy. *Circulation* 1979;60: 492–496.
65. Vanhoutte PM: Pharmacology of the blood vessel wall. *J Cardiovasc Pharmacol* 1981;3:1359–1369.
66. Voelkel N, Reeves JT: Primary pulmonary hypertension. In: Moser KM ed. *Pulmonary Vascular Disease.* New York-Basel: Marcel Dekker 1979: 573–628.
67. Fishman AP: Dietary pulmonary hypertension. *Circ Res* 1974;35:657–660.
68. Wagenvoort CA, Wagenvoort N: *Pathology of pulmonary hypertension.* New York-London: John Wiley and Sons, 1977.
69. Lopez-Sendon J, Coma-Canella I: Pulmonary hypertension following ingestion of toxic cooking oil. *Clin Resp Physiol* 1982;18:90P–91P (Abstract).
70. Fuchs J, Mlczoch J, Niessner H, et al.: Abnormal fibrinolysis in primary pulmonary hypertension. *Eur Heart J* 1981;2:Suppl A,168 (Abstract).

CHAPTER 10

EXPERIMENTAL MODELS OF PULMONARY HYPERTENSION

John T. Reeves and Jan Herget

It is nearly invariable in human disease that real advances in therapy follow rather than precede an understanding of the disease process. Our biggest obstacle in treating a disease is understanding its causes. Pulmonary hypertension is no exception, and much of what we do understand has come from studies in experimental animals. However, the use of animals in biologic research is coming under increasing scrutiny and even criticism. The thoughtful criticism has emphasized the responsibilities of the researcher to be sympathetic in his handling of research animals. However, restricting or abolishing animal research will limit inquiry into disease mechanisms and treatment.

A complete treatment of animal models in pulmonary hypertension has recently been published.[1] Here, in this chapter, we will emphasize causal mechanisms, and will focus on only a few experimental models, namely chronic hypoxic pulmonary hypertension, that caused by monocrotaline, hypertension from chronic elevation of pulmonary venous pressure, high flow induced pulmonary hypertension, and recurrent pulmonary embolism. Acute hypoxic vasoconstriction is considered in Chapter 6.

CHRONIC HYPOXIC PULMONARY HYPERTENSION

When the whole lung is chronically hypoxic, pulmonary hypertension develops. Persons who live at high altitude and those who hypoventilate may develop clinically significant pulmonary hypertension.

In these, hypoxic pulmonary hypertension threatens their health because the overall lung vasoconstriction does not benefit oxygenation, but does increase right ventricular pressure. In such cases, vasodilation could be beneficial by decreasing the pressure load on the right ventricle.

A second condition associated with hypoxic pulmonary hypertension is regional hypoxia, which results from the impairment of distribution of inspired air in lung disease. Here, the regional vasoconstriction has a regulatory effect and improves the blood oxygenation in the lungs. In such cases vasodilation potentially could impair blood oxygenation. These two effects of hypoxia should be kept in mind in studies dealing with the treatment of experimental pulmonary hypertension by vasodilator drugs. Whereas the animal models using generalized alveolar hypoxia (exposure of animals to hypoxic environment) are common, the attempts using experimental lung disease characterized by regional alveolar hypoventilation are rare (for review see Reference 1).

Hypoxia and Lung Development

Chronic hypoxic vasoconstriction in the whole lung is probably beneficial in the fetus, where as shown by work in Dawes' laboratory in Oxford,[2] hypoxia in the fluid filled lung helps direct the flow toward the fetal organ of oxygenation, the placenta. Then with the first breath, oxygenation of the alveoli helps establish the pulmonary blood flow which is necessary for survival at birth and thereafter. The frequency, severity, and importance of pulmonary hypertension in the newborn have caused investigators to look to animal models for help in understanding the factors causing the normal fall in pulmonary arterial pressure and those which might cause a fetal-type circulation to persist.

A potentially important factor is the number of vascular channels carrying blood through the lung. Levin showed that rapid growth in the number of fetal lung vessels occurs in the days just prior to birth.[3] This growth in the number of vessels probably continues for a few days after birth. For example, we considered that a part of the normal fall in lung vascular resistance in the first week after birth in the calf was related to the rapid increase in the number of lung vessels.[4] A subsequent count of arteries in the newborn piglet indicated that the number of arteries per alveolus increased during the first week after birth,[5] but decreased thereafter. This subsequent decrease in the number of muscular arteries may not reflect actual loss of channels, but rather a loss or atrophy of the medial layer in small arteries.[6] Thus, immediately after birth there normally may be an increase in the number of new vascular channels as well as regression of medial thickness in existing channels. The latter, once begun, continues throughout life.[6]

Alveolar hypoxia from birth retards the normal fall in lung vascular resistance in man (for a review see Reference 7). Newborn calves maintained from birth at 3,350 m altitude showed sustained pulmonary hypertension (Figure 1) which was not immediately reversed by acutely raising the inspired oxygen tension.[4] The fetus has existed in the relative hypoxia of the intrauterine environment, and at the time of birth has well developed vascular smooth muscle in pulmonary arterioles, and high pulmonary arterial pressure. Continuing the hypoxic environment after birth appeared to maintain both the muscularization of arterioles and the high lung blood pressure. It is also possible that chronic hypoxia from birth inhibited the normal post-natal increase in the number of lung vessels.[4]

The mechanisms involved in persistence of fetal pulmonary vascular morphology at high altitude[8] are probably not identical to mechanisms responsible for development of chronic hypoxic pulmonary hyperten-

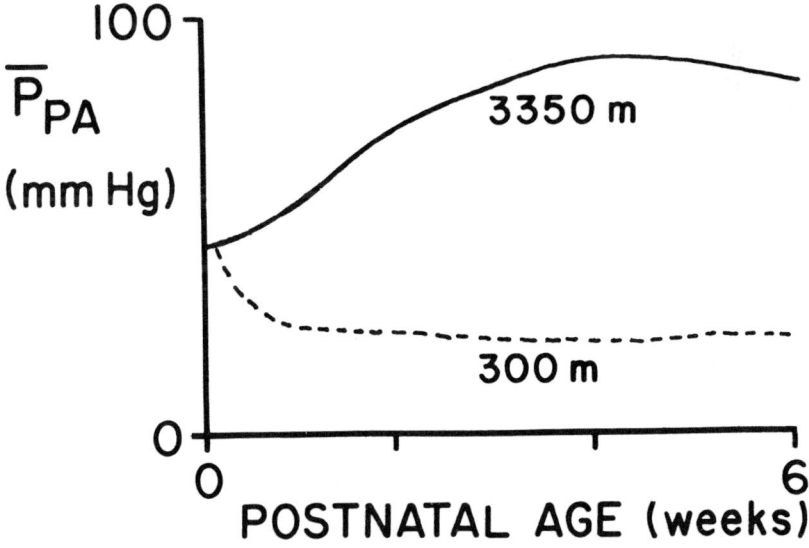

Figure 1. Mean pulmonary arterial pressure (Ppa) changes following birth of the calf. Shown by the unbroken line are pressures in calves maintained from birth at 3,350 m (11,000 ft.) in an altitude chamber. The broken line indicates pressures when calves are born and continue to reside at the low altitude of 300 m (1,000 ft).[7]

sion in adults. Turek et al.[9] showed twice as much right heart hypertrophy in rats which had been born in hypobaric hypoxia as in rats exposed to the same level of hypoxia at the age of 10 weeks. They did not provide, however, any measurements of pulmonary hemodynamics or morphometry of pulmonary vessels.

Even at low altitude where the alveolar oxygen tension is high, the atrophy of the vascular smooth muscle in the lung lags behind the fall in blood pressure. The persistence of this fetal vascular smooth muscle could cause the newborn, even at sea level, to have excessive pulmonary vascular responses to constrictor stimuli. In humans, pulmonary hypertension of the newborn is a particularly important problem. (See Chapter 2.)

Collateral Ventilation

What is repsonsible for the slow atrophy of vascular smooth muscle after birth? Wagner and his colleagues[10] have taken the view that matching of blood flow to oxygenated alveoli is not the purview of the vessels alone. For example, the adults of certain species—dog, sheep (and also man)—have rather well developed channels for collateral ventilation within the lung and they have relatively thin walled pulmonary arteries.[10] However, the adults of the bovine and porcine species do not have intrapulmonary channels for collateral ventilation. They have thickened coats of vascular smooth muscle and they are susceptible to pulmonary hypertension with chronic hypoxia. The concept is that when collateral channels for ventilation are available, local hypoxia within the lung does not occur and vascular smooth muscle undergoes diffuse atrophy. In the absence of such channels, as in the cow and pig, the only mechanism available for matching perfusion to oxygenated alveoli is local vasoconstriction, and the vascular smooth muscle remains thickened.

However, even in those species where collateral channels are present in the adult, they are absent at birth. Recent work in the newborn lamb suggests that the time course for the regression after birth of the vascular smooth muscle is the same as the time course of the development of collateral ventilation.[11] It might be argued that also in adults inflammatory changes in chronic lung disease might influence the pattern of lung collateral ventilation[12] and contribute in development of pulmonary hypertension.

Examination of animal models concerned with the development of the lung and its vessels after birth have indicated: 1) the fetal lung becomes much more vascular as term approaches, and the increase in vascularity continues in the early newborn period; 2) hypoxia after birth retards the normal regression of medial hypertrophy with the maintenance of a high lung resistance; 3) collateral ventilatory channels within the lung are usually absent at birth and when (or if) those channels develop, more complete regression of vascular smooth muscle may occur.

Arachidonic Acid Metabolism

Basic questions are "what is responsible for the high fetal pulmonary vascular resistance?" and, "what causes the resistance to fall after birth?" In addition to the factors mentioned above and to those discussed in earlier chapters of this book (Chapters 1 and 6), factors related to metabolism of arachidonate may be important. Arachidonic acid is an essential fatty acid found in the membranes of most cells in the body. When metabolized via the cyclo-oxygenase pathway prostaglandins and thromboxane are produced.[13] The cyclo-oxygenase enzyme may be inhibited by substances such as aspirin, indomethacin, or meclofenamate. Work from Cassin's laboratory has addressed the potential importance of this pathway for the fetal and neonatal circulation. They have found that indomethacin causes a 60% decrease in the rate of formation of fetal lung fluid.[14] The cyclo-oxygenase pathway may be controlled differently at different ages.[15] The goat fetus and newborn lungs preferentially produce PGE_2 compared to the adult.[16] In critical periods of life such as pregnancy, birth, weaning, or puberty, there are profound and rather sudden hormone changes which could alter metabolic pathways of vasoactive substances. Perhaps most important for the present discussion is the observation that indomethacin inhibits the decrease in pulmonary vascular resistance which normally occurs at birth[17,18] (Figure 2). Such observations suggest that arachidonate metabolism is involved somehow in the control and development of the lung circulation. (Arachidonate products in conjunction with oxygen tension are clearly important in controlling a neighboring vessel, the ductus arterious [for a review see Reference 19].)

Arachidonic acid can also be metabolized via another enzyme involving lipoxygenase.[20] Leukotrienes, formerly considered to be the slow reacting substances of anaphylaxis, are formed via this pathway. Although these substances are primarily involved in inflammation,

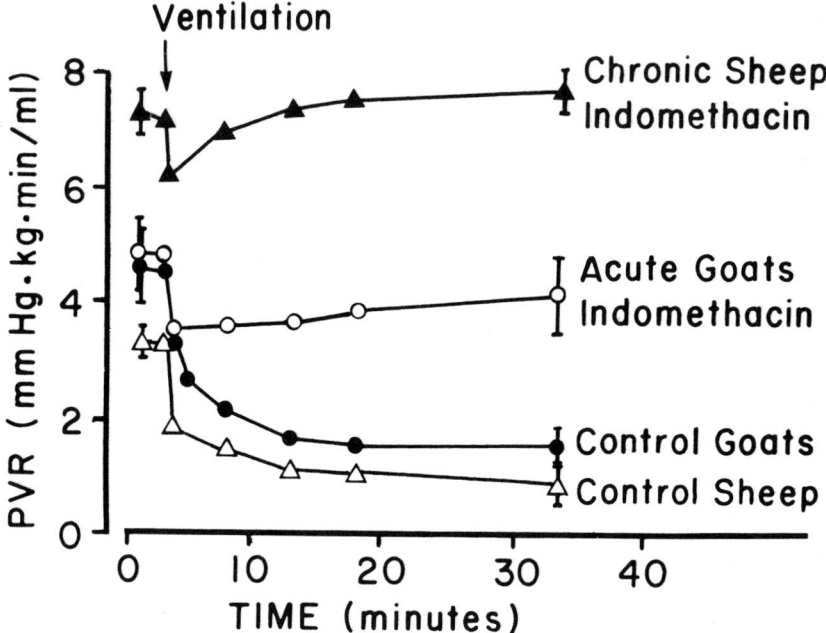

Figure 2. Effects of indomethacin (2 mg/kg) on decrease in pulmonary vascular resistance (PVR) of fetal goats and sheep following ventilation when given to fetal goats acutely or to ewes for 9 to 23 days during gestation. (Reproduced with permission from Reference 18.)

some of them promote pulmonary vasoconstriction and edema.[21] They have recently been found in the airways of children with a syndrome called *persistence of pulmonary hypertension of the newborn*.[22] It has been postulated that blockade of cyclo-oxygenase can shunt arachidonate metabolism to the lipoxygenase pathway.[23] If so, a possible interpretation of the pulmonary hypertensive effect of indomethacin in the newborn animal is that leukotriene formation has been augmented. Leukotriene C_4 given to rat lungs perfused with an albumin free solution causes prolonged vasoconstriction.[21]

The extent to which leukotrienes are involved, if at all, in the control of the fetal circulation remains to be investigated. However, the role of arachidonate metabolites in relation to oxygen tension is an extremely important question relating to circulatory control in the fetus and newborn. Involvement of the lipoxygenase pathway has recently been proposed as a component in the closure of the ductus arteriosus.[24]

Species Differences in the Adult

One of the important aspects of hypoxic vasoconstriction is that it is widespread in the animal kingdom (for a review see Reference 25), having been reported in fish, reptiles, birds, and mammals. The implication is that this is a primitive mechanism retained through evolutionary processes and that it has importance in maintaining a species. The concept might be that the body maintains in the oxygenating circuit an "oxygen sensor" which then directs the flow of oxygen-poor blood to the site of the most abundant oxygen supply. In a fish the oxygenating circuit is the gill, and the mechanism might direct flow to that gill, or portion thereof, which is exposed to the most oxygen-rich water. In an animal with a choice of oxygenating organs such as skin, gills, or lung, there is the obvious advantage of shunting blood to the organ best able to oxygenate the blood.[25]

The hypoxic vasoconstrictor response seems to be ubiquitous among adult mammals, and in most species reported, acute hypoxia approximately doubles pulmonary vascular resistance (Figure 3) (see Chapter 6). When hypoxia is maintained for more than a few minutes, adaptive mechanisms may come into play in some species but not in others. For

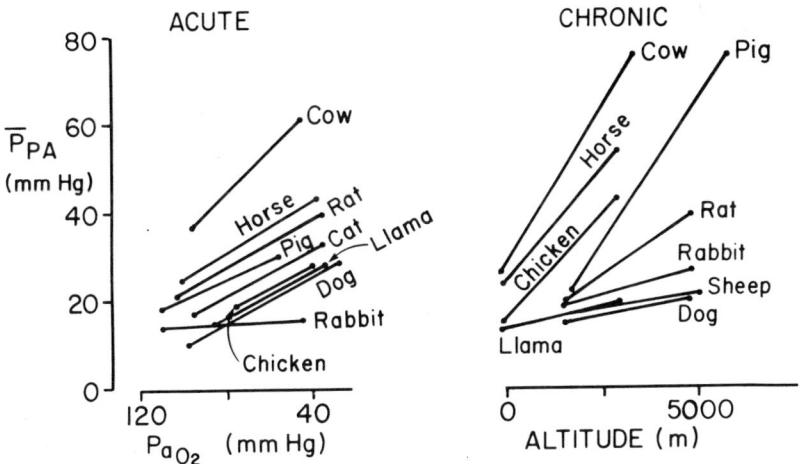

Figure 3. Mean pulmonary arterial pressure (Ppa) in response to acute lowered arterial oxygen partial pressure (PaO_2), left, and in response to several weeks' residence at high altitude, right, for a variety of animal species. (Mean pulmonary arterial pressure was estimated as $0.7 \times$ systolic pressure.)

example, the elevated pressure is not well sustained in the dog[26,27] but may be sustained in the calf.[28] After a few days the pulmonary vasopressor response to hypoxia in rats is decreased. After a few weeks of hypoxic exposure, a rather substantial variability in pulmonary arterial pressure is seen among the different species. The variability is greater than was present among these species during an acute hypoxic response.[29]

At one end of the spectrum are the bovine and porcine species where the pulmonary pressor response to acute hypoxia may predict rather well among individuals the response to chronic hypoxia[30] and where the pulmonary hypertension with chronic hypoxia substantially exceeds that with acute hypoxia, Figure 3. At the other end of the spectrum is the sheep or the dog where the pressure with chronic hypoxia is increased little or none above that with acute hypoxia (Figure 3). Thus, while hypoxic pulmonary pressor responses are ubiquitous among adult mammals, there are large interspecies differences in the pressure adaptation to chronic hypoxia. Tucker et al.[31] demonstrated a relationship between morphology of peripheral pulmonary arteries and sensitivity to chronic hypoxia. Species with abundant smooth muscle in media of pulmonary arterioles (calf and pig) develop more severe pulmonary hypertension when exposed to high altitude than species with thin pulmonary arterioles (dog and sheep). The most sensitive species also show absence of collateral ventilation as described above.

Perhaps the most dramatic expression of the adaptation to chronic hypoxia is that occurring in a population which remains for generations at high altitude. For example, Table 1, for 7 species that have been for many generations at high altitude, the right ventricular weight as a ratio to the total ventricular weight averaged 28 ± 2% (S.D.). This ratio, which is a sensitive measure of right ventricular hypertropy, was only slightly more than the ratio for individuals from low altitude populations of these species, 22 ± 1%. The small standard deviations in each instance indicated that there was not much variation for the various individuals within the species nor was there much variation between the species. By contrast, when individuals from the low altitude populations were brought for several weeks to high altitude, the average heart weight ratio was 49 ± 14% indicating right ventricular hypertrophy. No only did these newcomers have more right ventricular hypertrophy than did the natives of a particular species, but there was more variation between the species.

One example of adaptation to high altitude within a species is that which has occurred with the introduction of domestic cattle into Colo-

TABLE 1
Ratio of Right Ventricular to Total Ventricular Weights in 7 Species at Sea Level, Native to High Altitude, and when Brought from Low Altitude to High Altitude

			High Altitude Measurements			
		Sea Level Native RV/T		Native RV/T		Newcomers RV/T
Species	n	(Percent)	n	(Percent)	n	(Percent)
Man	12	21 ± 0.6	10	29 ± 1.5		
Guinea pig	12	20 ± 1.8	10	27 ± 2.3	5	39 ± 2
Rabbit	12	23 ± 1.1	10	31 ± 3	6	45 ± 2
Dog	25	24 ± 1.8	15	29 ± 1.4	5	38 ± 0.4
Sheep	11	22 ± 0.8	20	26 ± 3.9	6	39 ± 1
Pig	10	23 ± 1.9	12	27 ± 1.5	6	57 ± 2
Cow	10	22 ± 1.5	10	26 ± 1	5	76 ± 8

The high altitude native guinea pigs, rabbits, and dogs lived at 4,300 m. The pigs were native to 3,200 m, cattle to 3,600 m, and man to 3,750 m. The newcomers were residents of 1,600 m exposed for 3–8 weeks to 4,500 m. Mean ± standard deviation. (Adapted from reference 29).

rado within the last 100 years. Indeed, brisket disease was first recognized in cattle living at high altitude in 1915.[32] A subsequent series of investigations initiated by scientists from Colorado State University[33,34] showed that brisket disease was right heart failure from pulmonary hypertension. The heart failure fluid collected anterior to the sternum, in the brisket, because that was the most dependent area with tissue loose enough to allow fluid to collect. The incidence of brisket disease was found to be up to 50% in lowland cattle brought to the high pastures, but was as little as 1% in resident herds. A breeding program established one line of cattle which was susceptible and another which was resistant to chronic pulmonary hypertension.[34,35] The susceptible cattle developed pulmonary hypertension more quickly at high altitude,[34,35] and they had thicker pulmonary arterioles soon after birth even at low altitude.[36] When pregnant, the susceptible cows had more pulmonary hypertension than the resistant cows.[37] Resident herds over several generations developed less susceptibility to pulmonary hypertension[38] than did cattle brought in from low altitude.[37,39] Presumably many susceptible animals died prior to reaching reproductive age (natural selection). In addition, ranchers soon recognized the problem and transferred affected animals to low altitude herds. The genetic transmission of the susceptible trait was supported by experiments which transferred the embryos bred from susceptible bulls and cows to a non-susceptible host cow which became, in effect, a surrogate mother.[40] When born, the "susceptible" calves demonstrated an exaggerated pulmonary pressor response to high altitude confirming their susceptibility, whereas the surrogate mothers showed little pressor response, confirming their resistance to hypoxic pulmonary hypertension. Clearly, genetic factors allow a population evolving at high altitude to adapt by reducing its susceptibility to pulmonary hypertension.[38]

Thus far, we have indicated that the degree of pulmonary hypertension at high altitude depends upon several factors, such as pulmonary vascular reactivity of the species, the capacity of the species and of individuals to adapt to high altitude, and the postnatal age at which high altitude exposure begins. There are still additional factors such as the ventilatory response and the hematopoetic response to chronic hypoxia and the sex of the individual exposed. Increased ventilation at high altitude lowers the PCO_2 and increases PO_2 (for reviews see References 41 and 42). Hypocapnic alkalosis blunts the pulmonary vascular response to hypoxia (see Chapter 6). Thus, for a given altitude, increased ventilation may moderate the pulmonary hypertension observed, by minimizing the degree of alveolar hypoxia and by reducing the pulmonary vascular reactivity. Of the various species examined, cattle most consistently failed to hyperventilate at high altitude,[39] Table 2.

Increasing hematocrit increases blood viscosity which in turn increases resistance to blood flow through the lung. Barer et al.[45,46]

TABLE 2
Mean Values for Several Species at Low Altitude and after Several Weeks at High Altitude

Species (Reference)	Ppa Low	Ppa High	Hct Low	Hct High	PCO_2 Low	PCO_2 High
Cow (45)	29†	73†	39	40	40	40
Pig (43) (male)	21†	78†	40	65	37	31
Pig (42)	27†	72†	38	48	—	—
Rat (42)	37*	57*	48	64	36	31
Rabbit (42)	26*	35*	37	55	38	31
Rabbit (49)	24*	39*	34	56	—	—
Sheep (44)	21†	23†	35	38	40	40
Sheep (42)	20†	23†	36	44	42	32
Guinea pig (42)	18*	21*	47	60	37	35
Dog (42)	26†	28†	43	49	39	29

*systolic pressure
†mean pressure

showed that in the rat, polycythemia following exposure to chronic hypoxia contributed substantially to pulmonary hypertension. The hypoxic pressor response is potentiated in the presence of polycythemia.[47] Cattle among the species studied have the least hematopoetic response (Table 2). Thus, the bovine species develops severe pulmonary hypertension at high altitude despite the failure to develop polycythemia at high altitude. In the rabbit which has a modest response to acute hypoxia, the pulmonary hypertension which develops at high altitude has been attributed largely to the excessive polycythemia which occurs.[48]

Males appear to be more susceptible to pulmonary hypertension at high altitude than do females. Male swine maintained for 4 weeks at 5,490 m had more severe hypoxemia and more right ventricular hypertrophy than did female swine.[43] The male effect could be related to testosterone itself. When castrated male rats were given testosterone and then placed at high altitude for 5 to 6 weeks, they developed more right ventricular hypertrophy than rats not given testosterone or than those given estrogen or progesterone.[49]

Thus, the degree of pulmonary hypertension during chronic hypoxia is determined by the interaction of many factors. Even so, not all have been presented. For example, variables due to pulmonary blood flow,[50] sympathetic tone,[51] or even the degree of gastric distension[52] have not been discussed. Consideration of as many as possible of these factors will determine the choice of a particular animal model. There is also the consideration of size. Traditionally, large species such as cattle, pigs, goats, horses, and dogs have been chosen in part at least because of the convenient size for cardiac catheterization and ventilatory measurements. However, more recent advances in the study of small animals have allowed for high quality and continuous measurement of pulmonary hemodynamics in the awake rat.[53,54]

The medial hypertrophy of the small pulmonary arteries which occurs during chronic hypoxia is usually considered to be a result of hypoxic pulmonary vasoconstriction. However, there is circumstantial evidence that platelets may contribute to the medial hypertrophy. Platelets contain a substance which stimulates the growth of monkey[55,56] and human[57] arterial smooth muscle cells. The platelet-derived growth factor is located in the same granules as β-thromboglobulin and both are released together from the platelet.[57] Elevated plasma β-thromboglobulin levels have been measured in patients with chronic obstructive pulmonary disease and cor pulmonale, suggesting increased platelet activation.[58] Administration of dipyridamole (100 mg q.i.d. for 10 days) returned the values to normal levels. Another clinical study of 63 patients with pulmonary hypertension, secondary to a variety of causes, demonstrates a relationship between shortened platelet survival time and hypoxemia.[59] From the evidence cited above it appears that patients with hypoxic lung disease are likely to have increased platelet activation and shortened platelet survival. The missing link lies between these "in vivo" observations and the "in vitro" demonstration of platelet-derived smooth muscle growth factor.

Several animal experiments help to close this gap. Rats treated with the antiplatelet agents dipyridamole, or sulfinpyrazone, have less medial thickening in the small pulmonary arteries after 2 weeks of hypobaric hypoxia (520 mm Hg) than control rats.[60] Rats treated with aspirin to acetylate platelets have less pulmonary hypertension and less right ventricular hypertrophy than control rats.[61] Medial thickness was not measured in this study. While the changes induced by antiplatelet agents do not necessarily incriminate platelets, the evidence in aggregate suggests a connection between platelet activation and medial hypertrophy. The possibility that platelets may be involved in the pathophysiology of high-flow pulmonary hypertension[62] will be discussed below.

The animal models of chronic hypoxic pulmonary hypertension relate well to measurements made in man. For example, relatively low pulmonary arterial pressures have been reported from Peruvian populations which have lived at high altitude in the Andes for thousands of years. Pressures higher than in the Peruvians have been reported from the population of Leadville, Colorado (U.S.A.), which was first settled approximately 100 years ago (Figure 4). Thus, with man and other mammals natural selection at high altitude may favor lower pulmonary arterial pressure.

Chronic mountain sickness occurs both in the Andean population and in the residents of Leadville, Colorado. One manifestation is excessive polycythemia which appears to be rather common among middle-aged men in Leadville. An important etiologic factor may be hypoventilation,[64] especially during sleep (Chapter 8). Pulmonary arterial pressure measurements not available from Leadville have been reported from the Peruvian Andes in the patients with chronic mountain sickness. Pulmonary hypertension is present. There also is severe hypoxemia. The magnitude of the pulmonary hypertension appears to be approximately appropriate for the degree of hypoxemia present (Figure 4). It is as though the pulmonary hypertension is in response to the hypoxic stimulus. Persons with the obesity-hypoventilation syndrome (Pickwickian syndrome) have a similar pulmonary vascular response to hypoxia as do the chronic mountain sickness patients (Figure

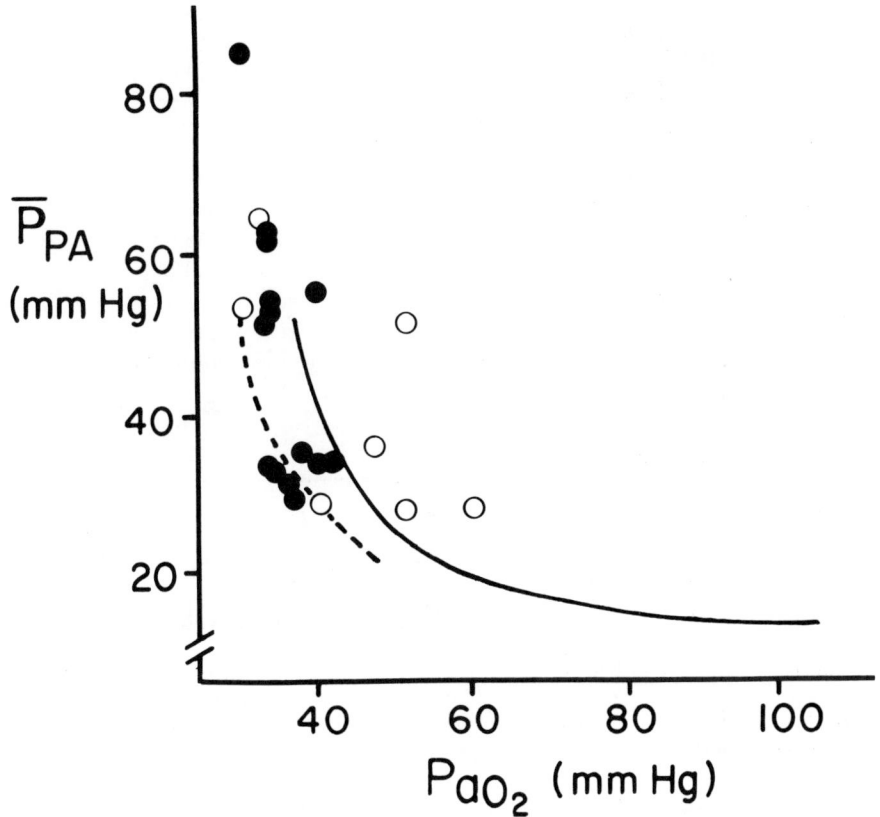

Figure 4. Mean pulmonary arterial pressure (Ppa) vs arterial oxygen tension (PaO$_2$) in man for residents of various altitudes. The unbroken curved line indicates the line of best fit for 124 persons living in North America. The open circles indicate subjects with Pickwickian syndrome. The broken curved line indicates the best fit for 124 measurements of pulmonary arterial pressure reported from Mexico and South America. The closed circles indicate persons from North and South America with chronic mountain sickness. (Adapted from Reference 63.)

4). In both disease syndromes profound chronic, alveolar hypoxia probably initiates the clinical disorder. When, in chronic mountain sickness, the hypoxia is relieved by the patient moving to sea level, regression of the pulmonary hypertension may take months (Figure 5).

Thus, in a sense man is also an experimental model of chronic hypoxic pulmonary hypertension. The experience gained from man has complemented and supported that from animals. Yet hypoxic pulmonary hypertension like systemic hypertension has proven to be a

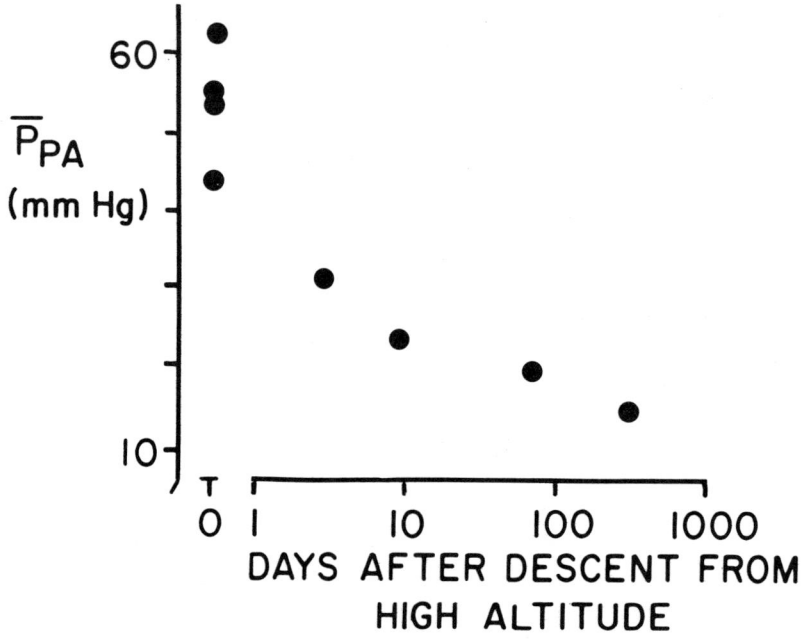

Figure 5. *Decrease in pulmonary hypertension in 4 high altitude residents after they moved to sea level. These were high altitude residents of Peru with chronic mountain sickness. One was a resident of Leadville who moved to low altitude because of pulmonary hypertension. (Adapted from Reference 63.)*

difficult problem. Also like systemic hypertension, it remains an important scientific frontier, where the various animal models will play a crucial role in increasing our future understanding.

LUNG INJURY-INDUCED PULMONARY HYPERTENSION

Some types of chronic lung injury in both man and animals are accompanied by chronic pulmonary hypertension. Several different chemical substances were used to produce chronic lung injury accompanied by pulmonary hypertension (for a review, see Reference 1). The best studied, by far, and considered here, is monocrotaline, a pyrrolizidine alkaloid found in the seeds of the plant *crotalaria spectabilis*. A detailed review of the substance and its effects are found elsewhere.[65] In intravenous doses it causes pulmonary edema within hours in a number of animal species.[66] However, when given subcutaneously, or by mouth to rats, progressive pulmonary hypertension develops after a delay of several days.[67] The rats die within a few weeks. In our experience (Sugita, Reeves, unpublished) mice, rabbits, and hamsters are relatively resistant to the pulmonary hypertensive effects of monocrotaline and dogs are only occasionally susceptible. The concept has been advanced that monocrotaline itself is inactive but must be metabolized, perhaps in the liver to an active compound.[68] The active compound often called monocrotaline pyrrole may be a dehydro form of the monocrotaline molecule. Perhaps only certain species such as the rat have the necessary enzyme to metabolize monocrotaline into its active form. A recent study indicates that even the monocrotaline pyrrole has no effect on the metabolism of lung slices, suggesting that it too is an intermediate in the pathogenetic process.[69]

A particularly interesting aspect is the delay between the administration of monocrotaline, or its pyrrole, and the beginning of the pulmonary hypertension. The delay of at least several days has been documented in terms of the development of right ventricular hypertrophy,[70] by the measurement at intervals of right ventricular pressure, and even by the continuous monitoring of pulmonary arterial pressure and flow in the awake chronically instrumented rat.[71] When the pressure does begin to rise, there is an accompanying increase in indices of protein synthesis and in dry lung weight.[72,73] There is hypertrophy and/or hyperplasia of many cell types within the lung including mast cells,[74] alveolar macrophages,[75] type II cells,[76] vascular smooth muscle cells,[77] and possibly alveolar and interstitial cells. Thus, although the pulmonary hypertension is severe and may be the mechanism of death, it occurs late in the natural history of the process and is accompanied by hyperplasia of many different cell types.

Because of the variety of doses, routes of administration, and chemical forms of monocrotaline, it is difficult to establish with certainty the sequence of events following monocrotaline administration. However, histologic evidence of lung edema, cited above, and physiologic evidence of lung vessel leak[72] suggest that endothelial injury may be an early or perhaps the earliest event after monocrotaline. Simultaneously, ornithine decarboxylase increases several fold within 24 hours of monocrotaline administration.[78] Ornithine decarboxylase is considered to be the rate limiting enzyme in the synthesis of polyamines which in turn are early indicators of increased protein synthesis.

The circulating platelet count falls 2 days after monocrotaline,[79] and there is the beginning of an inflammatory response.[80] By 5 days 5-hydroxytryptamine clearance is clearly reduced.[81] The decrease of

5-hydroxytryptamine uptake is regarded as a measure of activity of endothelial cells.[82] The decrease of serotonin uptake, however, can be also explained by decrease of vascular surface area in lungs, which was observed by Hislop and Reid[83] using the lung morphometry. After 7 days or more, as indicated above, there appears to be the simultaneous and progressive development of protein synthesis, cellular hyperplasia, increase in lung dry weight, and pulmonary hypertension. Evidence for the importance of protein synthesis in the genesis of the syndrome is supported by the finding that limiting food intake limits the response to monocrotaline.[84] Apparently increased lung collagen is not present[85] but there are IgG deposits extensively found in the alveolar walls and interstitium suggesting that the immune system has been activated.[86] If this sequence of events is approximately correct, then the monocrotaline response involves complex, multiple, and interacting mechanisms.

A schema proposing the monocrotaline action has been published.[87] If the responses are multifaceted, then it is not surprising that a large variety of inhibitors have provided only partial protection against the substance (Table 3). Some of the agents listed have been more effective than others but none have afforded complete protection. One innovative approach has been that of Sugita and his colleagues.[128] They gave rats unilateral pneumothorax followed by monocrotaline administration. The collapsed lung was relatively protected from monocrotaline effects, probably because blood flow to it was relatively low at the time monocrotaline or its metabolites were circulating. The other explanation might be that hypoxia in collapsed lungs was the protective factor.

TABLE 3
Substances Used in Attempts to Inhibit
Pulmonary Hypertension from Monocrotaline

Class of Drug	Drug Administered	Reference
Adrenergic blockade	Phenoxybenzamine	(92,96,97)
	6-OH dopamine	
	Zoxazolamine	
Calcium inhibitors	Cinnarizine	(96)
Converting enzyme inhibition	SQ 14225	(92,95)
	SQ 20881	
5-hydroxytrypamine inhibition	p-chlorophenylalanine	(92,94,97)
Platelet depletion	Platelet antiserum	(93)
Cyclo-oxygenase inhibitors	Indomethacin	(92)
Sedative	Phenobarbitone	(96)
Antihistamine		(92)

Radioprotective agents like mercaptoethylamine and also cysteine have been shown to have protective effects against monocrotaline lung injury.[88] Many radioprotective chemicals are potent oxygen radical scavengers. The possibility arises that oxygen radicals, which were shown to produce lung injury in acute experiments,[89] might be produced in the metabolism of monocrotaline. It would be consistent with findings that the most pronounced effects of monocrotaline are usually found in lungs, i.e., the organ with the highest tissue PO_2. Some support for this idea was that radiation (300 rads) did not protect the rats from monocrotaline injury.[90] In fact, the injury may have been both accelerated and augmented. The above experiments point to the burgeoning interest in the mechanism of monocrotaline action.

While the mechanism remains elusive, we have gained some valuable general insights into the pulmonary hypertensive process. Perhaps the most important lesson from monocrotaline is that we cannot consider pulmonary vascular abnormalities apart from the environment in which they exist. That is, monocrotaline does not cause just a vascular disorder. Although one may speculate that the initial insult is to the vascular endothelium, the subsequent events involve the interstitium of the alveolar walls, the macrophages in the alveolar lumen, the circulating blood, and the immune response. Regional changes in lung compliance will result in uneven distribution of inspired air and mismatching of ventilation/perfusion relationships in the injured lungs. The excessive lipid accumulation in the alveoli[90] could be an important clue that ultimately relates to vascular function. Thus monocrotaline induced pulmonary hypertension, as well as that induced by carrageenan, another inflammatory substance,[91] ties together several aspects of lung function and metabolism. Aspects of this animal model possibly relate to pulmonary hypertension in pulmonary interstitial disease, pulmonary fibrosis, cystic fibrosis, and certain collagen vascular diseases in man.

CHRONIC VENOUS PULMONARY HYPERTENSION

The high frequency of pulmonary venous hypertensive disorders makes high left atrial pressure a common cause of pulmonary hypertension. Patients with mitral valve disease, either stenosis or insufficiency, and those with left heart failure from any cause are at risk for pulmonary hypertension. When left atrial pressure is raised acutely, pulmonary arterial pressure rises. However, veins and arterioles dilate and capillaries are recruited (for a review, see Reference 98) leading to a decrease in pulmonary vascular resistance. When the high left atrial pressure is chronic, the pulmonary hypertension is chronic and is accompanied by hypertrophy of vascular smooth muscle, hyperplasia of other lung cells, and pulmonary hypertension which is out of proportion to the elevated pressure (see Figure 5, Chapter 1). The chronically increased pulmonary vascular resistance leads to right heart failure which in turn increases the morbidity and mortality from heart disease. Despite the frequency and importance of this form of pulmonary hypertension, relatively little attention experimentally has been paid to it.

Most of the experiments causing chronic pulmonary venous hypertension have been conducted in dogs. Van Bogaent[99] increased left atrial pressure surgically by an anastomosis between the aorta and the left atrium. Kinoshita and Rodbard[100] invaginated the left atrium by implanting a silastic ball and thereby produced chronic pulmonary venous hypertension. Wallace and Hamilton[101] found mild pulmonary hypertension in dogs with spontaneous mitral insufficiency, and Zook[102] reported pulmonary hypertension in a cat with acquired stenosis of pulmonary veins. These reports described pulmonary hypertension ranging from mild to severe and in some of the animals pulmonary vascular changes were described.

Perhaps the most successful model for chronic venous pulmonary hypertension was developed in the calf.[103] In the bovine species, the left atrium receives only one pulmonary vein from the left and one from the right lung. When those were surgically narrowed, pulmonary hypertension occurred in 11 of 20 calves and in 2 the pressure approached systemic levels. These two had marked hypoxemia. The histologic changes in the vessels related well to the level of the pressure and showed medial hypertrophy and intimal thickening as has been reported in human pulmonary venous disease. What we have learned from these reports is that indeed chronic elevation of pulmonary venous pressure causes secondary changes on the arterial side of the vascular bed.

Unfortunately, we do not have reports of studies investigating directly the link by which chronic elevation of pulmonary venous pressure in some individuals causes a marked reactive pulmonary arterial hypertension. However, we can look at the matter from a slightly different perspective. Elevation of microvascular pressure increases fluid filtration from vessels into lung interstitium; we might inquire as to the effect of chronic or repeated leak of vascular endothelium. Recent studies in rats which survived administration of a pulmonary edema-producing dose of placidyl® showed that on recovery there was a surge of protein synthesis which became maximum within 24 hours of recovery, but which persisted for 8 days.[104] Repeated bouts of sublethal pulmonary edema by weekly doses of thiourea have caused mild but definite chronic pulmonary hypertension in rats.[105]

From the collected experience in humans with left heart disease, from the animal models of chronic pulmonary venous hypertension, and from the experiments with leak in pulmonary vessels, one wonders if there is a relation between vascular leak and chronic pulmonary hypertension. From a teleological view, the lung must stay relatively "dry" to effectively oxygenate blood. Possibly the body mounts a hyperplasic response to "wall off" leaking vessels. One "cost" of such an effort could be pulmonary hypertension. An alternative concept which relates lung edema to lung vessel resistance is that of West and Dollery.[106] With elevation of pulmonary venous pressure there occurs precapillary edema which collects around arterioles and impedes the flow through them. In addition, the edema may stimulate vasoconstriction, further increasing resistance. Since this process occurs in edematous areas, flow is thereby redistributed to areas without edema, thus preserving oxygenation. Clearly, further work is justified to determine what factors are responsible for causing excessive pulmonary hypertension with chronic elevation of pulmonary venous pressure and to investigate the possible mechanisms. Transvascular leak is a characteristic feature of many lung injuries and might be present even in chronic exposure to hypoxia.[107] Increase of fluid filtration into lung interstitium might comprise the common link between different types of pulmonary hypertension.

HIGH FLOW PULMONARY HYPERTENSION

One of the most distressing findings for patients and physicians is that of irreversible pulmonary hypertension in a child or young adult with a congenital cardiac defect which otherwise would be amenable to surgical correction. Occasionally young children with patent ductus arteriosus or perhaps with ventricular septal defects have been found some years later to have fixed inoperable pulmonary hypertension. More than 50 years ago Moschowitz[108] recognized that the hyperdynamic hypertensive state of the lung circulation caused the pulmonary vascular obstructive lesions. Subsequently, investigators have developed animal models with high blood flow to simulate human pulmonary hypertension.[109]

Simple ligation of the pulmonary artery to one lung[110] or lung removal,[111] which approximately doubles the flow through the other lung, causes minimal elevation of pulmonary arterial pressure. Even when the pulmonary artery to one lung is ligated at birth in mammals at sea level, or is congenitally absent in man, there is usually little or no pulmonary hypertension. However, the combination of ligation plus hypoxia does result in pulmonary hypertension.[111] When bilateral femoral arterial-to-venous shunts were surgically created in adult dogs to increase pulmonary flow by 2-to-3 fold for more than 4 months, the absolute mean pulmonary arterial pressure was raised only from 15 to 25 mm Hg.[112] When the aorta was connected side-to-side distal to a band in the left main pulmonary artery, the pressure observed after 10 to 20 months was 70/20 in 1 dog and 50/30 in 2 others.[113] In all 3 dogs the pulmonary vascular histology was normal. (However, when a Potts or Waterston anastomosis [aorta side to side with left or right pulmonary artery] is made in children, pulmonary hypertension is a well recognized complication). In the adult dog only when a systemic artery was connected to a lobar artery could systemic level pressure be observed in the pulmonary artery and could histologic changes of severe pulmonary hypertension be observed.[113] It seems that the lung of the adult mammal, particularly the dog, has a great capacity to adapt to high flow such that severe pulmonary hypertensive vascular changes can only be reproduced when a rather large systemic vessel is connected to a lobar or sublobar unit of lung.

An interesting observation was reported by Ferguson and Varco.[114] The morphological changes of pulmonary vessels were more pronounced when a systemic-to-pulmonary shunt was performed by an end-to-end anastomosis than when the anastomosis was made end-to-side, although the initial pressures and pulmonary blood flows were identical in both cases. Kinetic energy of the blood is likely to be greater in the former than in the latter. Therefore, it might be concluded that the kinetic energy of blood flow may play a part in development of vascular lesions.

One wonders by what mechanism the high flow, high pressure might induce the vascular changes which largely affect the arterial side of the pulmonary circulation, particularly at branching points. The concept has been advanced[115,116] that under the conditions of high pressure and high flow the endothelial surface of the lung arterial bed is subjected to inordinate shear stress which is the "drag force" of fluid flow on a stationary wall. The endothelium of blood vessels is a highly complex structure possibly with numerous projections.[117] Further, it

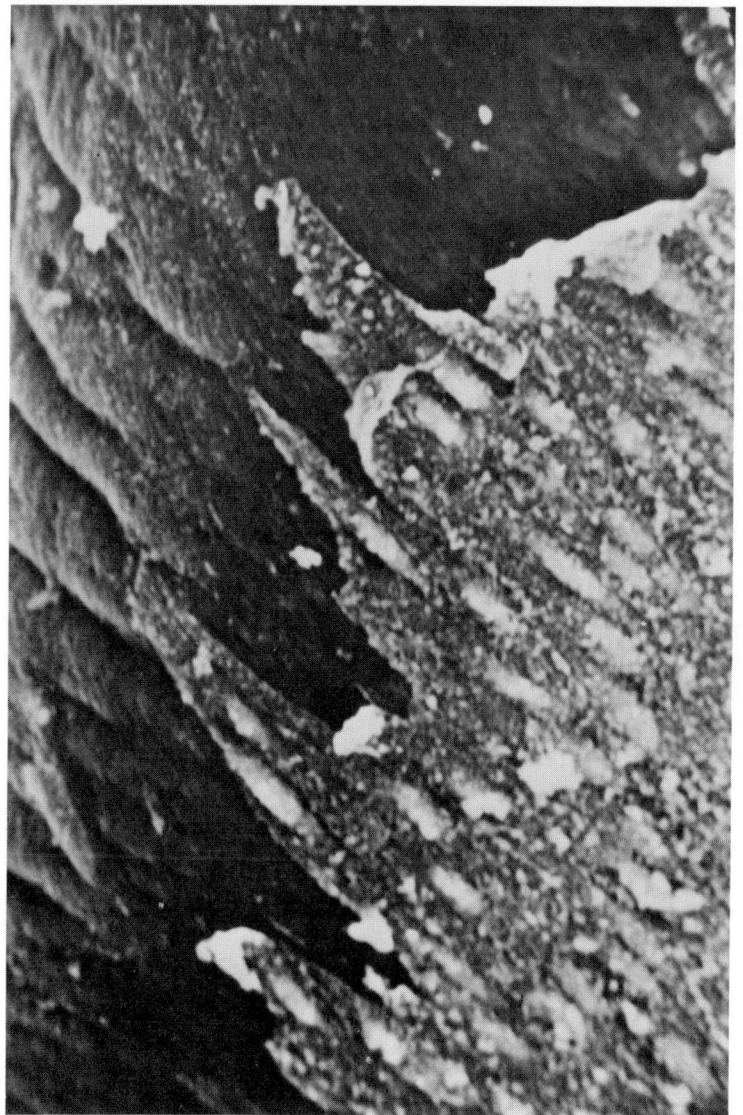

Figure 6. Scanning electron micrograph × 800 showing sloughing of endothelium at branch point in a pulmonary artery of a dog 5 months after creation of a shunt from the brachiocephalic artery to the left upper lobe. (Reproduced with permission from Van Benthuysen et al. from Reference 115.)

may have a protective layer of complex glycoprotein.[117] The delicate endothelial cell vascular interface can be relatively susceptible to damage by shear stress from high blood flow and large pressure drop along a vascular segment.[118]

The role of shear stress was examined in dogs having the left brachiocephalic artery anastomosed to the left upper lobe artery.[116] After 5 months the mean pulmonary arterial pressure in the shunted lobe was 80 mm Hg and after 10 months it was 95 mm Hg. Vascular abnormalities by light microscopy confirmed earlier observations[119] and included medial hypertrophy and intimal proliferation, which in some dogs was marked. Scanning electron micrographs showed markedly distorted and thickened endothelium and in some dogs loss of endothelium from the luminal surface, particularly at branch points (Figure 6). The authors considered that when the endothelium is damaged, platelets are likely to become activated and to adhere to the damaged endothelial surface. Platelet derived growth factor and other factors liberated by platelets may stimulate a hyperplasic reaction and also may stimulate the migration of smooth muscle cells to the area of the damaged endothelium. Such a mechanism which has been proposed for other vascular beds[120] may also be operative for the lung.

VanBenthuysen in subsequent experiments in this shunt model[121] found platelet survival was decreased and platelet consumption was increased by 72%. Pulmonary vascular resistance in the shunted lobe was nearly 4 times normal. Antiplatelet therapy was associated with nearly normal platelet activity and nearly normal pulmonary vascular resistance. These experiments have suggested that high pressure and flow may damage endothelium and activate platelets. The combination of damaged endothelium and activated platelets may in turn lead to the development of intimal fibrosis and irreversible pulmonary hypertension. Platelet adherence also has been considered to be important in the development of vascular lesions in another example of pulmonary hypertension, that which occurs in experimental infestation of dogs with the heart worm, *dirofilaria immitis*.[122] Both of these models focus attention on the role of the endothelium in the maintenance of a functional pulmonary circulation. If the shear stress concept is valid, the implication is that an increased pressure drop above some threshold value along a vascular segment can cause continued endothelial damage, which in turn leads to endothelial replacement by fibrous tissue. Further, endothelial loss or damage may deprive the vessel of potent pulmonary vasodilator substances.[123]

CHRONIC EMBOLIC PULMONARY HYPERTENSION

Pulmonary embolism is a major cause of morbidity and mortality. Recurrent pulmonary embolism, although less common, can lead to disabling pulmonary hypertension (Chapter 5). Establishing a satisfactory animal model has been surprisingly difficult (for a review, see Reference 1). When very small autologous clots were used in the dog,[124] significant pulmonary hypertension was not produced, even though up to a total of 452 ml of clot was injected in divided doses over a 19-week period. Eccentric fibrous plaques were found in some pulmonary arteries. Pulmonary hypertension has been produced in dogs[125] and in rabbits[126] with repeated doses of larger blood clots. In each instance many injections were required. A variety of material has been embolized including lycopodium spores, starch, and air. Some pulmonary hypertension has been produced, but in each instance multiple injections over many weeks have been required and mortality has been high.

Recently, an attempt has been made to develop a canine model of pulmonary hypertension using sephadex beads of known diameter, 280 ± 70.[127] The number of beads required to cause an elevation of pressure or resistance in 20 kg dogs was a threshold dose of approximately 10^6 beads given over a span of 16 to 30 weeks. The number of beads was several fold greater than the number of vessels of comparable diameter likely to be present in the dogs. The histological sections of lung showed clustering of beads in the vessels. At present, the chronic embolic model of pulmonary hypertension is time consuming and difficult. However, once established, pulmonary hypertension has appeared to be persistent at least for several months and was well tolerated by the dogs. It is not clear what mechanism the body has to maintain lung blood flow in the presence of such a large burden of relatively inert embolic material. Such a mechanism may be protective in human recurrent pulmonary thromboembolism where months or years may be required for persistent pulmonary hypertension to become established. This is a potentially useful model for the examination of questions such as: the natural history of embolic pulmonary hypertension; respiratory gas exchange abnormalities in embolism; and ventricular function in developing pulmonary hypertension.

CONCLUSIONS

Our knowledge of the regulation of pulmonary circulation in disease was for years restricted almost solely to the role of airway hypoxia. The animal models of experimental pulmonary hypertension focused our attention on additional mechanisms. First is the importance of several vasoactive substances, in particular the metabolites of arachidonic acid. Second are the consequences of damage of pulmonary endothelial cells and transvascular leak which appear to be a common feature of most models studied. Third is the role of blood components in the pathophysiology of the pulmonary vascular bed. The finding that active vasoconstriction is an important feature of many types of experimental chronic pulmonary hypertension provides an opportunity for the study of pulmonary vasodilation pharmacology.

REFERENCES

1. Herget J, Palecek F: Experimental chronic pulmonary hypertension. *Int Rev Exper Path* 1978;18:347–406.
2. Dawes GS: *Foetal and Neonatal Physiology*. Chicago: Year Book Publishers, 1968.
3. Levin DL, Rudolph AM, Heymann MM, Phibbs RH: Morphological development of the pulmonary vascular bed in fetal lambs. *Circulation* 1976;53:144–151.
4. Reeves JT, Leather JE; Postnatal development of pulmonary and bronchial arterial circulations in the calf and the effects of chronic hypoxia. *Anat Record* 1967;157:641–656.
5. Rendas A, Branthwaite M, Reid L: Growth of pulmonary circulation in normal pig—structural analysis and cardiopulmonary function. *J Appl Physiol* 1978;45:806–817.
6. Takahaski T, Wagenvoort N, Wagenvoort CA: The density of muscularized pulmonary arteries in normal lungs. *Arch Pathol Lab Med* 1983;107:19–22.
7. Reeves JT: Pulmonary vascular response to high altitude residence. In: *Cardiovascular Clinics*. Vol. 5. Brest AN, ed. Clinical Pathologic Correlation 2, Philadelphia: F.A. Davis Co., 1973:81–95.
8. Arias-stella J, Saldana M: The terminal position of pulmonary arterial tree in people native to high altitude. *Circulation* 1963;28:915–925.
9. Turek Z, Ringalda BEM, Gardtner M, Kreutzer F: Myoglobin distribution in the heart of growing rats exposed to simulated altitude of 3,500 m in their youth or born in the low pressure chamber. *Pflugers Arch* 1973;340:1–10.

10. Kuriyama T, Wagner WW: Collateral ventilation may protect against high-altitude pulmonary hypertension. *J Appl Physiol* 1981;51:1251–1256.
11. Petrun MD, Herget J, Wagner WW Jr: The development of collateral ventilation parallels the regression of the foetal vascular pattern. *Fed Proc* 1983;42:489.
12. Berend N, Skoog C, Thurlbeck WM: Collateral ventilation in excised human lungs. *J Appl Physiol* 1981;50:927–930.
13. Hyman AL, Spannhake EW, Kadowitz PW: Prostaglandins and the lung. *Am Rev Resp Dis* 1978;117:111–136.
14. Cassin S, Tod ML: Indomethacin and fetal lung formation. *Fed Proc* 1982;41:1128.
15. Cassin S, Tod ML, Kuck H: Arachidonic acid and the perinatal pulmonary pressor response to hypoxia. *Physiologist* 1982;25:271.
16. McNamara DB, Laird M, Hyman AL, Kadowitz PJ, Cassin S: Prostaglandin H_2 metabolism by fetal, newborn and adult goat lung. *Fed Proc* 1982;41:1125.
17. Leffler CW, Tyler TL, Cassin S: Effect of indomethacin on pulmonary vascular response to ventilation of fetal goats. *Am J Physiol* 1978;234:H346–H351.
18. Cassin S: Humoral factors affecting pulmonary blood flow in the fetus and newborn infants. In: *Report of the 83rd Ross Conference on Pediatric Rsch.; Cardiovascular Sequalae of Asphyxia in Newborn.* Columbus, Ohio: Ross Laboratories, 1982:10-26.
19. Coceani F, Olley PM: Considerations on the role of prostaglandins in the ductus arteriosus. In: *Advances in Prostaglandin and Thromboxane Research* Samuelsson B, Wamwell PW, Paoletti R, eds. 1980;7:871–877.
20. Samuelson B: Leukotrienes: Mediators of immediate hypersensitivity reactions and inflammation. *Science* 1983;20:568–575.
21. Voelkel NF, Murphy RC, Reeves JT: Non-anaphylactic leukotriene production in isolated perfused rat lungs. *Fed Proc* 1982;41:993.
22. Stenmark K, James S, Voelkel N, Murphy RC, Reeves JT: Recovery of leukotriene C_4 and D_4 from the airway lavage of newborns with severe hypoxemia and pulmonary hypertension. *N Engl J Med* 1983, (in press).
23. Piper PJ, Letts LG, Galton SA: Generation of a leukotriene-like substance from porcine vascular and other tissues. *Prostaglandins* 1983;25:591–599.
24. Needleman P, Halmberg S, Mandlebaum B: Ductus arteriosus closure may result from suppression of prostacyclin synthesis by an intrinsic hydroperoxy fatty acid. *Prostaglandins* 1981;22:675–682.
25. Johansen K: Cardiovascular support of metabolic functions in vertebrates. In: *Lung Biology in Health and Disease*. Vol. 13. Evolution of respiratory processes, Wood SC, Lenfant C, eds. New York: Marcel Dekker, 1979:107–192.
26. Malik AB, Kidd BSL: Time course of pulmonary vascular response to hypoxia in dogs. *Am J Physol* 1973;224:1–6.
27. Tucker A, Reeves JT: Nonsustained pulmonary vasoconstriction during acute hypoxia in anesthetized dogs. *Am J Physiol* 1975;228:756–761.
28. Reeves JT, Leathers JE: Circulatory changes following birth of the calf and the effect of hypoxia. *Circ Res* 1964;15:343–354.

29. Reeves JT, Wagner WW, McMurtry IF, and Grover RF: Physiologic effects of high altitude on the pulmonary circulation. In: Robertshaw D, ed. *International Review of Physiology. Environmental Physiology III*, Vol. 20, Chap. 6, Baltimore: University Park Press, 1979;289-310.
30. Will DH, Hicks JL, Card CS, Reeves JT, Alexander AF: Correlation of acute with chronic hypoxic pulmonary hypertension in cattle. *J Appl Physiol* 1975;38:495-498.
31. Tucker A, McMurtry IF, Reeves JT, Alexander AF, Will DH, Grover R: Lung vascular smooth muscle as determinant of pulmonary hypertension at high altitude. *Am J Physiol* 1975;228:762-767.
32. Glover GH, Newsome IE: Brisket disease. *Colo Agric Expt Sta Bull* 1915; 204:Jan.
33. Will DH, Alexander AF, Reeves JT, Grover RF: High altitude induced pulmonary hypertension in normal cattle. *Circ Res* 1962;10:172-177.
34. Will DH, Hicks JL, Card CS, Alexander AF: Inherited susceptibility of cattle to high altitude pulmonary hypertension. *J Appl Physiol* 1975;38: 491-494.
35. Weir EK, Tucker A, Reeves JT, Will DH, Grover RF: The genetic factor influencing pulmonary hypertension in cattle at high altitude. *Cardiovasc Res* 1974;8:745-749.
36. Weir EK, Will DH, Alexander AF, McMurtry IF, Looga R, Reeves JT, Grover RF: Vascular hypertrophy in cattle susceptible to hypoxic pulmonary hypertension. *J Appl Physiol* 1979;46:517-521.
37. Moore LG, Reeves JT, Will DH, Grover RF: Pregnancy-induced pulmonary hypertension in cows susceptible to high mountain disease. *J Appl Physiol* 1979;46:184-188.
38. Will DH, Hornell JF, Reeves JT, Alexander AF: Influence of altitude and age on pulmonary arterial pressure in cattle. *Proc Soc Exp Biol Med* 1975;150:564.
39. Grover RF, Reeves JT, Will DH, Blount SG Jr: Pulmonary vasoconstriction in steers at high altitude. *J Appl Physiol* 1963;18:567-574.
40. Cruz JE, Reeves JT, Russell BE, Alexander AF, Will DH: Embryo transplanted calves: The pulmonary hypertensive trait is genetically transmitted. *Proc Soc Exp Biol Med* 1980;164:142-145.
41. Lenfant C, Sullivan K: Adaptation to high altitude. *N Engl J Med* 1971; 284:1298-1309.
42. Dempsey JA, Forster HV: Mediation of ventilatory adaptations. *Physiol Rev* 1982;62:262-331.
43. McMurtry IF, Frith CH, Will DH: Cardiopulmonary responses of male and female swine to simulated high altitude. *J Appl Physiol* 1973;35: 459-462.
44. Reeves JT, Grover EB, Grover RF: Pulmonary circulation and oxygen transport in lambs at high altitude. *J Appl Physiol* 1963;18:560.
45. Barer GR, Finlay M, Bee D, Wach RA: Pulmonary hypertension of chronic hypoxia in rat model. Anatomical and theological factors. *Bull Eur Physiopath Resp* 1982;18:69-73.
46. Barer GR, Bee D, Wach R: Continuation of polycythaemia to pulmonary hypertension in simulated high altitude in rats. *J Physiol* 1983;336: 27-38.

47. McGrath RL, Weil JV: Adverse effects of normovolemic polycythemia and hypoxia on hemodynamics in the dog. *Circ Res* 1978;43:793–798.
48. Reeves JT, Grover EB, Grover RF: Circulatory response to high altitude in the cat and rabbit. *J Appl Physiol* 1963;18:575–579.
49. Moore LG, McMurtry IF, Reeves JT: Effects of sex hormones on cardiovascular and hemotologic responses to chronic hypoxia in rats. *Proc Soc Exp Biol Med* 1978;158:658–662.
50. Tucker A, Reeves JT, Jackson DL, Grover RF: Decreased pulmonary vascular responses in dogs with increased pulmonary blood flow. *Scand J Physiol Pharmacol* 1978;56:1011–1016.
51. Harris P, Heath D: *The Human Pulmonary Circulation*, New York: Churchill Livingstone, 1977:467–469.
52. Jensen R, Pierson RE, Braddy PM, Sanri D, Benitez A, Horton DP, Laverman LH, McChesney AE, Alexander AF, Will DH: Brisket disease in yearling feedlot cattle. *J Am Vet Med Assoc* 1976;169:515–517.
53. Rabinovich M, Gamble W, Nadas AS, Miettinen OS, Reid L: Rat pulmonary circulation after chronic hypoxia haemodynamic and structural features. *Am J Physiol* 1979;236:H818–H828.
54. Stanbrook HS, Morris KG, McMurtry IF; Chronic hypoxic pulmonary hypertension in rats is reduced by calcium channel blockers. *Fed Proc* 1983;43:596.
55. Rose RJ, Glomset J, Kariya B, Harker L: A platelet-dependent serum factor that stimulates the proliferation of arterial smooth muscle cells in vitro. *Proc Natl Sci USA* 1974;71:1207–1210.
56. Rutherford RB, Ross R: Platelet factors stimulate fibroflasts and smooth muscle cells quiescent in plasma serum to proliferate. *J Cell Biol* 1976;69:196–203.
57. Witte LD, Kaplan KL, Nossel H, Lages BA, Weiss HJ, DeWitt SC: Studies of the release from human platelets of the growth factor for cultured human arterial smooth muscle cells. *Circ Res* 1978;42:402–409.
58. Nenci GG, Berrettini M, Todisco T, Costantini V, Grasselli S: Platelet activation in hypoxic pulmonary hypertension. *Bull Eur Physiopath Resp* 1982;18:115P.
59. Steele P, Ellis JH Jr, Weily HS, Genton E: Platelet survival time in patients with hypoxemia and pulmonary hypertension. *Circulation* 1977;55:660–662.
60. Keith IM, Will JA, Weir EK: Pharmacologic attenuation of hypoxia-induced arterial hypertrophy in rat lungs. *Fed Proc* 1982;41:1686.
61. Kentera D, Susic D, Zdravkovic M: Effects of verapamil and aspirin on experimental chronic hypoxic pulmonary hypertension and right ventricular hypertrophy in rats. *Respiration* 1979;37:192–196.
62. VanBenthuysen KM, Dauber IM, Hyers TA, Steele PP, Weil JV: The role of platelets in hypertensive pulmonary vascular disease. *Fed Proc* 1982;40:3210.
63. Reeves JT, Grover RF: High altitude pulmonary hypertension and edema. In: *Progress in Cardiology*. Vol. 4. Yu P, Goodwin JF, eds. Philadelphia: Lea and Febiger 1975:99–118.
64. Kryger MH, McCullough RB, Collins D, Scoggins CH, Weil JV, Grover RF: Treatment of excessive polycythemia of high altitude with respiratory stimulant drugs. *Am Rev Resp Dis* 1978;117:455–464.

65. Kay JM, Heath D: *Crotalaria Spectabilis, The Pulmonary Hypertension Plant.* Springfield, Ill.: Thomas, 1969.
66. Hurley JV, Tago MV: Pulmonary oedema in rats given dehydromonocrotaline: A topographic and electron microscope study. *J Path* 1975; 117:23–82.
67. Kay JM, Harris P, Heath D: Pulmonary hypertension produced in rats by ingestion of crotalaria spectabilis seeds. *Thorax* 1967;22:176.
68. Mattock AR: Toxicity of pyrrolipidine alkaloids. *Nature* 1968; 217: 217–223.
69. Roth RA, Dotzlaf LA, Baranyi B, Kud CH, Hook JB: Effect of monocrotaline ingestion on liver, kidney and lung of rats. *Tox Appl Pharmacol* 1981;60:193–203.
70. Hayashi Y, Hussa JF, Lalich JJ: Cor pulmonale in rats. *Lab Invest* 1967; 16:875–881.
71. Meyrick B, Gamble W, Reid L: Development of crotalaria pulmonary hypertension: Hemodynamic and structural study. *Am J Physiol* 1980; 239:H692–H702.
72. Sugita T, Hyers TM, Dauber IM, Wagner WW, McMurtry IF, Reeves JT: Lung vessel leak precedes right ventricular hypertrophy in monocrotaline treated rats. *J Appl Physiol* 1983;54: 371–374.
73. Lafranconi M, Huxtable RJ: The time course of lung hyperplasia and right heart hypertrophy produced by the pyrrolizidine alkaloid monocrotaline. *Fed Proc* 1981;40:629.
74. Takeoka O, Angeuine DH, Lalich JJ: Stimulation of mast cells in rats fed various chemicals. *Am J Pathol* 1962;40:545–554.
75. Sugita T, Henson PM, Henson JE, Hyers TM, Wagner WW, Reeves JT: Abnormal alveolar macrophages in monocrotaline induced pulmonary hypertension. *Fed Proc* 1982;41:1609.
76. Butler WH: An ultrastructural study of the pulmonary lesion induced by pyrrole derivatives of the pyrrolizidine alkaloids. *J Pathol* 1970;102: 15–19.
77. Kay JM, Heath D: Observations on the pulmonary arteries and heart weight of rats fed on crotalaria spectabilis seeds. *J Pathol Bacteriol* 1966; 92:385–394.
78. Gillespie MN, Altiere RJ, Olson JW: Prolonged elevation of lung ornithine decarboxylase (ODC) activity during development of monocrotaline (MCT)-induced pulmonary hypertension in rats. *Fed Proc* 1983; 42:800.
79. Hilliker KS, Roth RA: Monocrotaline toxicity. Development of pulmonary effects and thrombocytopenia in rats. *Fed Proc* 1981; 40:647.
80. Kuriyama T, Sugita T, Takizawa H, Watanabe S, Ogata T: Experimental study of pulmonary hypertension. Correlation between histopathological changes of pulmonary vasculature and elevation of pulmonary arterial pressure. *J Jpn Thorac Soc* 1976; 14:496–505.
81. Hilliker KS, Garcia CM, Roth RA: Effect of monocrotaline pyrrole on 5-hydroxytryptamine and paraquat uptake by rat lung slices. *Fed Proc* 1982;41:1579.
82. Junod AF: Metabolism of vasoactive agents in lung. *Am Rev Resp Dis* 1977;115:51–57.
83. Hislop A, Reid L: Arterial changes in crotalaria spectabilis-induced pulmonary hypertension in rats. *Br J Exp Pathol* 1974; 55:153–163.

84. Garey DE, Roth RA: Dietary restriction and cardiopulmonary toxicity of monocrotaline pyrrole. *Fed Proc* 1983;42:353.
85. Lafranconi WM, Duhamel R, Brendel K, Huxtable RJ: Analysis of collagen content of lung and heart from monocrotaline treated rats. *Fed Proc* 1982;41:1579.
86. Brunner LH, Bell TG, Bull RW, Roth RA: Is the immune system involved in the pneumotoxicity of monocrotaline pyrrole in the rat? *Fed Proc* 1983;42:799.
87. Meyric RB, Reid L: Development of pulmonary arterial changes in rats fed crotalaria spectabilis. *Am J Pathol* 1979;94:37−50.
88. Hayashi Y, Lalich JJ: Protective effect of mercaptoethylamine and cysteine against monocrotaline intoxication in rats. *Toxicol Appl Pharmacol* 1968;12:36−43.
89. Tate RM, vanBenthuysen KM, Shasby DM, McMurtry IF, Repine JE: Oxygen radical mediated permeability edema and vasoconstriction in isolated perfused rabbit lungr. *Am Rev Resp Dis* 1982;126:802−806.
90. Sugita T, Stenmark KR, Wagner WW, Henson P, Henson J, Hyers TM, Reeves JT: Abnormal alveolar cells in monocrotaline induced pulmonary hypertension. *Exp Lung Res* (in press).
91. Herget J, Palecek F, Preclik P, Cermakova M, Vizek M, Petrovicka M: Pulmonary hypertension induced by repeated pulmonary inflammation in the rat. *J Appl Physiol Respirat Environ Exercise Physiol* 1981;51: 755−761.
92. Kuriyama T, Sugita T, Watanabe S: Metabolism of vasoactive substances and pulmonary hypertension. *J Jpn Thorac Soc* 1978; 16:418−424.
93. Roth RA, Hilliker KS, Bell TG: Effects of thrombocytopenia on the cardiopulmonary responses to monocrotaline pyrrole. *Fed Proc* 1983;42: 489.
94. Kay JM, Suyama KL, Keane PM: Monocrotaline-induced and hypoxia-induced pulmonary hypertension are reduced by P-chlorophenylanine (PCPA). *Fed Proc* 1983;42:778.
95. Molenti A, Salliday N, Port C, Ward WF: Partial prevention of monocrotaline induced pulmonary arterial changes by the angiotensin-1-converting enzyme CA-1-CE inhibitor SQ 14225. *Fed Proc* 1982;41:451.
96. Kay JM, Smith P, Heath D, Will J: Effects of phenobarbitone, cinnarizine, and zoxazolamine on the development of right ventricular hypertrophy and pulmonary vascular disease in rats treated with monocrotaline. *Cardiovasc Res* 1976;10:200−205.
97. Tucker A, Bryant SE, Frost HH, Migally N: Monocrotaline induced right ventricular hypertrophy is reduced by pre-treatment with 6-hydroxydopamine (6-OHDA) or p-chlorophenylalanine (PCPA). *Fed Proc* 1982; 41:1609.
98. Grover RF, Wagner WW, McMurtry IF, Reeves JT: The pulmonary circulation. In: *Handbook of Physiology, Peripheral Circulation and Organ Blood Flow*, 1983 (forthcoming).
99. VanBogaert A, Tosetti R: Experimental pulmonary hypertension. *Br Heart J* 1963;25:774−783.
100. Kinoshita Y, Rodbard S: Hemodynamic and pathologic changes following introduction of an endothelial lined mass into the atrium. *Proc Soc Exp Biol Med* 1966;121:902−098.
101. Wallace CR, Hamilton WF: Study of spontaneous congestive heart failure in the dog. *Circ Res* 1962;11:301−314.

102. Zook BC: Some spontaneous cardiovascular lesions in dogs and cats. *Adv Cardiol* 1974;13:148−168.
103. Silove ED, Tavernor WD, Berry CL: Reactive pulmonary arterial hypertension after pulmonary venous constriction in the calf. *Cardiovasc Res* 1972;6:36−44.
104. Fricke RF, Secker-Walker RH: Recovery from ethclorxynol-induced pulmonary edema in the rat. *Am Fed Clin Res* April 1980, p. 45.
105. O'Brien RF, Hill NS, Rounds S: Right ventricular hypertrophy and increased pulmonary vasoreactivity induced by chronic α-napthyl-thiourea (ANTU) in rats. *Clin Res* 1982;30:435A.
106. West JB, Dollery TC, Heard BE: Increased pulmonary vascular resistance in the dependent zone of isolated lung in dog caused by perivascular lung edema. *Circ Res* 1965;17:191−206.
107. Bartlett D, Remmers JE: Effects of high altitude exposure on the lungs of young rats. *Respir Physiol* 1971;13:116−125.
108. Moschowitz E: Hypertension of the pulmonary circulation; its causes, dynamics and elevation to circulatory states. *Am J Med Sci* 1927;179:388−406.
109. Levy SE, Blalock A: Experimental observations on the effects of connecting by suture the left main pulmonary artery to the gasteric circulation. *J Thorac Surg* 1939;8:525−530.
110. Kato H, Kidd L, Olley PM: Effects of hypoxia on pulmonary vascular reactivity in pneumoectomized puppies and minipigs. *Circ Res* 1971;28:394−402.
111. Vogel JHK, McNamara DG, Hallman G, Rosenberg H, Jamieson G, McGrady JD: Effects of mild chronic hypoxia on the pulmonary circulation in calves with reactive pulmonary hypertension. *Circ Res* 1967;21:661−669.
112. Hopkins RA, Hammon JW, McHale PA, Smith PK, Anderson RW: Pulmonary vascular impedance analysis of adaptation to chronically elevated blood flow in the awake dog. *Circ Res* 1979; 45:267−274.
113. Geer JC, Glass BA, Albert HM: The morphogenesis and reversibility of experimental hyperkinetic pulmonary vascular lesions in the dog. *Exper Molec Path* 1965;4:399−415.
114. Ferguson DJ, Varco RL: The relation of blood pressure and flow to the development and regression of experimentally induced pulmonary arteriosclerosis. *Circ Res* 1955;3:152−158.
115. Esterly JA, Glagow S, Ferguson DJ: Morphogenesis of intimal obliterative hyperplasia of small arteries in experimental pulmonary hypertension. An ultrastructual study of the role of the smooth muscle cells. *Am J Pathol* 1968;52:325−347.
116. VanBenthuysen KM, Hammon JW, Mitchner JS, Anderson RW: Electron microscopic alterations in experimental pulmonary hypertension. *J Surg Res* 1977;22:398−418.
117. Ryan US, Ryan JW: Surface properties of pulmonary endothelial cells. In: *Annals of N.Y. Acadamy Science. Surface Phenomena in Hemorheology: Their Theoretical, Experimental and Clinical Aspects.* 1983 (in press).
118. Fry DL: Acute vascular endothelial changes associated with increased blood velocity gradients. *Circ Res* 1968;22:165−197.

119. Muller WH, Damman JF, Head WH: Changes in the pulmonary vessels produced by experimental pulmonary hypertension. *Surgery* 1973;39:365–375.
120. Unni KK, Kottke BA, Titus JL, Frye RL, Wallace RB, Brown AL: Pathologic changes in autocoronary saphenous vein grafts. *Am J Cardiol* 1979;34:526–532.
121. VanBenthuysen KM, Dauber IM, Hyers TA, Steele PP, Weil JV: The role of platelets in hypertensive pulmonary vascular disease. *Fed Proc* 1981;40:794.
122. Schaub RG, Rawlings CA, Keith JC: Platelet adhesion and myointimal proliferation in canine pulmonary arteries. *Am J Pathol* 1981;104:13–22.
123. Van Grondelle A, Voelkel NF, Mathias M, Reeves JT: Lung prostacyclin production with change in shear stress and vascular distention. *Fed Proc* 1982;41:1749.
124. Geer JC, Glass BA, Albert HM: Pulmonary vascular lesions in the dog produced by autogenous clot embolism. *Exper Molec Pathol* 1965;4:391–398.
125. Jacqes WE, Hyman AL: Experimental pulmonary embolism in dogs. *Arch Pathol* 1957;64:487–493.
126. Olsen EGJ: Repeated pulmonary thromboembolism in rabbits. *Lab Invest* 1975;32:323–329.
127. Sheulub I, van Grondelle A, McCullough R, Hofmeister S, Reeves JT: An embolic model of chronic pulmonary hypertension in the dog. *J Appl Physiol* (in press).
128. Sugita T, Sawada A, Kuriyana T, Watanabe S, Okagata T: Experimental study of pulmonary hypertension: Protective effects of artificial unilateral pneumothorax on the development of monocrotaline-induced pulmonary hypertension. *Ann. Report of the Ministry of Health and Welfare-Respiratory Failure Research Committee of Japan.* 1979:153–159 (Japanese).

CHAPTER 11

LUNG BIOPSIES and PULMONARY VASCULAR DISEASE

C. A. Wagenvoort

INTRODUCTION

As has been shown in previous chapters, there is a variety of mechanisms that may induce elevation of pulmonary arterial pressure and an even far greater array of etiologic agents by which these mechanisms may be set into motion. The morphology of the hypertensive pulmonary vascular lesions is closely related to the mechanisms, rather than to the causes, of pulmonary hypertension. This means that widely differing conditions like rheumatic mitral stenosis, left atrial myxoma, and mediastinal fibrosis, may produce the same pattern of changes in lung vessels, since they all may result in obstruction to the pulmonary venous flow. The pathologist, who is acquainted with the various morphologic types of pulmonary vascular disease, is in a position to identify the type of pulmonary hypertension, but with regard to its etiology he can only indicate a group of causes rather than one specific cause. Even so, this may be very helpful if the pulmonary hypertension is unexplained clinically and lung tissue should become available during life.

Much has been learned with regard to the alterations in the pulmonary vasculature by using autopsy material. It is only in more recent years that the study of lung biopsies from patients with pulmonary hypertension has considerably added to our knowledge.

Apart from the benefit to the patient with regard to diagnosis, prognosis, and therapy, the additional advantage of a lung biopsy in these instances pertains to a better understanding of the evolution of hypertensive pulmonary vascular disease. The early alterations can be found in these biopsy specimens more often than at autopsy, in some instances progression or regression of lesions can be studied and, in addition, adequate material may become available for electronmicroscopy, histochemistry, and immunopathology.

Lung tissue may be obtained either during cardiac surgery, or separately as an open lung biopsy. In the first situation the risk for the patient is virtually nil. When the thorax is already open, the taking of a small piece of lung tissue is a minor procedure. In several centers such biopsies have been performed routinely during surgery for acquired or congenital heart disease.[1-6] We ourselves have collected over 2,000 lung biopsy specimens in this way. It is clear that the benefit for the patients is limited in those instances in which corrective surgery was carried out, since the evaluation of pulmonary vascular disease is usually only significant in terms of the prognosis. On the other hand, the systematic study of these biopsies has certainly contributed to our knowledge and understanding of the various lesions, particularly when studied in relation with clinical and hemodynamic data.

There have been two situations in which lung biopsies during cardiac surgery have had a special significance. In one group of patients with pulmonary hypertension, in whom banding of the pulmonary artery was performed, it was possible to compare the specimen with one taken several years later during corrective surgery. In this way one may study the eventual regression or progression of pulmonary vascular disease.[7]

There was also a small group of patients, usually with congenital heart disease, in whom the exact nature of the cardiac condition remained in doubt even during heart operation. In these instances the pattern of pulmonary vascular lesions sometimes provided valuable information and allowed the clinical diagnosis to be confirmed or refuted.

Open lung biopsies for evaluation of pulmonary vascular disease are carried out, either in patients with unexplained pulmonary hypertension to establish the type of vascular disease, or in patients with known congenital heart disease to establish the severity of pulmonary vascular disease. In the latter instances the question posed to the pathologist is whether the extent and degree of the vascular alterations will allow corrective surgery or not.

RISK

There is an understandable hesitation to perform a biopsy in patients with pulmonary hypertension. It is a separate procedure that is not without risk, particularly in those with severe pulmonary hypertension. There are many reports in the literature of adverse reactions and even sudden death in such patients, notably when they suffer from the classical or vasoconstrictive form of primary pulmonary hypertension.[8-12] Nowadays, with modern anesthesia and careful monitoring of the patient, the risk apparently is not very great. As far as we could ascertain, in none of 55 patients with unexplained pulmonary hypertension from whom we received an open lung biopsy, could death be attributed to this procedure.

IS A LUNG BIOPSY REPRESENTATIVE?

Whether the vascular lesions in a biopsy specimen are representative from the lungs as a whole, depends in the first place on the size of the biopsy. The most significant alterations are found in muscular pulmonary arteries accompanying bronchi and bronchioles and in pulmonary veins lying in the interlobular fibrous septa. It is clear that these arteries and veins, that is with a diameter in the range of 100 μm, are not evenly distributed over the lung tissue, in contrast to alveolar capillaries, arterioles, and venules. It is also evident that no reliable judgment is possible on the basis of a few vessels. An adequate size of the specimen is therefore imperative, but what is adequate? In our experience, when a biopsy specimen from an adult lung measures approximately $2.5 \times 2.0 \times 1.0$ cm, it will rarely fail to give a reliable impression of the type, the severity, and the extent of the pathology in the vasculature of the lungs as a whole. For a child or an infant, this biopsy may of course be proportionally smaller since here the arteries and veins are lying more closely together. From a comparison of the lung vessels in a biopsy specimen with those in lung tissue obtained at a subsequent autopsy, it appears that the chance for errors in this respect increases rapidly when the biopsy is smaller than the thumb nail of the patient. Haworth and Reid[13] demonstrated that small pieces of lung tissue generally provide adequate representation of the lung vessels.

It is obvious, therefore, that if a biopsy is envisaged, it should be an open lung biopsy and not a transbronchial or transthoracic needle biopsy of the lung. Although the fragments of tissue obtained in this way may contain a few vessels, the chances for a correct diagnosis with regard to pulmonary vascular disease are extremely small.

There are some situations in which even a biopsy specimen of adequate size may turn out not to reflect the picture in other lung areas. This may happen with regard to lesions that are widely scattered. Generally, when there are plexiform lesions (p. 407), these will be found in a biopsy specimen, particularly when a search for them is made in serial sections. Sometimes, however, when they are scarce, they may not be present in the available specimen. As a rule, however, other arterial changes will indicate not only the type of hypertensive pulmonary vascular disease but also its severity. More important are conditions in which there is a regional distribution of vascular lesions, in the sense that they differ in one part of a lung as compared to other parts, or in one lung as compared to the other lung.

This brings us to the question of whether there is a *site of preference* for the taking of a lung biopsy. It has been maintained that the lingula of the left lung is not suitable, since the vascular changes here can be more severe than elsewhere in the lungs.[14] This may apply to the utmost tip of the lingula since the immediate subpleural region often shows fibrosis of lung tissue with concomitant vascular changes. We could not confirm, however, that a lingula biopsy of adequate size would be unsuitable for an evaluation. In our experience in the vast majority of cases, the site of the biopsy is irrelevant, since almost always the changes in the lung vessels tend to be evenly distributed. The exceptions are of course related to the regional distribution just mentioned. This applies particularly to pulmonary venous hypertension where, as we will see, the changes in the upper parts of the lungs often differ from those at the lung bases. The medial changes are more prominent in the lower parts of the lung, while intimal lesions more pronounced in the upper parts (p. 421). As a rule, a single biopsy will give an impression of the type as well as of the severity of vascular disease as long as the pathologist is aware from which area of the lungs it has been taken.

While multiple biopsies are generally unnecessary, therefore, there are some conditions in which a single biopsy may give an erroneous impression. This applies particularly to those instances in which the hemodynamic situation differs in various parts of the lungs, such as in the presence of a stenosis of one pulmonary artery or one vein. A biopsy from both lungs may then be necessary.

PROCESSING THE LUNG TISSUE

If electronmicroscopy is required, small pieces may be cut from the unfixed specimen for fixation in Karnovsky's fixative and further processing for ultrastructural evaluation. Similarly, a small piece of unfixed material may be frozen for immunologic studies. This should only be done if an adequate amount of lung tissue remains available for light microscopy, since the other methods of study tend to contribute less to the actual diagnosis. The biopsy specimen is cut in slices of 3 to 4 millimeters thick, parallel to the plane of surgical resection. (Figure 1). These pieces are subsequently fixed in 4% neutral formalin. This is done under vacuum for two reasons. First, because in this way air bubbles are removed from the tissue. Otherwise, the bubbles may damage the histologic sections when these are cut from the paraffin embedded blocks. A second reason is that vacuum fixation provides a very adequate and natural expansion of the collapsed lung tissue. Not only the air spaces but also the vessels tend to dilate in this way. Others have inflated the lungs in situ, placed two clamps on the lungs thus isolating a piece of lung tissue, and incised the tissue between the clamps.[4] In this way well inflated lung tissue is obtained, but the vacuum method has the additional advantage of removing the air.

After paraffin embedding, histologic sections are cut at 5 μm and routinely stained with hematoxylin and eosin, elastic-van Gieson stain, and Perl's iron stain. It is not possible to give a reliable judgment of the alterations in the lung vessels based upon a hematoxylin-stained section only because the degree as well as the type of intimal fibrosis and the severity of medial hypertrophy cannot be judged adequately. On the other hand, changes like vasculitis and plexiform lesions may be difficult to detect in an elastic stain. The iron stain is often indispensable for assessing the degree of hemosiderosis. Other histologic stain-

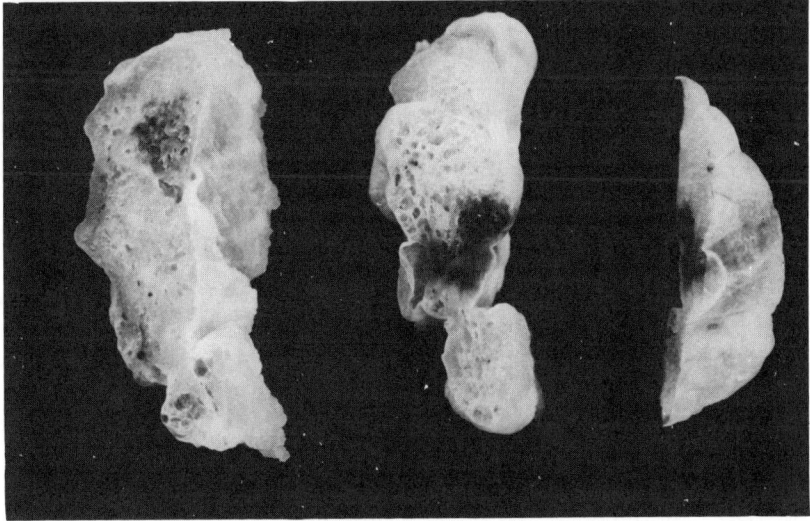

Figure 1. Lung biopsy specimen cut in three slices each of approximately 4 mm thick.

ing methods are sometimes necessary, depending on the microscopic findings.

In many cases serial sections of the biopsy specimen are necessary. Often in a single section there is a suggestion of a particular lesion that may easily be confirmed or refuted by studying multiple sections. Usually a series of approximately 20 slides will suffice.

When studying the sections under the microscope, all aspects of the vessels, that is arteries, veins, capillaries, and lymphatics, as well as the lung tissue, like fibrosis or hemosiderosis, should be taken into account. Since this is fairly time-consuming and since multiple staining methods, additional sections, and eventually serial sections may be required, we are not in favor of using frozen sections for immediate evaluation of the pulmonary vasculature during cardiac surgery. This was advocated by Rabinovitch et al.[15] However, the advantage of avoiding an open lung biopsy, in our opinion, is more than annulled by the possible inaccuracy of a diagnosis thus obtained. Moreover, the evaluation of the pulmonary vasculature may lead to the conclusion that a different type of cardiac operation is indicated, or even that surgery should not be attempted at all. Such a realization should not come at the time that the thorax has already been opened.

REPORTING ON LUNG BIOPSIES

As mentioned above, all aspects pertaining not only to various lung vessels and their layers but also to the lung tissue itself should be described, and our conclusion should be based on an evaluation of all these features. Sometimes cardiac surgeons express a preference for a concise answer in the form of a single grade. However, serious objections can be made to the use of a grading system in general and particularly for assessing the pulmonary vasculature in an individual patient in this way.[16] Grading systems like the one used by Heath and Edwards[17] were essentially devised for the pattern of vascular lesions now known as plexogenic arteriopathy and denoted certain qualitative aspects of the arterial alterations. The quantitative aspects, which of course are at least as important, are not taken into account. If there is intimal fibrosis of pulmonary arteries, the verdict, "grade III," leaves in abeyance whether this intimal change is mild or obstructive. Also, as we will see, there are various types of intimal fibroses with different implications with regard to prognosis of therapy. This is also an advantage of the open lung biopsy over microradiology[18,19] in which the degree of arterial obstruction, but not the type of vascular disease, can be identified. The aim of the final conclusion of our report should be to indicate the type of pulmonary vascular disease, its severity, and eventually advice concerning the possibility of corrective surgery.

INDICATIONS FOR LUNG BIOPSIES IN PULMONARY VASCULAR DISEASE

Unexplained (Primary) Pulmonary Hypertension

The first open lung biopsy specimens generally were from patients with unexplained pulmonary hypertension. Often these specimens were submitted with the suggested clinical diagnosis of primary pulmonary hypertension, clearly meant as the classical or vasoconstrictive form of primary pulmonary hypertension. In 1975 a World Health Organization (WHO) Committee[20] drew attention to the fact that unexplained pulmonary hypertension usually appeared to be one of three forms that clinically may be very difficult to tell apart. There are pulmonary hypertension due to chronic silent thromboembolism, pulmonary venoocclusive disease, and the classical type of primary pulmonary hypertension, for which this report suggested the name "primary plexogenic arteriopathy." In this condition the pattern of vascular lesions is essentially the same as in congenital heart disease with a left-to-right shunt (p. 400). Primary pulmonary hypertension has hence been defined as "clinically unexplained pulmonary hypertension." It stands to reason and it is our own experience[12] that other forms of pulmonary hypertension than the three mentioned in the WHO report, sometimes remain clinically unexplained.

Whereas various forms of pulmonary hypertension may present unsolvable diagnostic problems to the clinician, for the pathologist it is usually not difficult to tell them apart since the morphology is very distinctive. Of course the question arises whether it is worthwhile taking an open lung biopsy since the prognosis in most forms of unexplained pulmonary hypertension is poor and therapy usually ineffective. It is difficult to answer that question categorically, although there is no doubt that thus far the ultimate gain for the patient has been limited. In recurrent thromboembolic pulmonary hypertension, positive results have been reported from anticoagulant therapy[21] that is ineffective in plexogenic arteriopathy. In the latter condition vasodilator therapy has been tried extensively (see Chapter 4) but the overall results have not been encouraging. To a large extent it will depend on the state to which pulmonary vascular disease has progressed and unfortunately, as a rule, the first symptoms appear, and consequently the diagnosis is made when the lesions have become advanced and irreversible.

There is, however, little doubt that if any attempt to influence the course of the disease process is to be made at all, its eventual success will depend on a definite diagnosis of the nature of the pulmonary vascular disease, which generally can be made only by open lung biopsy.

Congenital Heart Disease

In congenital heart disease with a left-to-right shunt, pulmonary hypertension is almost always associated with a pattern of vascular lesions designated "plexogenic arteriopathy." Therefore, if a lung biopsy is taken in these instances, it is done not so much to establish the nature of the vascular disease as to assess the degree to which it has progressed. Generally, clinical and hemodynamic studies will ascertain whether the alterations within the pulmonary vasculature are limited, so that they will not stand in the way of a correction of the cardiac defect, or that they are so advanced that corrective surgery is no longer advisable. As can be expected, there are cases in which such a decision is difficult either because of technical problems with catheterization studies or because, as in borderline cases, the results of such studies are ambiguous. In these instances a pre-operative lung biopsy may indicate whether a corrective operation has a chance of being successful or not. This indication has produced lung biopsies in rapidly increasing numbers in recent years.

Uncertain Diagnosis in Heart Disease

Occasionally the exact nature of a heart condition, particularly a congenital cardiac anomaly, remains in doubt despite extensive clinical and hemodynamic evaluation, or even surgical exploration. A lung biopsy taken during heart operation or as a pre-operative lung biopsy may contribute to the diagnosis of the cardiac disease, for instance by indicating the likelihood of an as yet unsuspected obstruction in the pulmonary arterial pathway or in the pulmonary venous outflow.

MORPHOLOGIC VARIETIES OF PULMONARY VASCULAR DISEASE

Where to Look for Changes

Since these biopsies are submitted for evaluation of the pulmonary vasculature, all lung vessels should be studied carefully, not only pulmonary arteries but also arterioles, veins and venules, capillaries, bronchial vessels, collaterals, and lymphatics. Attention should also be paid to the lung tissue itself and to the pleura. As we will see, some parenchymal alterations may point to hemodynamic disturbances. Occasionally, however, lesions unrelated to the pulmonary circulation may happen to be observed and may give valuable information about the patient's condition. A single vessel or a few vessels will almost never allow a reliable histologic diagnosis; this is also the reason why too small a biopsy specimen is often unsatisfactory. It is the total picture that should be judged.

Elastic arteries, that is vessels with a diameter of over 500 or 1,000 μm, are not often present in a peripheral biopsy specimen. If they are, there is usually thickening of the media, sometimes with atherosclerotic changes, in pulmonary hypertension. Various post-thrombotic lesions, similar to those in the muscular arteries (p. 416) may occur in recurrent thromboembolism.

Within the muscular arteries, in the great majority of the cases, one of the known morphologic varieties of pulmonary vascular disease, to be discussed hereafter, will emerge. Sometimes a combination of two patterns is found. There remains a small group of cases in which the interpretation of the findings is ambiguous or impossible, although even then some useful suggestions can sometimes be made.

Normal Pulmonary Vasculature

The transition of the larger elastic pulmonary arteries to the muscular arteries takes place in adults at a diameter between 1,000 and 500 μm. In infants this transition is usually at a smaller diameter.[22]

These muscular arteries, in which the most characteristic alterations may be expected in pathologic conditions, normally have a thin media and a relatively wide lumen. The medial thickness, when measured in a cross-section, is in the range of 5% of the external vascular diameter.

The muscular coat is bounded by internal and external elastic laminae. The intima consists mainly of an endothelial layer overlying the internal elastic lamina, but in adults over the age of 20 and particularly over the age of 40 years, mild intimal fibrosis as an age change is very common (Figure 2). Moreover, there is a fairly thin adventitia. The arterial branches tend to lose their muscular coat gradually at a diameter between 100 and 70 µm, so that the small arterioles may be partly muscular as well as non-muscular (Figure 3).

The pulmonary veins and venules are normally even more thin-walled than the arteries. Their media is composed of irregularly arranged elastic fibers interspersed between scarce smooth muscle cells. As in the arteries, their intima is thin and is also subject to mild intimal fibrosis with increasing age.

Bronchial arteries are uncommonly encountered in peripheral lung biopsies. As a rule they will not be confused with pulmonary arterial branches because their caliber in relation to the bronchi they accompany is much smaller and they usually lack a distinct external elastic lamina.[22]

Plexogenic Arteriopathy

This is a term introduced by a WHO committee[20] to designate a characteristic pattern of pulmonary vascular lesions occurring in patients with pulmonary hypertension, most commonly due to a left-to-right shunt. This generally results from a congenital cardiovascular anomaly such as atrial or ventricular septal defect, patent ductus arteriosus, persistent truncus arteriosus, etc. (see Chapter 3). The same pattern may be observed in a sequestered lobe of a lung, in which the pulmonary arteries are supplied by a branch from the aorta. It is a known complication in patients with tetralogy of Fallot in whom too large a shunt between the systemic and pulmonary circulations, especially the Pott's shunt, causes secondary pulmonary hypertension. Experimentally it is somewhat difficult to produce, but various attempts in dogs have been successful.[23,24]

A less common condition associated with plexogenic arteriopathy is the classical or vasoconstrictive form of primary pulmonary hypertension. This primary plexogenic arteriopathy occurs mainly in children and young adults. In individuals over the age of 60 years it is rare. In adults there is a female/male ratio of approximately 4; in children it is equal[12] (see Chapter 4).

The cause of primary plexogenic arteriopathy is by definition unknown. There has, however, been one situation in which there is a very strong suspicion that this "primary" form was caused by the oral ingestion of the anorectic drug aminorex or menocil. The drug was associated with an epidemic of "primary" pulmonary hypertension in Switzerland, Austria, and Western Germany between 1967 and 1970[25-27] (see Chapter 9).

Uncommonly, plexogenic arteriopathy is associated with portal hypertension due to cirrhosis of the liver or other hepatic injury, or to portal vein thrombosis.[28,29] Finally, lesions of this pattern may be observed in patients who have pulmonary schistosomiasis. The mechanism in the latter two conditions remains subject to speculation.

Morphology

In the muscular pulmonary arteries the most common, and earliest lesion, is *medial hypertrophy* (Figure 4). Thickening of the media is brought about in part by an increase in thickness of individual muscle fibers but particularly by an increase in their number. This is especially obvious when we look at the small branches. Normally, arterioles of a caliber below 100 or 70 μm are devoid of muscle fibers. In pulmonary hypertension these small vessels acquire a complete muscular coat sometimes at a caliber of 30 or 20 μm (Figure 5). This *muscularization* of arterioles may be very widespread.

Not uncommonly, medial hypertrophy of arteries and muscularization of arterioles (Figure 6) are extremely severe in very young infants with congenital heart disease.[30,31] Although at that age other vascular lesions are usually absent, it is advisable to give a warning to the clinicians if such a situation is found in a preoperative lung biopsy specimen, because severe vasoconstriction of the pulmonary arterial tree often complicates the outcome of a surgical correction of the cardiac defect.

At a later state *cellular intimal proliferation* develops. It primarily affects small branches that may be narrowed or virtually obstructed by loosely proliferating intimal cells without significant deposition of collagen or elastic fibers (Figure 7). This deposition occurs at a somewhat later stage and then results in a peculiar type of intimal fibrosis with an onion-skin arrangement (Figure 8). This *concentric-laminar intimal fibrosis* has a tendency to lead to complete occlusion of the lumen.[22] In the long run this leads to a retraction of the obliterated vessel. In these instances the onion-skin appearance is no longer recognizable (Figure 9). In the more advanced states of this form of

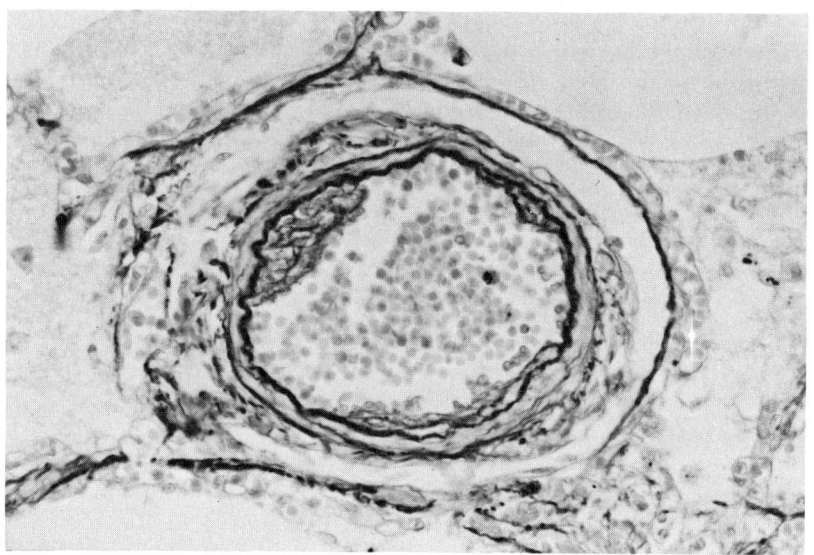

Figure 2. Normal muscular pulmonary artery with thin media and mild intimal fibrosis as an age change. Man, 42 years. Elastic-van Gieson stain (El.v.G.), × 230.

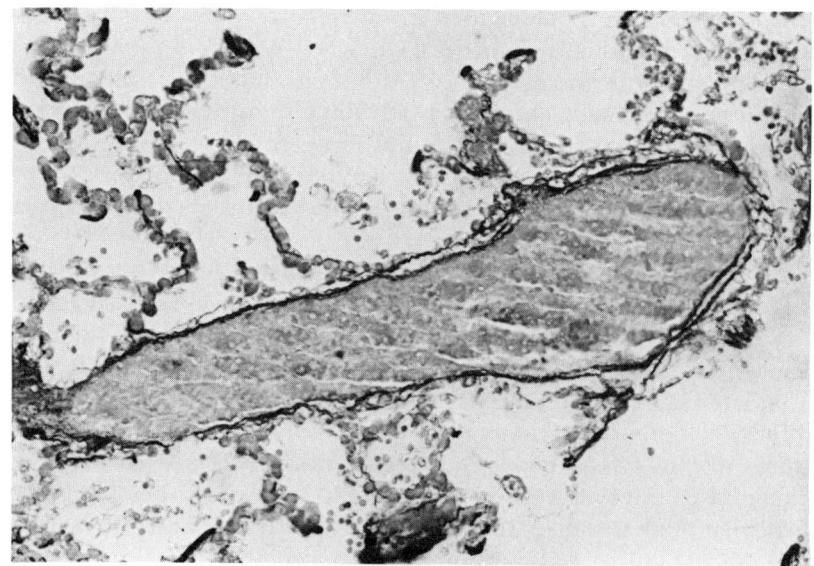

Figure 3. Normal pulmonary arteriole with alternating muscular and non-muscular portions. Man, 25 years. El.v.G., × 230.

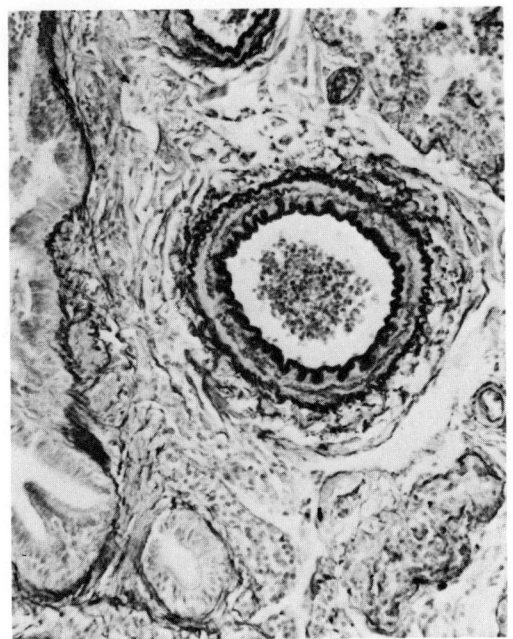

Figure 4. Muscular pulmonary artery with medial hypertrophy. Boy, 4 years with ventricular septal defect (V.S.D.) El.v.G., × 140.

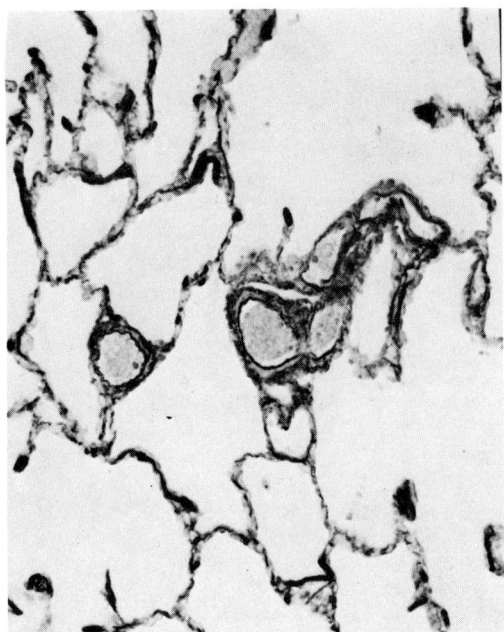

Figure 5. Muscularization of small pulmonary arterioles. Boy, 6 years with single ventricle. El.v.G., × 140.

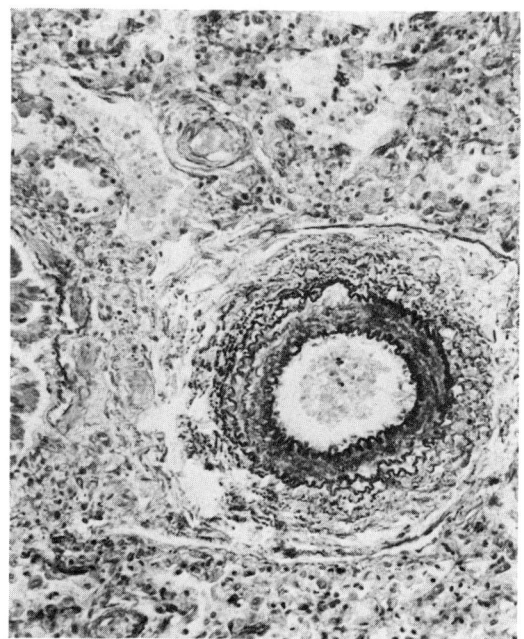

Figure 6. Severe medial hypertrophy of pulmonary artery. Male infant, 3 months with V.S.D. El.v.G., × 140.

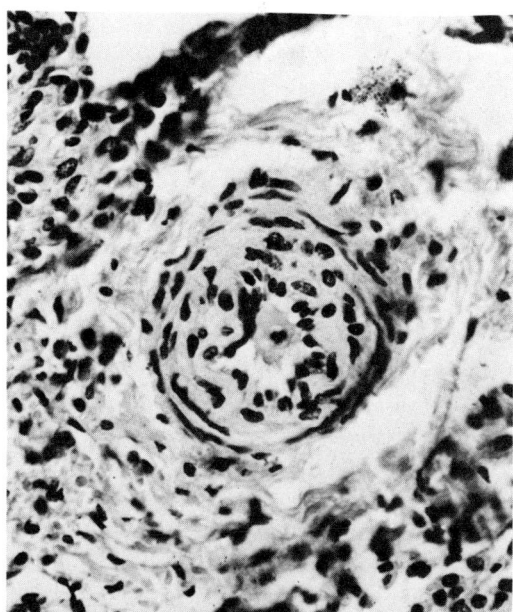

Figure 7. Cellular intimal proliferation of pulmonary artery. Boy, 1½ years with V.S.D. Hematoxylin and eosin (H.E.), × 140.

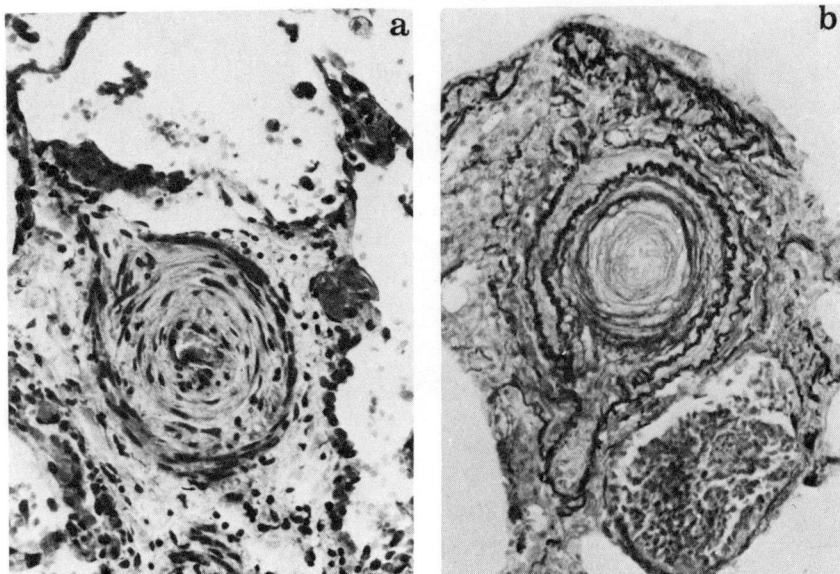

Figure 8. Concentric-laminar intimal fibrosis with obstruction of lumen of pulmonary artery. (a) Girl, 6 years with primary plexogenic arteriopathy (P.P.A.) H.E., × 230. (b) Girl, 2½ years with V.S.D. El.v.G., × 230.

hypertensive pulmonary vascular disease, three types of lesions may be observed.

The arterial media may give way to the increased pressure so that *dilatation lesions* develop in the form of clusters of very thin-walled branches (Figure 10). Focal areas of necrosis of the media occur usually in a short segment of a branch immediately after its origin from a larger artery. The necrosis goes along with imbibition of fibrin by the wall and with formation of a fibrin clot in the lumen (Figure 11). This *fibrinoid necrosis* is sometimes associated with arteritis (Figure 12). It may be followed by the so-called *plexiform lesions* that develop in the same areas.[22] These consist of a dilated arterial segment with destruction of its wall, often with remnants of fibrinoid necrosis and a plexus of capillary-like channels which occurs as a result of recanalization of the fibrin clot (Figures 13 and 14).

Both morphologic and experimental evidence[24,32,33] suggest that the plexiform lesions develop in areas affected by fibrinoid necrosis. Originally the plexiform lesions were included in the group of dilatation lesions[17] and, as we have seen, dilatation is one of their essential features. For practical reasons, however, it is advisable to separate them as distinctive lesions, not only because of their characteristic morphology that make them far more readily identifiable than for

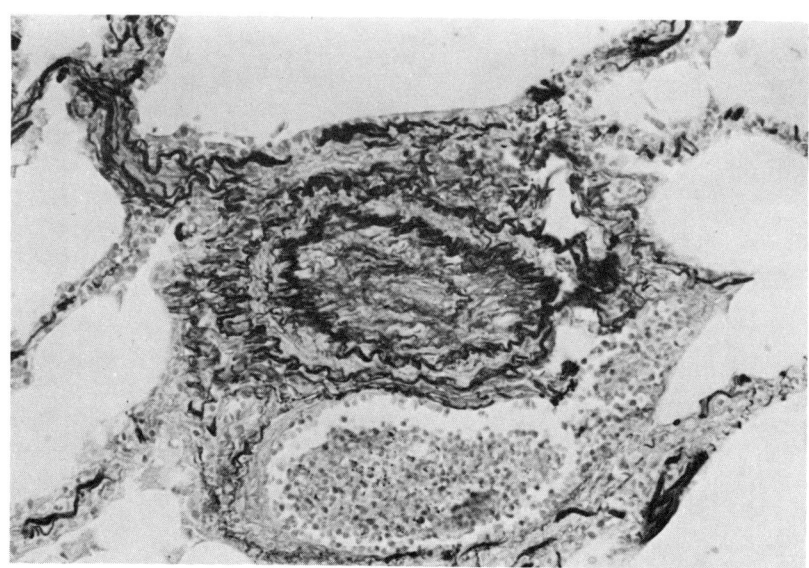

Figure 9. Obliteration by intimal fibrosis with retraction of pulmonary artery. The type of intimal fibrosis is no longer recognizable. Woman, 26 years with P.P.A. El.v.G., × 230.

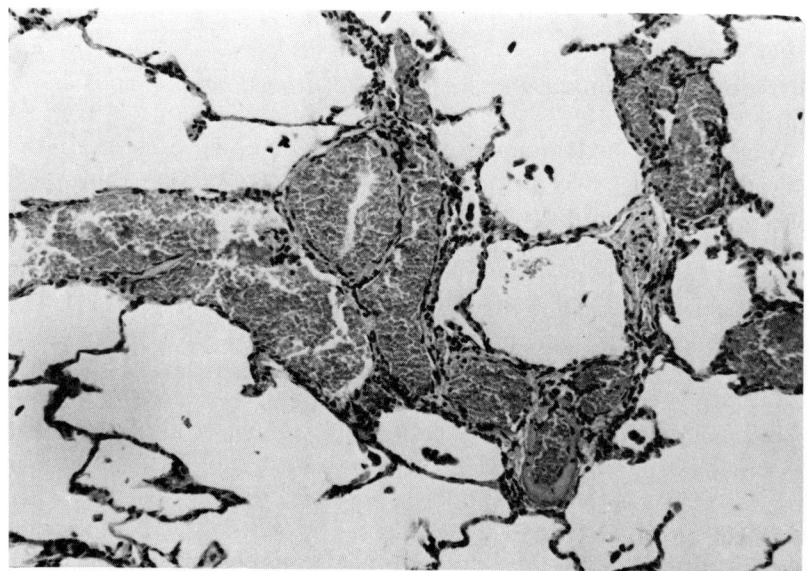

Figure 10. Dilatation lesion in the form of a cluster of thin-walled arterial branches. Boy, 10 years with complete transposition of great arteries (T.G.A.) and V.S.D. H.E., × 140.

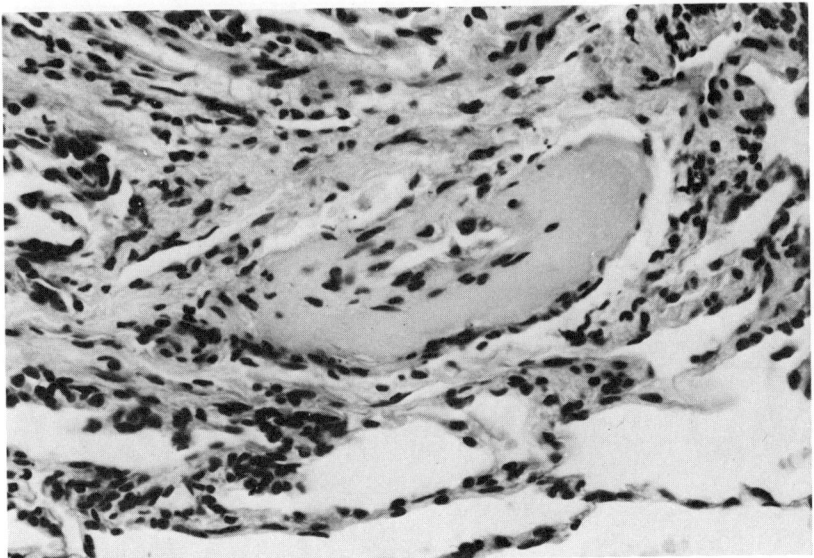

Figure 11. Fibrinoid necrosis of pulmonary artery. Boy, 10 years with T.G.A. and V.S.D. H.E., × 140.

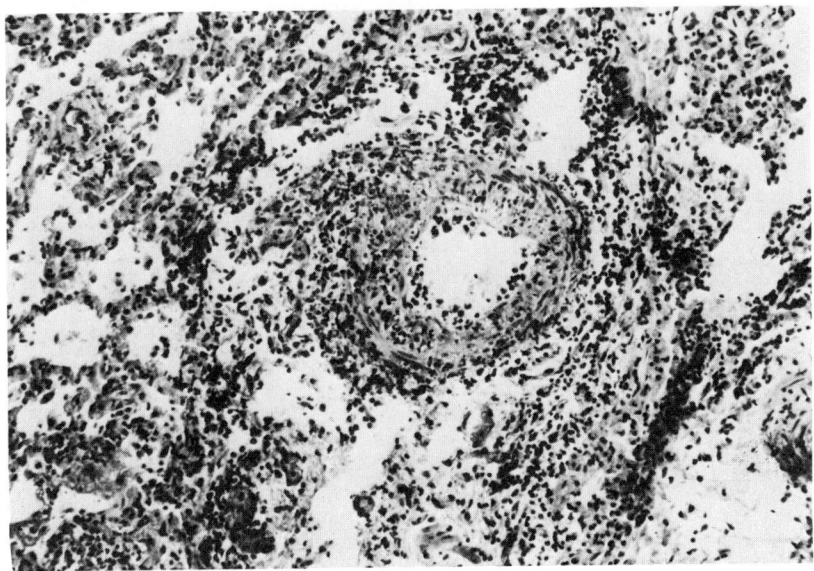

Figure 12. Acute pulmonary arteritis. Girl, 6 years with P.P.A. H.E., × 140.

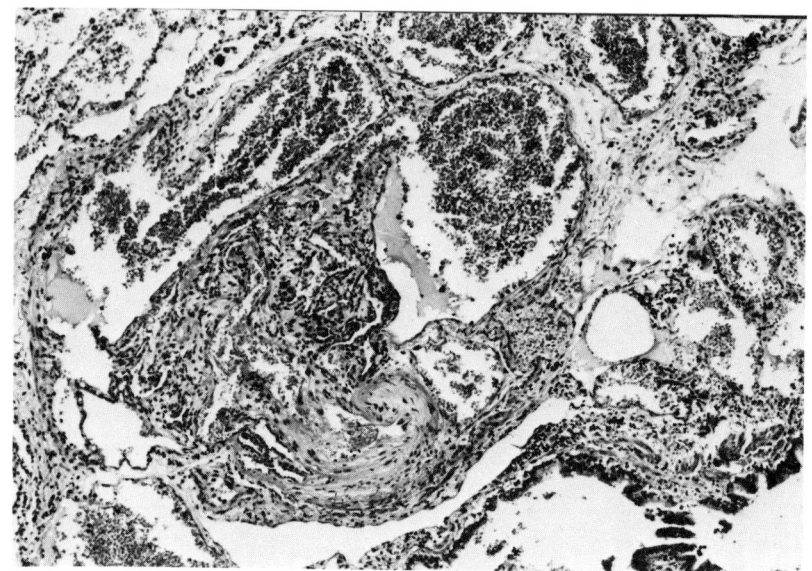

Figure 13. Plexiform lesion of pulmonary artery. Man, 32 years with P.P.A. H.E., × 90.

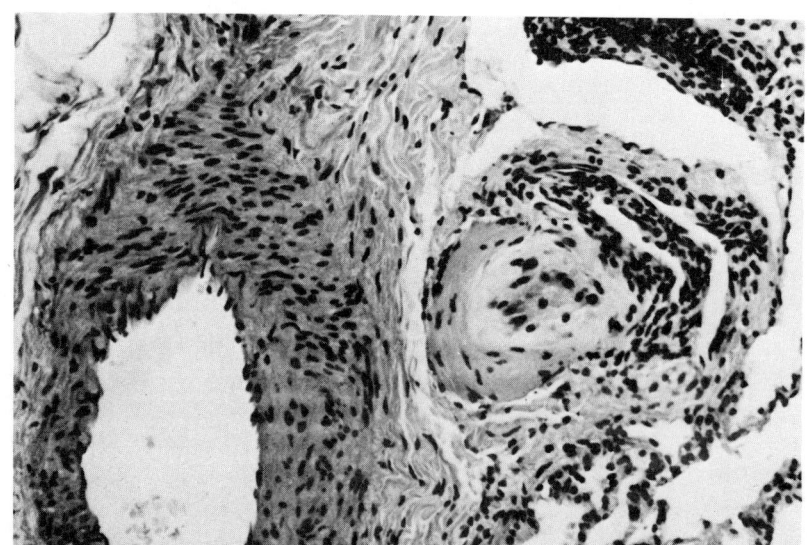

Figure 14. Pulmonary artery with fibrinoid necrosis and early plexiform lesion. Girl, 2½ years with V.S.D. H.E., × 140.

instance the so-called "vein-like branches,"[17] but also because it is likely that their prognostic significance is somewhat different. The presence of fibrinoid necrosis and/or plexiform lesions in a lung biopsy specimen in our experience indicates invariably a poor prognosis for the patient.[34] It is not certain whether the same is true for dilatation lesions, although they are usually found only in advanced disease. Also their place in the sequence of development of pulmonary vascular alterations is somewhat ambiguous. Most probably they develop ahead of fibrinoid necrosis and plexiform lesions, although they can occur simultaneously or later.

Reversibility

Of paramount importance is the question whether, and to what extent in a given case, plexogenic arteriopathy is reversible. The point is hardly relevant with regard to primary plexogenic arteriopathy. As long as the cause is unknown, it is unlikely to be removed and regression of pulmonary vascular disease is not to be expected. The only exception to this rule apparently is "primary" pulmonary hypertension associated with aminorex. As shown above, the use of this anorectic agent resulted in plexogenic arteriopathy, and it has now become clear that discontinuation of the drug may be followed by regression, if the vascular disease is not too advanced. Approximately half of these patients died as a result of pulmonary hypertension, but the other half recovered while their pulmonary arterial pressures decreased to normal or near normal.[35]

A similar course of events is seen in plexogenic arteriopathy due to congenital heart disease with a shunt. Surgical correction of the defect results in regression of the vascular lesions and restoration of normal or near normal pressures as long as pulmonary hypertension has not become "fixed." In most instances data derived from clinical and hemodynamic studies will decide whether a patient with congenital heart disease is a candidate for corrective surgery or not. There are, however, many exceptions in the sense that these data are ambiguous or borderline.

This became evident when we studied lung biopsies taken during cardiac surgery. In many instances it could be predicted that the outlook for the patient was dim in view of the severity of the hypertensive pulmonary vascular disease, even though the operation was successful and the initial post-operative course encouraging. Conversely, it seems likely, although this could never be proven, that corrective surgery was inappropriately withheld from some patients who might have done well.

In these borderline cases the direct morphologic evaluation of the lung vessels in an open biopsy specimen may give an unequivocal answer,[34] as long as we are able to decide which lesions or combinations of lesions are reversible and which are not. For that purpose it is useful to compare lung biopsies taken at the time of a banding of the pulmonary artery in patients with congenital heart disease and pulmonary hypertension, with biopsies taken several years later when corrective surgery was carried out in the same patients.[7] It appears that medial hypertrophy has a strong tendency to regress, if not to normal then at least to a distinctly lesser degree (Figure 15).

Cellular intimal proliferation was remarkably reversible, even when in the first biopsy specimen it caused pronounced narrowing of pulmonary arterial branches (Figure 16). In the later biopsy specimens only remnants, in the form of a thin dense layer of intimal fibrosis, could be found (Figure 17). The same applied to concentric-laminar intimal fibrosis as long as it was mild. If severe, there was not only no regression but, as a rule, distinct progression of vascular disease. Fibrinoid necrosis and plexiform lesions had the same predictive value. From these findings it evolves that the onion-skin type of intimal

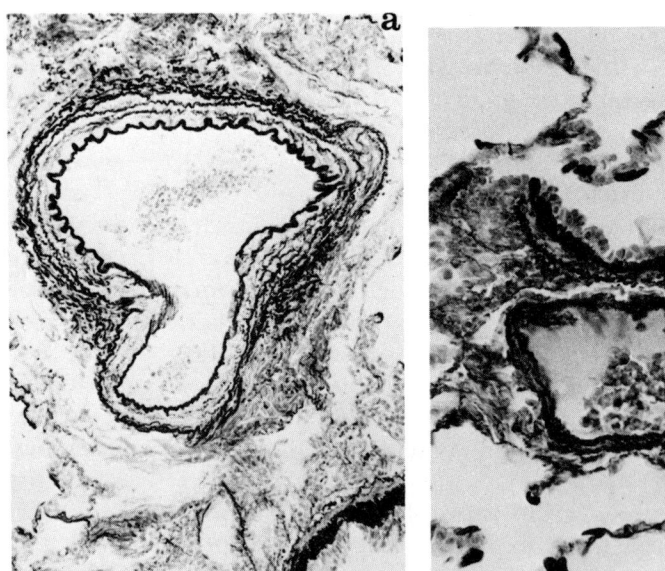

Figure 15. (a) Muscular pulmonary artery with medial hypertrophy. Boy, 1 year with V.S.D. Lung biopsy specimen taken during banding procedure. El.v.G., × 140. (b) Artery with normal media from same patient. Biopsy specimen taken 5 years later during closure of V.S.D. El.v.G., × 140.

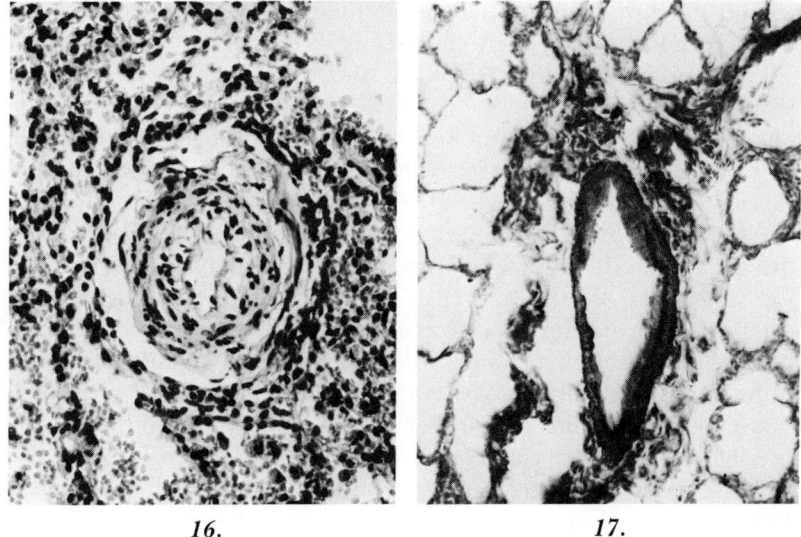

Figure 16. Cellular intimal proliferation of pulmonary artery with narrowing of lumen. Boy, 4 years with T.G.A. and V.S.D. Lung biopsy specimen taken during banding procedure. H.E., × 230.

Figure 17. Pulmonary artery with thin layer of dense intimal fibrosis. Same patient as the one from Figure 16. Biopsy specimen taken 7 years later at time of correction of cardiac defect. El.v.G., × 140.

fibrosis is a critical criterion for the feasibility of surgical intervention. Somewhere between mild and severe intimal fibrosis lies the "point of no return," assuming that the more advanced changes are absent. The preliminary results indicate that the chance for regression is great when less than one-fifth of the average luminal diameter is obstructed and very small when this exceeds one-third.

It is clear that even a preoperative open lung biopsy may not give an unequivocal answer with regard to operability under all circumstances, but the number of borderline cases in which such operability is considered doubtful, is greatly reduced. Of 76 open lung biopsies from patients in whom we could obtain a follow-up of 1 year or more, positive advice with regard to operation was given in 42 cases, negative in 24 cases, and "doubtful" in 10 cases. This last group, however, included 2 cases from an early period in which only an occasional artery contained fibrinoid necrosis or a plexiform lesion, so that it was thought that this did not necessarily stand in the way of a favorable outcome for correction. Since that time we have come to the conclusion, on the basis of the available evidence, that corrective surgery should not be attempted whenever these lesions are present, even when very few vessels are thus affected.

Preliminary results of a follow-up study on the patients from whom biopsy specimens were judged, indicate that this method of evaluation of pulmonary vascular pathology provides an important contribution to the decision whether corrective surgery of a cardiac defect should be carried out or not.

An entirely different aspect of hypertensive pulmonary vascular disease applies to underdevelopment of the pulmonary arterial bed in the sense that the size as well as the numbers of small pulmonary arteries are considerably decreased.[31,36-38] This concept has of course important implications as it means that a high and irreversible pulmonary resistance may occur in the absence of any obstructive intimal lesions. It also means that attention has to be paid to size and number of pulmonary arteries in a lung biopsy specimen.

However, doubts have been raised whether this concept is valid, at least in the sense of a regular occurrence in congenital heart disease. Others could not find any decrease in arterial numbers in congenital heart disease when compared to normal controls.[39,40] Using the same technique, diminished numbers of pulmonary arteries have been found in experimental animals subjected to either hypoxia[41,42] or to Crotalaria administration.[43,44] But Kay et al.[45] could not confirm this, while Mooi and Wagenvoort[46] questioned the validity of the methods used by previous investigators. Although there is reason to believe that an underdevelopment of the pulmonary arterial tree may occur, it is likely that this is very rare and far from being a regular incidence.

It is not at all uncommon that in plexogenic arteriopathy a different type of arterial intimal fibrosis is observed. This may be due to complicating thromboembolism, notably when there is valvular endocarditis. Far more often it is due to organization of primary thrombi. This is particularly seen in cases of complete transposition of the great arteries, which have an increased tendency to thrombus formation (Figure 18).

Pulmonary venous changes do not belong to the pattern of plexogenic arteriopathy, but such changes may be observed whenever left heart failure develops or when there are complicating anomalies that form an impediment to the pulmonary venous outflow (p. 419).

Embolic and Thrombotic Pulmonary Vascular Lesions

The importance of post-thrombotic vascular changes in the evaluation of lung biopsy specimens is twofold. First, we can identify the

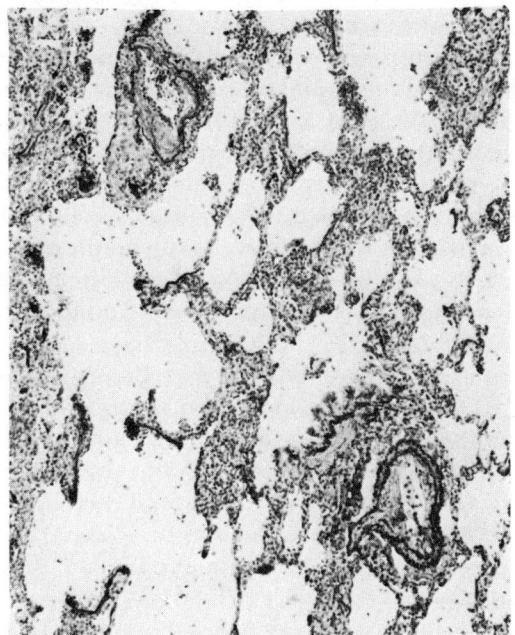

Figure 18. Eccentric postthrombotic intimal fibrosis of pulmonary arteries. Woman, 18 years with T.G.A. and V.S.D. El.v.G., × 90.

nature of an unexplained pulmonary hypertension, if it is due to silent thromboembolism. Second, we will have to realize that post-thrombotic intimal fibrosis in patients with congenital cardiac disease does not have the same ominous prognostic significance that must be attributed to the concentric-laminar intimal fibrosis. The latter would constitute a contraindication for corrective surgery, but the former does not necessarily stand in the way of a successful operation. (Also see Chapter 5.)

Morphology

If changes in the lung vessels are based upon thromboembolism or primary thrombosis, their morphologic aspects are fairly characteristic. These lesions are particularly numerous in chronic pulmonary hypertension due to recurrent thromoembolism. In spite of the elevation of pressure in the pulmonary circulation, medial hypertrophy of the muscular pulmonary arteries is often not a prominent feature. In about 20% of these cases, the average thickness of the pulmonary arterial media is markedly increased; in others, it is not or hardly so.

Thrombi lodged in the lung vessels following embolism become incorporated into the vascular wall by organization. In this way eccentric plaques of post-thrombotic intimal fibrosis are formed (Figure 19). This intimal fibrosis lacks the laminar arrangement of that observed in plexogenic arteriopathy. It very often causes complete obliteration (Figure 20). Moreover, in contrast to plexogenic arteriopathy, it has a focal distribution. An artery may be completely occluded in one area but without any alterations in its further course. If the degree of intimal fibrosis is assessed morphometrically on the basis of obstruction of vessels in cross-section, the average value is often fairly low, in spite of the fact that numerous arteries are totally occluded, if only in one spot.

Recanalization occurs regularly (Figure 21) with a tendency of the recanalizing channels to widen so that the remnants of the organized thrombi stand out as sometimes coarse, sometimes thin, septa of connective tissue. In elastic arteries, where they are recognized on gross inspection, these are known as "bands and webs"[47] (Figure 22), in muscular arteries as "intravascular fibrous septa" (Figure 23). These lesions are pathognomonic for recanalization of thrombi, whether embolic or primary.[22]

Recent thrombi are not necessarily present. In fact, there are many cases of chronic embolic pulmonary hypertension in which no or hardly any recent thrombi can be found. Occasionally, infected emboli may have given rise to purulent arteritis. If this is unexpectedly found in a lung biopsy from a patient with congenital heart disease, its source, for instance a valvular endocarditis or an infected aneurysm of a pulmonary artery (Figures 24 and 25), may be detected in this way.

Reversibility

Obliteration of the artery with retraction of its wall is an irreversible alteration. If recanalization occurs, some restoration of blood flow is possible, although it is doubtful whether the functional significance of these channels is as great as their sizes might suggest. If a lumen is partially obstructed by an eccentric plaque, shrinkage of the plaque will cause some secondary widening of the lumen. Although regression of embolic hypertensive pulmonary vascular disease is thus limited, there is no progression as sometimes occurs in plexogenic arteriopathy, that is if further embolism can be prevented.

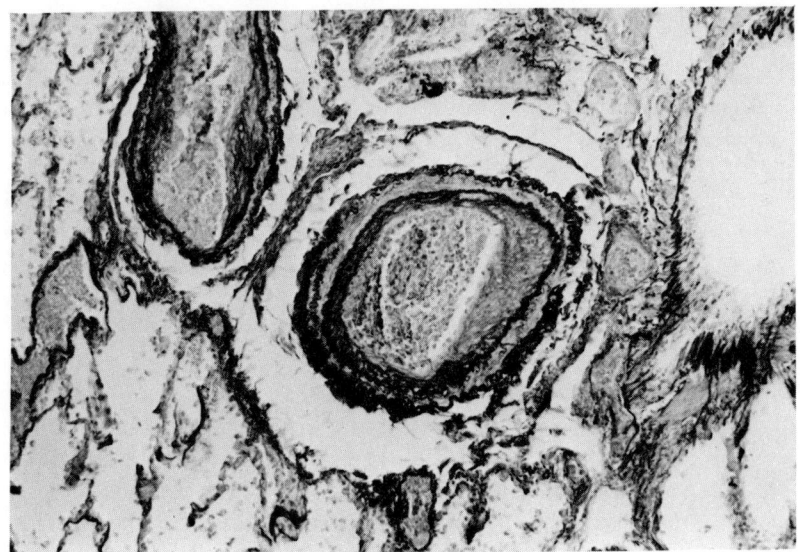

Figure 19. Pulmonary artery with eccentric plaque of intimal fibrosis, resulting from organization of thromboembolus. Woman, 29 years with chronic recurrent pulmonary thromboembolism. El.v.G., × 140.

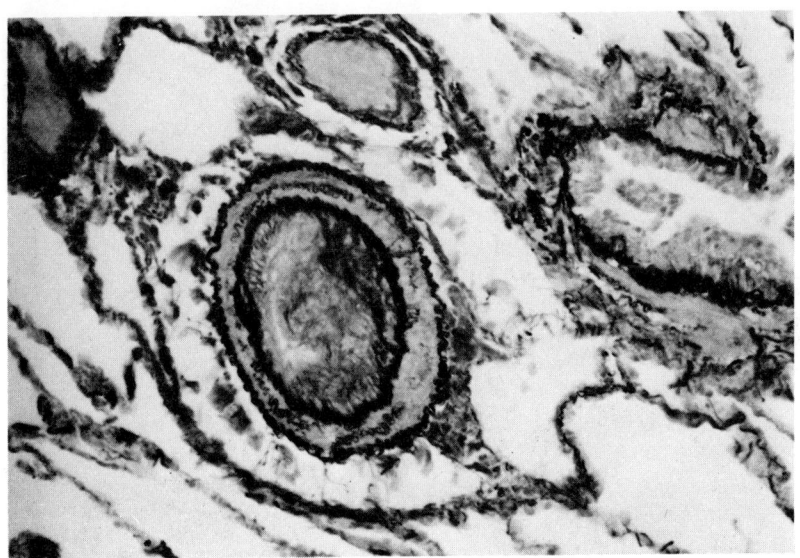

Figure 20. Virtually complete obliteration of pulmonary artery due to organized thromboembolus. Woman, 66 years with chronic recurrent pulmonary thromboembolism. El.v.G., × 230.

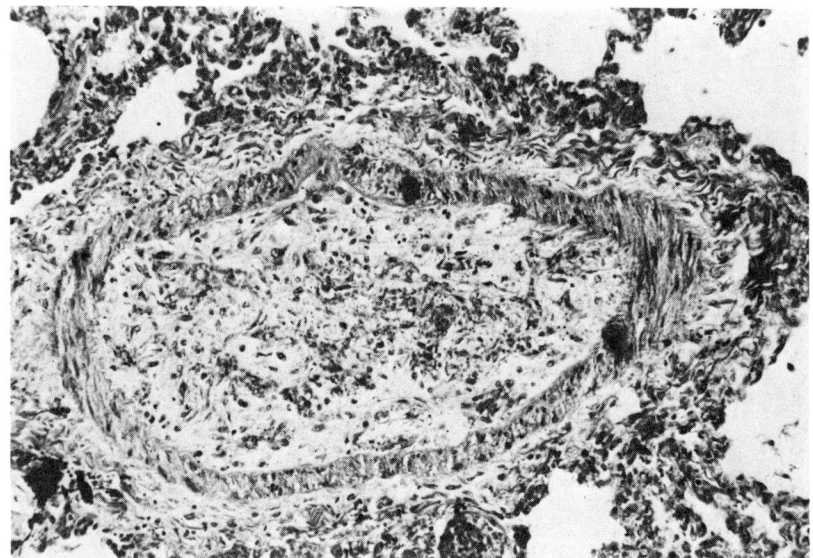

Figure 21. Early recanaliation of thromboembolus in pulmonary artery. Woman, 43 years with chronic recurrent pulmonary embolism. H.E., × 140.

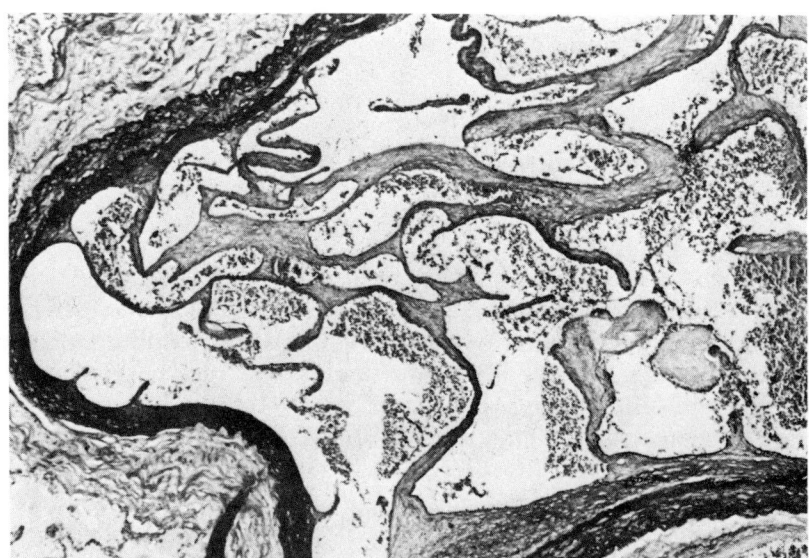

Figure 22. Large elastic pulmonary artery with weblike structure as a result of recanalization of thromboembolus. Man, 70 years with chronic recurrent pulmonary embolism. El.v.G., × 55.

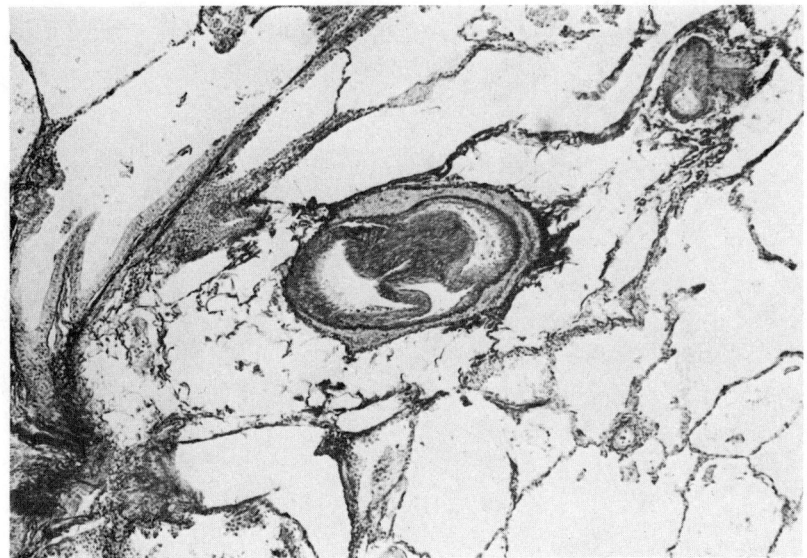

Figure 23. Intravascular fibrous septa in pulmonary artery due to recanalization of thromboembolus. Woman, 29 years with chronic recurrent pulmonary embolism. El.v.G., × 90.

Vascular Lesions in Pulmonary Venous Hypertension

Any impediment to the pulmonary venous outflow will cause essentially the same pattern of pulmonary vascular lesions. Thus, left ventricular failure, mitral valve disease, whether acquired or congenital, stenosis of large pulmonary veins, left atrial myxoma and even non-cardiovascular conditions like mediastinal fibrosis, all give rise to similar alterations in the lung vessels, making this the most common pattern of hypertensive pulmonary vascular disease.

Lung biopsies have often been taken during cardiac surgery for one of these conditions. Preoperative lung biopsies, however, are unusual. Even so, the pathologist who judges lung biopsies should be familiar with this type of pulmonary vascular disease since it is often found as a complicating factor, sometimes entirely unexpected. In that case the findings in the biopsy specimen may well lead to the detection of an additional cardiovascular malformation.

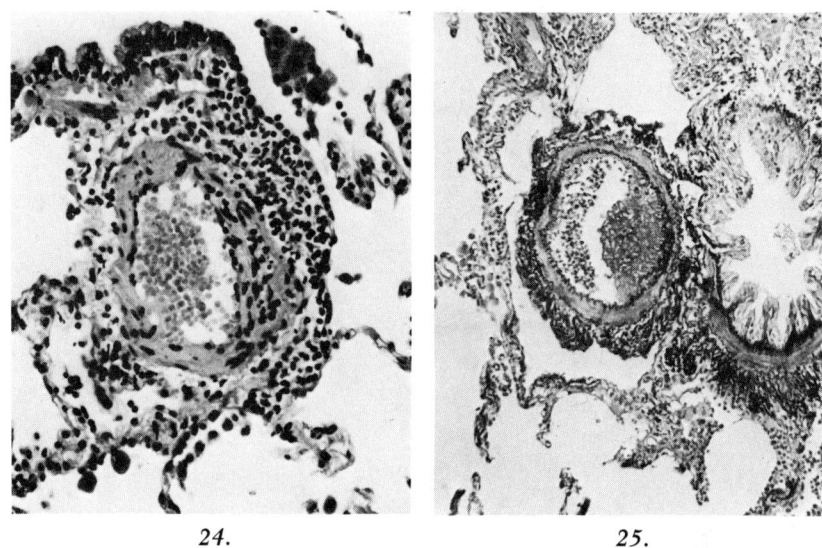

Figure 24. Muscular pulmonary artery with active vasculitis. Woman, 29 years with atrial septal defect. Since these changes were found in multiple arteries in a lung biopsy taken during closure of the defect and since there were also indications of chronic embolism, it was suggested that the changes were due to infected emboli. Later she appeared to have a mycotic aneurysm of a lobar pulmonary artery supplying the lobe from which the biopsy was taken. H.E., × 230.

Figure 25. Eccentric patch of intimal fibrosis resulting from organization of thromboembolus. Same patient as the one from Figure 24. El.v.G., × 140.

Morphology

This is a complicated pattern because not only arteries and arterioles but also pulmonary veins and lymphatics, and even the lung tissue, tend to show alterations attributable to this form of pulmonary hypertension.

In most instances medial hypertrophy of muscular pulmonary arteries is a striking feature, as is muscularization of arterioles[48] (Figure 26); the increased thickness of the media, however, is not only due to multiplication of smooth muscle cells but to a large extent to an increase of edematous intercellular ground substance and collagen.[49] This may explain the observation that the secondary thinning of the media in areas of severe intimal fibrosis, which is commonly observed in plexogenic arteriopathy, is rarely seen in pulmonary venous hypertension.

Intimal fibrosis is often widespread and severe (Figure 27). It is usually eccentric but even when it is circumferential it does not have the

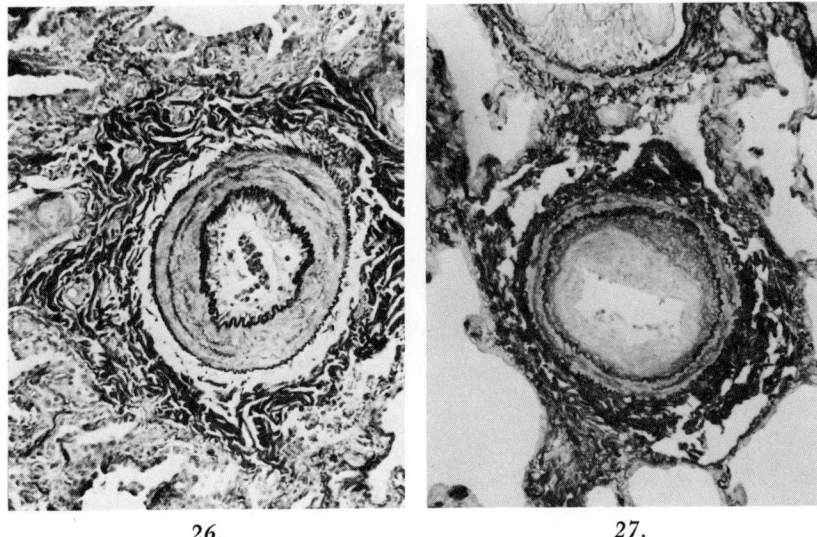

Figure 26. *Severe medial hypertrophy of pulmonary artery with muscularization of arterioles. Woman, 18 years with rheumatic mitral stenosis. El.v.G., × 140.*
Figure 27. *Severe irregular intimal fibrosis of pulmonary artery. Woman, 39 years with rheumatic mitral stenosis. El.v.G., × 140.*

onion-skin appearance of that seen in plexogenic arteriopathy. While it may resemble the intimal thickening due to organization of thromboemboli, it tends to occur over long distances in the arteries and not as isolated patches. Fibrinoid necrosis and arteritis are exceptional and dilatation lesions and plexiform lesions do not belong in this pattern.

As may be expected, in pulmonary venous hypertension the pulmonary veins are affected as well.[50] Their media is increased in thickness and gradually adopts a configuration resembling that of an artery, in that more or less distinct internal and external elastic laminae are formed on either side of the muscular coat (Figure 28). Commonly there is some intimal fibrosis as well (Figure 29).

In the lung tissue in about half of the cases, there is interstitial fibrosis usually in association with hemosiderosis (Figure 30). The iron pigment is predominantly found in macrophages and its distribution is usually focal but may be diffuse. Pulmonary lymphatics are markedly dilated.

In contrast to other forms of pulmonary hypertension where the vascular lesions are generally equally distributed over the lungs, in pulmonary venous hypertension there are differences according to their localization. Medial hypertrophy is more severe in the lower part of the lung. On the other hand, intimal fibrosis is usually more marked

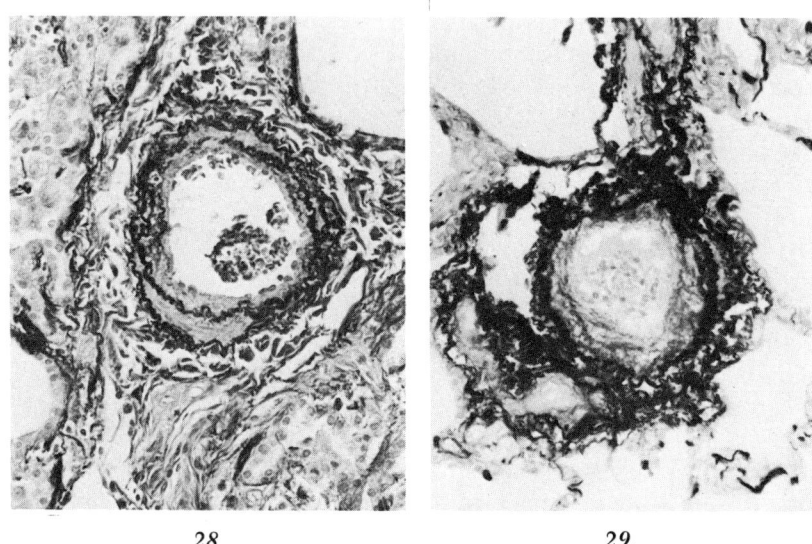

Figure 28. Pulmonary vein with medial hypertrophy and arterialization. Woman, 18 years with rheumatic mitral stenosis. El.v.G., × 350.
Figure 29. Pulmonary vein with intimal fibrosis. Woman, 39 years with rhematic mitral stenosis. El.v.G., × 230.

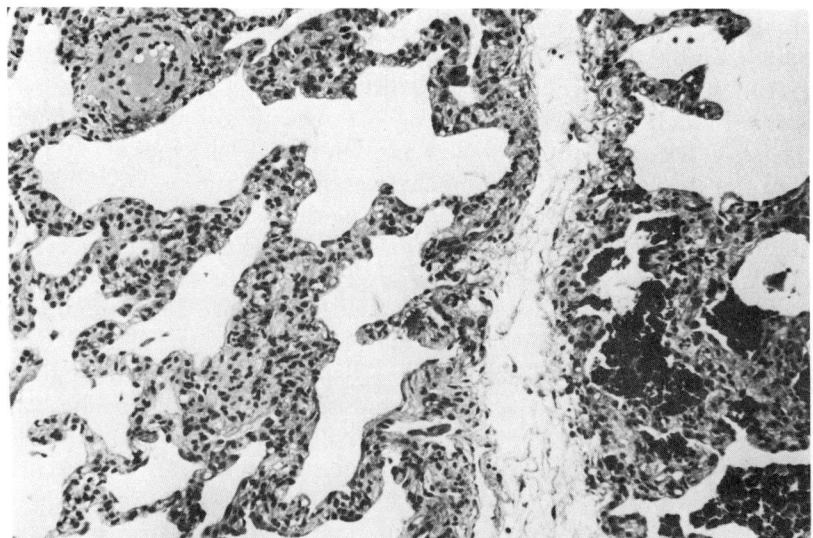

Figure 30. Interstitial fibrosis of lung tissue with hemosiderosis. Woman, 39 years with rheumatic mitral stenosis. H.E., × 140.

in the apex. This aspect has to be taken into account whenever a lung biopsy is studied. It is imperative that the site from which the biopsy specimen is taken is known to the pathologist (p. 396).

Reversibility

The severity of pulmonary vascular disease in pulmonary venous hypertension does not correlate well with the elevation of pulmonary arterial pressure, as it does in other forms of pulmonary hypertension. It is likely that edema of both medial and intimal layers, which is responsible for part of the thickening, contributes to this discrepancy. This may also explain that severe vascular lesions that would constitute a contraindication for a repair of a cardiac defect in congenital heart disease, are often readily reversible in a patient with mitral valve disease after commissurotomy or valve replacement. There are few opportunities to demonstrate this but its occurrence has been well documented.[22,51]

Pulmonary Veno-occlusive Disease

This is a rare disease, but the number of reports has increased rapidly in recent years. It is not clear whether this is due only to a better recognition of the condition or whether there is an actual increase in incidence. It occurs mainly in children and young adults but older individuals are not exempt. In contrast to primary plexogenic arteriopathy (p. 402), men and women are equally affected. Its etiology is obscure. Viral respiratory infections[52,53] and intoxications by household cleanser[54] or drugs[55] have been implicated, but it is likely that there is not a single etiologic agent.[56]

The clinical diagnosis is difficult and the condition is often confused with other forms of hypertensive pulmonary vascular disease. Morphologically the picture is easily identified and an open lung biopsy will rarely fail to provide the correct diagnosis. Unfortunately, up to now therapeutic success has been very limited.

Morphology

Pulmonary veins and venules are narrowed or occluded by intimal fibrosis. This is sometimes paucicellular and of a loose texture (Figure 31) but may also be rich in collagen, suggesting a later stage (Figure 32).

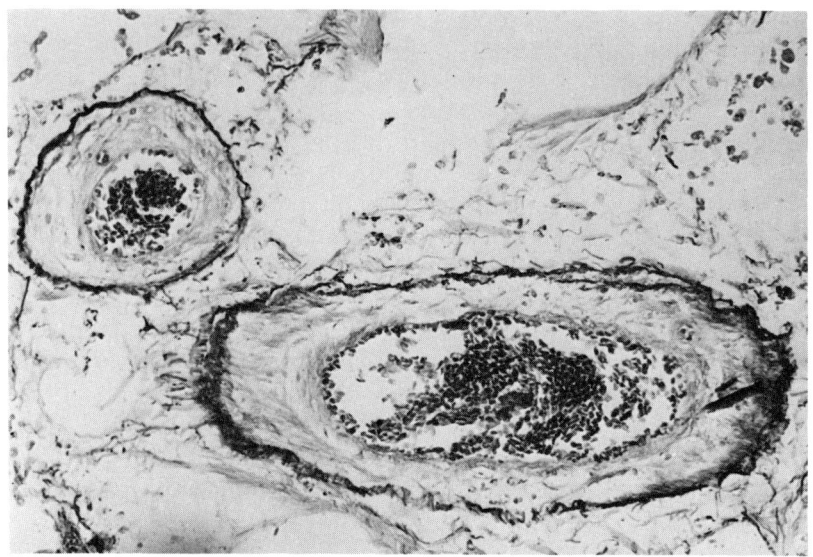

Figure 31. Pulmonary veins narrowed by loose, paucicellular intimal fibrosis. Man, 41 years with pulmonary veno-occlusive disease (P.V.O.D.) El.v.G., × 140.

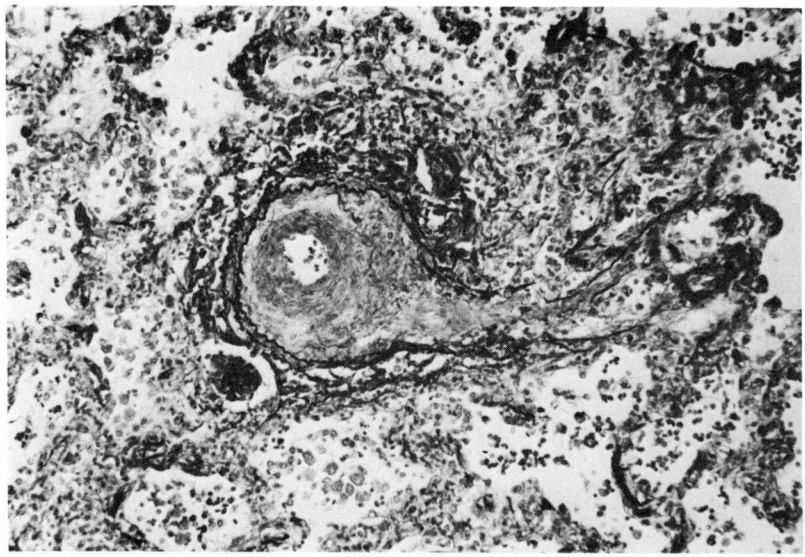

Figure 32. Pulmonary vein occluded by dense, collagen-rich intimal fibrosis. Boy, 6 years with P.V.O.D. El.v.G., × 140.

These features as well as the occasional occurrence of recent thrombi and the development of intravascular fibrous septa as a result of recanalization (Figure 33) all strongly suggest that thrombosis of pulmonary veins is involved in the pathogenesis of the disease. Usually there are distinctive circumscribed areas of congestion with interstitial fibrosis and pronounced hemosiderosis[57] (Figure 34).

The pulmonary arteries usually show secondary medial hypertrophy but are otherwise unremarkable, although they may contain some thrombi, with or without organization. There are, however, some cases in which exactly the same type of fibrotic occlusion is observed in arteries (Figure 35) as in veins,[58] suggesting a universal tendency to thrombosis.

Vascular Lesions in Hypoxic Pulmonary Hypertension

Hypoxic pulmonary hypertension may result from chronic bronchitis and emphysema, upper airway obstruction, Pickwickian syndrome, kyphoscoliosis etc. (see Chapters 7 and 8). It also occurs in residents of high altitude areas (see Chapter 10). The pattern of vascular lesions to be found under these circumstances is rarely observed in a lung biopsy. Wagenvoort[34] described two patients known to suffer from chronic bronchitis in whom a primary form of pulmonary hypertension was suspected, because there seemed to be a discrepancy between the relative mildness of the chronic bronchitis and the marked elevation of pulmonary arterial pressure. However, when open lung biopsies were taken, these specimens revealed only features indicative of hypoxic pulmonary hypertension.

Morphology

The changes in pulmonary vasculature are mainly confined to the smaller vessels.[59] The larger muscular arteries may be normal or show only mild medial hypertrophy. There is, however, distinct muscularization of small arteries and arterioles (Figure 36). Moreover, there is a development of bundles or layers of longitudinal smooth muscle cells in the intima of these small vessels (Figure 37). Similar changes can be found in the small pulmonary veins.[60]

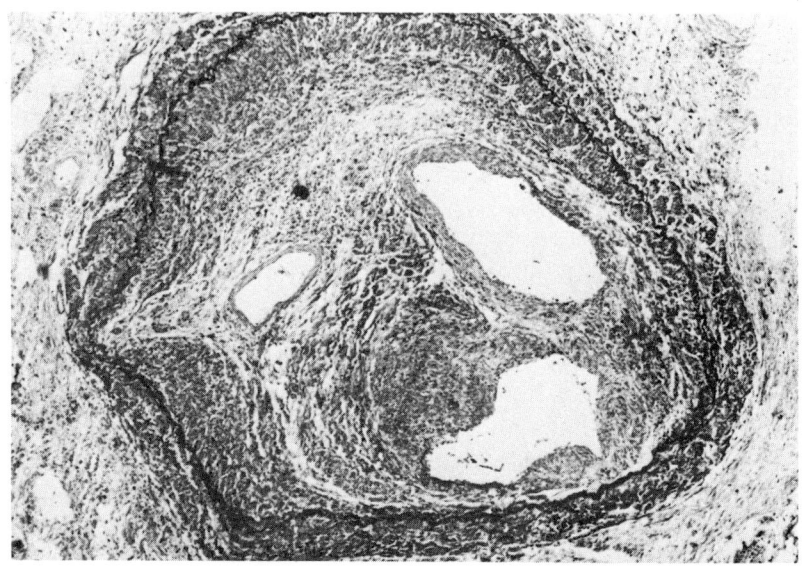

Figure 33. Pulmonary vein with intimal fibrosis and formation of intravascular septa due to recanalization. Woman, 33 years with P.V.O.D. El.v.G., × 55.

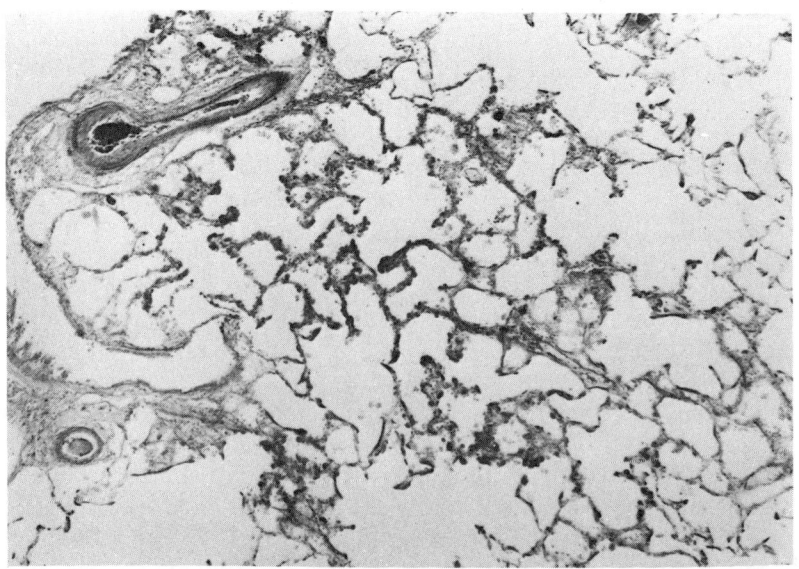

Figure 34. Focal interstitial fibrosis of lung tissue with hemosiderosis. Girl, 13 years with P.V.O.D. El.v.G., × 55.

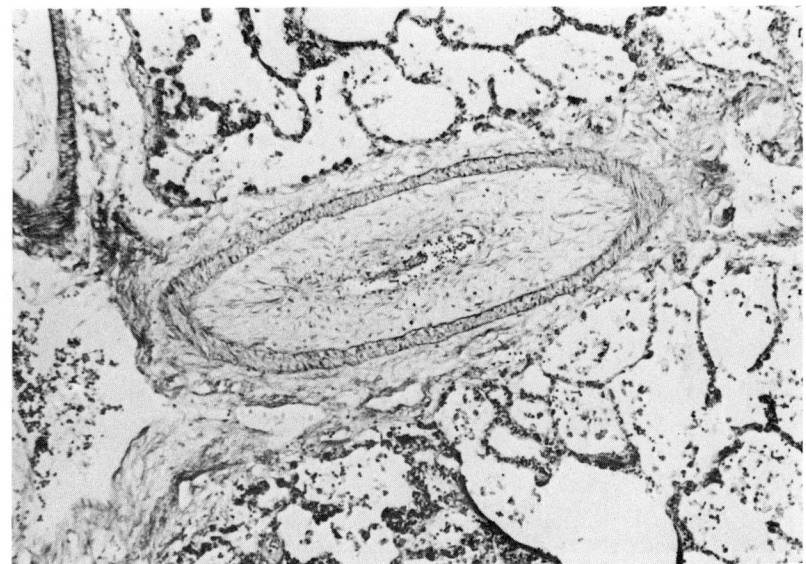

Figure 35. Obstruction of muscular pulmonary artery by intimal fibrosis. Boy, 9 years with P.V.O.D. El.v.G., × 90.

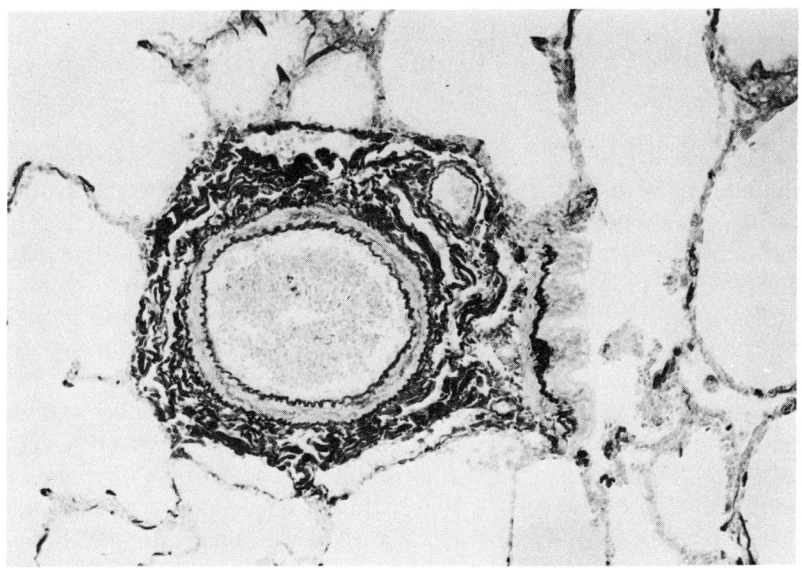

Figure 36. Normal pulmonary artery with muscularized arteriole. Man, 37 years with Pickwickian syndrome and hypoxic pulmonary hypertension. El.v.G., × 140.

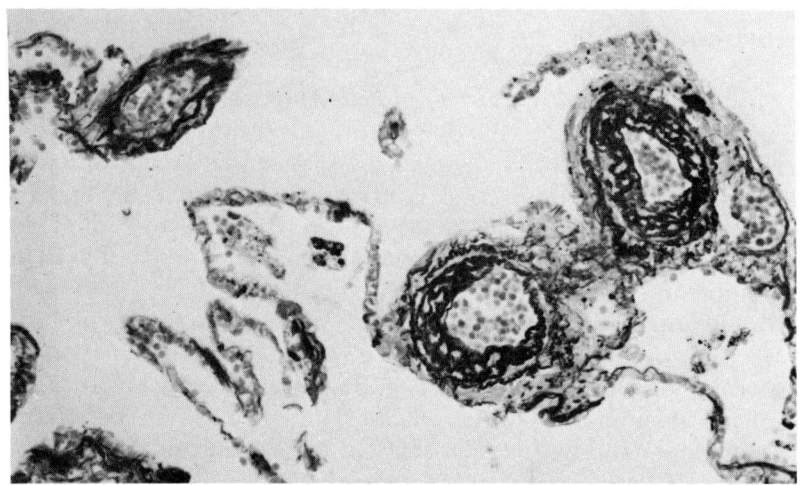

Figure 37. Muscularized pulmonary arterioles with longitudinal smooth muscle cells in intima. Man, 62 years with chronic bronchitis and emphysema. El.v.G., × 230.

Vascular Lesions in Lung Disease

Various diseases of the lung may cause pulmonary hypertension. The mechanisms by which an elevation of pulmonary arterial pressure is brought about may be completely different, and the same is true for the morphologic changes to be found in the lung vessels. In many instances, notably in chronic bronchitis and emphysema, these changes will correspond to those induced by chronic hypoxia as outlined above. In the presence of lung fibrosis or granulomatosis the picture is completely different.

The pathologist may be faced with this type of pulmonary vascular disease in lung biopsies, taken for various purposes. Often the purpose of performing a biopsy is to establish the diagnosis of a lung disease of which the nature is obscure, rather than the evaluation of pulmonary vascular disease. Even so, he will be confronted with prominent changes in the lung vessels and he should interpret their implications correctly. Sometimes, in patients with unexplained pulmonary hypertension, the biopsy is taken primarily for the assessment of the vascular disease since the underlying parenchymal changes were either undetected or considered unrelated to the pulmonary hypertension.

Morphology

In some conditions, such as disseminated lupus erythematosus, rheumatoid disease or Wegener's disease, pulmonary vasculitis is a characteristic feature. Whenever there is granulomatosis or fibrosis of the lung tissue, whether this is focal or diffuse and interstitial, both pulmonary arteries and veins usually exhibit severe alterations.[61-63] These changes are non-specific, that is, they are unrelated to the underlying condition and occur only in affected areas of the lungs.

In pulmonary arteries medial hypertrophy is pronounced and so is intimal fibrosis. The latter is of the eccentric, non-laminar type and very commonly leads to (sub)total occlusion of the vessel (Figure 38). Similarly, the pulmonary veins exhibit severe medial hypertrophy and arterialization and also very prominent intimal fibrosis (Figure 39).

There are two aspects that the pathologist must realize in reporting on such changes. First, he should not jump to the conclusion that these severe vascular changes are necessarily an expression of pulmonary hypertension. Even the most impressive and obstructive alterations may be associated with a normal pressure in the pulmonary circulation. As a rule it will appear that, in such instances, portions of the lungs that are not diseased contain normal lung vessels. In a lung biopsy specimen, however, there is often only fibrotic lung tissue and that may well give rise to the conviction that an elevated pressure is inevitably present.

The second difficulty is to differentiate between these vascular alterations and those found in pulmonary venous hypertension, and often this is not possible. As one may realize, arteries as well as veins are affected in both conditions and in a very similar way. The presence of interstitial fibrosis may not help us since this can also occur in both conditions. In a lung biopsy of adequate size it may help if there is some normal, non-fibrotic lung tissue adjacent to areas of fibrosis. If vascular lesions are limited to the fibrotic areas and absent in normal lung tissue, it is unlikely that they resulted from pulmonary venous hypertension. In mitral stenosis, for instance, medial hypertrophy and intimal fibrosis tend to be just as severe in fibrotic as in non-fibrotic parenchyma.

In our experience it is often possible to decide from the lung biopsy specimen whether the lesions are due to an impediment to the pulmonary venous flow or to fibrosis of lung tissue. This distinction has obvious clinical importance.

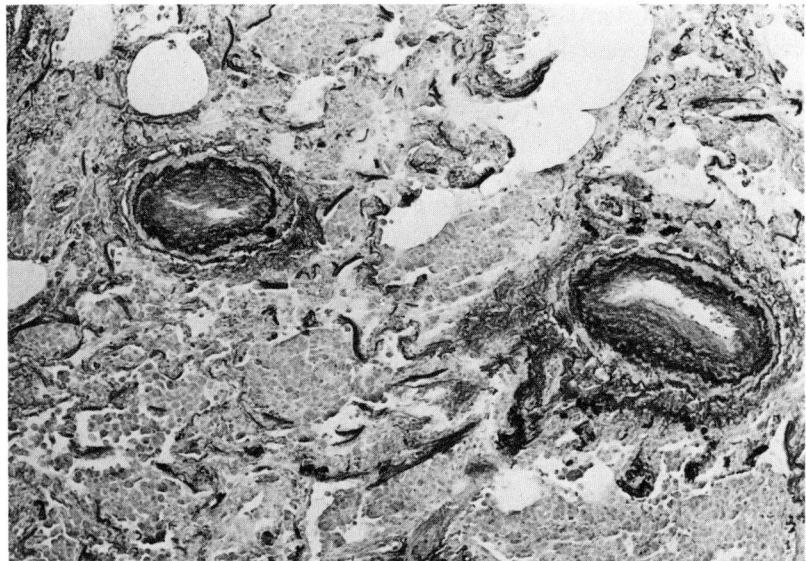

Figure 38. Severe medial hypertrophy and intimal fibrosis of pulmonary arteries lying in fibrotic lung tissue. Woman, 58 years with desquamative interstitial pneumonitis and extensive interstitial fibrosis of lung tissue. El.v.G., × 90.

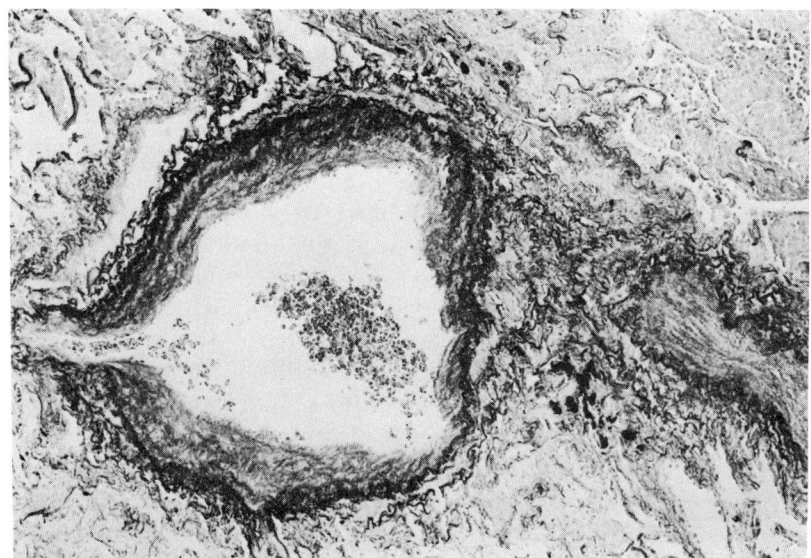

Figure 39. Medial hypertrophy, arterialization and intimal fibrosis of pulmonary veins. Same patient as the one from Figure 38. El.v.G., × 90.

Vascular Lesions in Diminished Pulmonary Flow

In patients with tetralogy of Fallot or tricuspid atresia, another characteristic pattern of changes in the lung vessels is presented. Now the pulmonary arterial pressure is not elevated and is often slightly lower than normal. Since there is an increased hematocrit in these cases, there is often a marked tendency to thrombosis of lung vessels. Some of the changes, although often to a lesser extent, may also be observed in isolated pulmonic stenosis.

Lung biopsy specimens have been studied when taken during cardiac repair.[2] Pre-operative open lung biopsies are unlikely to be submitted but sometimes the alterations of this pattern are found unexpectedly, for instance when there is a clinically undiagnosed stenosis of a pulmonary artery.

Morphology

In contrast to the various forms of pulmonary hypertension, where there is almost universally a hypertrophy of the media of the muscular pulmonary arteries, in diminished pulmonary flow the media tends to be thinner than normal. Sometimes medial atrophy is so prominent that arteries of a size of 100 to 150 μm have lost their muscular coat completely or almost completely (Figure 40). This feature, although often less conspicuous, is also common in isolated pulmonic stenosis or in the presence of a congenital stenosis of one or more larger pulmonary arteries. We have observed several cases in which the evaluation of an open lung biopsy specimen provided the clue to the detection of such a stenosis.

Other changes are related to the marked tendency to thrombosis. Recent thrombi may be found but are scarce. Organization of thrombi leads to eccentric patches of intimal fibrosis (Figure 41) and recanalization to the formation of intravascular fibrous septa[62] (Figure 42). In this respect the changes resemble those in other cases of primary or embolic thrombosis (p. 414) but apart from the medial atrophy, the septa tend to be more delicate in a patient with tetralogy of Fallot than in a patient with recurrent thromboembolism. This is probably related to another characteristic feature of diminished pulmonary flow. All vessels, arteries as well as veins, tend to be wide. The arterial diameter is often wider than that of the accompanying bronchus or bronchiole. This widening of lumina very likely applies also to channels of recanalization, which in turn leads to the thinness of the septa between these channels.

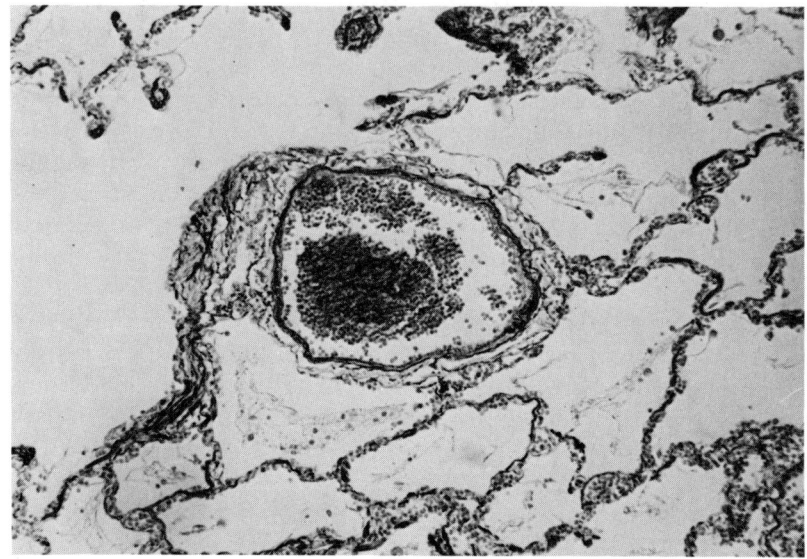

Figure 40. Muscular pulmonary artery with the wide lumen and distinct medial atrophy. Girl, 12 years with tetralogy of Fallot. El.v.G., × 140.

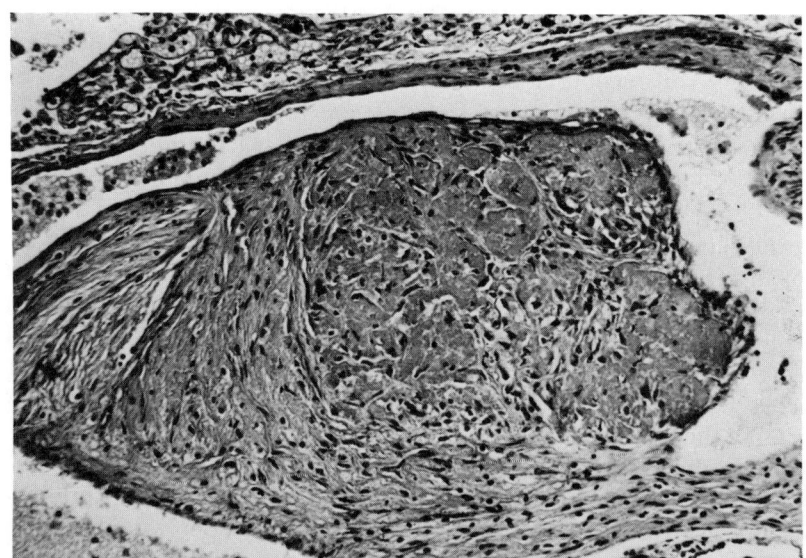

Figure 41. Organization of thrombus in thin-walled pulmonary artery. Woman, 19 years with tetralogy of Fallot. H.E., × 140.

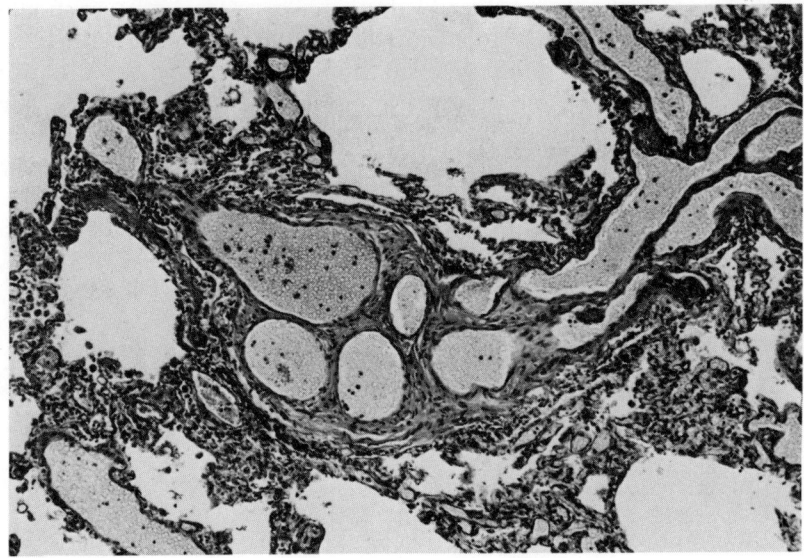

Figure 42. Multiple intravascular septa resulting from recanalization of thrombus in pulmonary artery. Woman, 19 years with tetralogy of Fallot. H.E., × 90.

CONCLUSION

The recent practice of open lung biopsy has, in many cases of pulmonary hypertension, provided clues as to etiology and has assisted in decisions regarding therapy. The risks of open lung biopsy need to be determined by careful prospective clinical studies, but with an experienced surgeon the risk may be less than previously thought. For example, as far as we could ascertain, in none of the 55 patients with unexplained pulmonary hypertension from whom we received a lung biopsy, could death be attributed to this procedure. A biopsy from a single site is usually representative of the vascular disease. In the adult, a specimen 2.5 × 2.0 × 1.0 cm will rarely fail to give a reliable impression of the type and the severity of lung vessel pathology. With regard to type, the eventual success of any attempt to influence the course of the pulmonary hypertensive disease will depend upon a definitive diagnosis, which generally can only be made by open lung biopsy.

The importance of establishing severity has been shown in congenital heart disease in the presence of a shunt. In many instances evaluation of the lung biopsy predicted the long-term outlook for the patient after closure of the shunt. We now think that corrective surgery should not be undertaken when, following biopsy, the vessels show fibrinoid necrosis or a plexiform lesion, even though very few vessels are thus affected. Also, severe and widespread intimal fibrosis of the onion-skin type should be regarded as a contraindication. Thus lung tissue, from open lung biopsy, when properly prepared and examined, has the potential for providing information concerning diagnosis and prognosis at a time when such information is still useful for the management of the individual patient.

REFERENCES

1. Wagenvoort CA, Nauta J, Van der Schaar PJ, Weeda HWH, Wagenvoort N: Effect of flow and pressure on pulmonary vessels. *Circulation* 1967; 35:1028.
2. Wagenvoort CA, Nauta J, Van der Schaar PJ, Weeda HWH, Wagenvoort N: Vascular changes in pulmonic stenosis and tetralogy of Fallot in lung biopsies. *Circulation* 1967;36:924.
3. Wagenvoort CA, Nauta J, Van der Schaar PJ, Weeda HWH, Wagenvoort N: The pulmonary vasculature in complete transposition of the great vessels judged from lung biopsies. *Circulation* 1968;38:746.
4. Rabinovitch M, Haworth SG, Castaneda AR, Nadas AS, Reid L: Lung biopsies in congenital heart disease: A morphometric approach to pulmonary vascular disease. *Circulation* 1978;58:1107.
5. Rabinovitch M, Haworth SG, Vance Z, Vawter G, Castaneda AR, Nadas AS, Reid L: Early pulmonary vascular changes in congenital heart disease studied in biopsy tissue. *Human Pathol* 1980;11:499.
6. Ogawa K, Ito H, Toryama A, Yamamoto T, Yamaguchi M, Horikoshi K, Asada S: Lung pathology in infants with severe pulmonary hypertension and cardiac disease. *J Thorac Cardiovasc Surg* 1979;77:728.
7. Wagenvoort CA, Wagenvoort N, Draulans-Noe Y: Reversibility of plexogenic pulmonary arteriopathy following banding of the pulmonary artery. Unpublished data, 1983.
8. Berthrong M, Cochran TH: Pathological findings in nine children with "primary" pulmonary hypertension. *Bull J Hopk Hosp* 1955;97:69.
9. Cawley LP, Stofer BE: Pulmonary arteriosclerosis of unknown origin. *Arch Path* 1957;64:270.
10. Caldini P, Gensini GG, Hofman MS: Primary pulmonary hypertension with death during right heart catheterization. *Am J Cardiol* 1959;4:519.
11. Sleeper JC, Orgain ES, McIntosh HD: Primary pulmonary hypertension. Review of clinical features and pathologic physiology with a report of pulmonary hemodynamics and derived from repeated catheterization. *Circulation* 1962;26:1358.
12. Wagenvoort CA, Wagenvoort N: Primary pulmonary hypertension: A pathologic study of the lung vessels in 156 clinically diagnosed cases. *Circulation* 1970;42:1163.

13. Haworth SG, Reid L: A morphometric study of regional variations in lung structure in infants with pulmonary hypertension and congenital cardiac defects. *Br Heart J* 1978;40:825.
14. Heath D, Best PV: The tunica media of the arteries of the lung in pulmonary hypertension. *J Path Bact* 1958;76:165.
15. Rabinovitch M, Castaneda AR, Reid L: Lung biopsy with frozen section as a diagnostic aid in patients with congenital heart defects. *Pediatr Cardiol* 1981;47:77.
16. Wagenvoort CA: Grading of pulmonary vascular lesions: A reappraisal. *Histopathol* 1981;5:595.
17. Heath D, Edwards JE: The pathology of hypertensive pulmonary vascular disease. A description of six grades of structural changes in the pulmonary arteries with special reference to congenital cardiac septal defects. *Circulation* 1958;18:533.
18. Reeves JT, Tweedale D, Noonan J, Leathers JE, Quigley MB: Correlations of microradiographic and histologic findings in the pulmonary vascular bed. *Circulation* 1966;34:971.
19. Reeves JT, Noonan JA: Microarteriographic studies of primary pulmonary hypertension. *Arch Path* 1973;95:48.
20. World Health Organization: *Primary Pulmonary Hypertension. Report on a WHO Meeting.* Hatano S, Strasser T, (Eds.) Geneva: 1975.
21. Wilhelmsen L, Selander S, Soderholm B, Paulin S, Vernauskas E, Werko L: Recurrent pulmonary embolism. *Am Heart J* 1966;71:206.
22. Wagenvoort CA, Wagenvoort N: *Pathology of Pulmonary Hypertension.* New York: J. Wiley & Sons, 1977.
23. Heath D, Donald DE, Edwards JE: Pulmonary vascular changes in a dog after aorto-pulmonary anastomosis for four years. *Br Heart J* 1959;21:187.
24. Downing SE, Vidone RA, Brandt HN, Liebow AA: The pathogenesis of vascular lesions in experimental hyperkinetic pulmonary hypertension. *Am J Path* 1963;43:739.
25. Gurtner HP: Atiologie und haufigkeit der primar vaskularen formen des chronischen cor pulmonale. *Dtsch Med Wsch* 1969;94:850.
26. Kaindl F: Primare pulmonale hypertension. *Wien Zsch Inn Med* 1969;50:451.
27. Gahl K, Fabel H, Greiser E, Harmjanz D, Ostertag H, Stender HS: Primar vaskulare pulmonale hypertension. *Z Kreislaufforsch* 1970;59:868.
28. Naeye RL: "Primary" pulmonary hypertension with coexisting portal hypertension. A retrospective study of six cases. *Circulation* 1960;22:376.
29. Levine OR, Harris RC, Blanc WA, Mellins RB: Progressive pulmonary hypertension in children with portal hypertension. *J Pediatr* 1973;83:964.
30. Wagenvoort CA: The pulmonary arteries in infants with ventricular septal defect. *Med Thorac* 1962;19:162.
31. Haworth SG, Sauer U, Buhlmeyer K, Reid L: Development of the pulmonary circulation in ventricular septal defect: A quantitative structural study. *Am J Cardiol* 1977;40:781.
32. Harley RA, Friedman PJ, Saldana M, Liebow AA, Carrington CB: Sequential development of lesions in experimental extreme pulmonary hypertension. *Am J Path* 1968;52:52a.
33. Saldana ME, Harley RA, Liebow AA, Carrington CB: Experimental extreme pulmonary hypertension and vascular disease in relation to polycythemia. *Am J Path* 1968;52:935.

34. Wagenvoort CA: Lung biopsy specimens in the evaluation of pulmonary vascular disease. *Chest* 1980;77:614.
35. Gurtner HP: Personal communication, 1982.
36. Hislop A, Reid L: Pulmonary arterial development during childhood: Branching pattern and structure. *Thorax* 1973;28:129.
37. Reid L, Ryland D: The pulmonary circulation in cystic fibrosis. In: Mangos JA, Talamo RC, Eds. *Fundamental Problems of Cystic Fibrosis and Related Diseases.* New York: Intercontinental Medical Book Corp.,1973:195.
38. Hislop A, Haworth SG, Shinebourne EA, Reid L: Quantitative structural analysis of pulmonary vessels in isolated ventricular septal defect in infancy. *Br Heart J* 1975;37:1014.
39. Takahashi T, Wagenvoort N, Wagenvoort CA: The density of muscularized pulmonary arteries in normal lungs. A morphometric study. *Arch Pathol Lab Med* 1983;107:19.
40. Takahashi T, Wagenvoort CA: Density of muscularized arteries in the lung. *Arch Pathol Lab Med* 1983;107:23.
41. Hislop A, Reid L: Changes in the pulmonary arteries of the rat during recovery from hypoxia-induced pulmonary hypertension. *Br J Exp Pathol* 1977;68:653.
42. Meyrick B, Reid L: Hypoxia and incorporation of ^{3}H-thymidine by cells of the rat pulmonary arteries and alveolar wall. *Am J Pathol* 1979;96:51.
43. Meyrick B, Reid L: Development of pulmonary arterial changes in rats fed Crotalaria spectabilis. *Am J Pathol* 1979;94:37.
44. Meyrick B, Reid L: Crotalaria-induced pulmonary hypertension. Uptake of ^{3}H-thymidine by the cells of the pulmonary circulation and alveolar walls. *Am J Pathol* 1982;106:84.
45. Kay JM, Suyama KL, Keane PM: Failure to show decrease in small pulmonary blood vessels in rats with experimental pulmonary hypertension. *Thorax* 1982;37:927.
46. Mooi W, Wagenvoort CA: Decreased number of pulmonary blood vessels: Reality or artifact. *J Path* 1983 (in press).
47. Vanek J: Fibrous bands and networks of postembolic origin in the pulmonary arteries. *J Path Bact* 1961;81:537.
48. Heath D, Edwards JE: Histological changes in the lung in diseases associated with pulmonary venous hypertension. *Br J Dis Chest* 1959;53:8.
49. Wagenvoort CA, Wagenvoort N: Smooth muscle content of pulmonary arterial media in pulmonary venous hypertension compared with other forms of pulmonary hypertension. *Chest* 1982;81:581.
50. Wagenvoort CA: Morphologic changes in intrapulmonary veins. *Human Path* 1970;1:205.
51. Ramirez A, Grimes ET, Abelmann WH: Regression of pulmonary vascular changes following mitral valvuloplasty. An anatomic and physiologic case study. *Am J Med* 1968;45:975.
52. Liebow AA, McAdams AJ, Carrington CB, Viamonte M: Intrapulmonary veno-obstructive disease. *Circulation* (Supp II) 1967;35:36, 172.
53. Wagenvoort CA, Losekoot G, Mulder E: Pulmonary veno-occlusive disease of presumably intrauterine origin. *Thorax* 1971;26:429.
54. Liu L, Sackler JP: A case of pulmonary veno-occlusive disease. *Angiology* 1972;23:299.
55. Joselson R, Warnock M: Pulmonary veno-occlusive disease after chemotherapy. *Human Path* 1983;14:88.

56. Wagenvoort CA. Pulmonary veno-occlusive disease. Entity or syndrome? *Chest* 1976;69:82.
57. Wagenvoort CA, Wagenvoort N: The pathology of pulmonary veno-occlusive disease. *Virch Arch A Path Anat Histol* 1974;364:69.
58. Pääkkö P, Sutinen S, Remes M, Paavilainen T, Wagenvoort CA: A case of pulmonary vascular occlusive disease: Comparision of post-mortem radiography with histology. Unpublished data, 1983.
59. Hasleton PS, Heath D, Brewer DB: Hypertensive pulmonary vascular disease in states of chronic hypoxia. *J Path Bact* 1968;95:431.
60. Wagenvoort CA, Wagenvoort N: Pulmonary veins in high-altitude residents: A morphometric study. *Thorax* 1982;37:931.
61. Naeye RL: Pulmonary vascular lesions in systemic scleroderma. *Dis Chest* 1963;44:374.
62. Wagenvoort CA, Wagenvoort N: Pulmonary vascular bed. Normal anatomy and responses to disease. In: Moser KM, Ed. *Pulmonary Vascular Diseases*. New York, Basel: M. Dekker, Inc., 1979.
63. Heath D, Smith P: Pulmonary vascular disease secondary to lung disease. In: Moser KM, Ed. *Pulmonary Vascular Diseases*. New York, Basel: M. Dekker, Inc., 1979.
64. Rich AR: A hitherto unrecognized tendency to the development of widespread pulmonary vascular obstruction in patients with congenital pulmonary stenosis (tetralogy of Fallot). *Bull J Hopk Hosp* 1948;82:389.

Index

Acetyl gylceryl ether phosphorylchlorine, 196
Acetylcholine, 121
Acetylsalicylic acid, 108
Acidemia, 60, 62
Acute thromboembolic pulmonary hypertension, 172–174
Adenosine, 252–254
α-adrenergic blockers, 149–150
Alpha-sympathicomimetics, 351
Aminorex, 125, 142, 342–348, 407
Anesthetics, 259–260
Angina, 8
Angiotensin II, 57, 263
Angiotensin converting enzyme, 57
Anorexigens, 125, 342–350
Anticoagulation, 144, 230–231
Antiplatelet agents, 144
Aortic valve heart disease, 5, 78
Apgar scores, 61–62
Apnea, 328, 330
Arachidonic acid metabolism, 264–267, 365–366 see also Prostaglandins; Thromboxane
Arterial blood gases, 208
Aspirin, 365
Atelectasis, 206, 277
ATP, 252–253, 268–271
Auto-immune disease, 122–123
Autonomic nervous system 52–53
Azathioprine, 155

Barbiturates, 144
β-adrenergic stimulators, 148–149
Biopsy see Lung biopsy
Bleomycin, 123
Bradycardia, 65
Bradykinin, 57, 121, 195, 260
Brisket disease, 368–371
British Medical Research Council study, 307
Bronchiectasis, 292

Calcium, 271–273
Calcium blockers, 150–151
Captopril, 148, 154
Cardiopulmonary disease, preexisting, 193
Catheterization, 4, 19–37
  evaluation, 28–34
  exercise testing, 34–37
  indications, 19–22
  quality control, 22–25
  risks, 24–25
  technique, 25–28
Chlorphentermine, 348
Choriocarcinoma, 140
Chronic hypoxic pulmonary hypertension, 361–374
Chronic mountain sickness, 292, 372–373
Chronic obstructive airways disease see Lung disease
Chronic thromboembolic pulmonary hypertension, 176–179, 383
Chronic venous pulmonary hypertension, 377–379
Cimetidine, 144
Cinnarizine, 376
Circulation, fetal and neonatal, 45–46
Cirrhosis, 126–127, 142
Citric acid cycle, 268
Coarctation of the aorta, 77–78
Collateral ventilation, 364–365
Congenital heart disease, 73–114, 400
  clinical syndromes, 77–80, 96–99, 104–108
  definition, 73–75
  diagnostic assessment, 77, 93–96, 103, 394–395, 400
  pathology, 402–414, 431
  pathophysiology, 75–77, 80, 99–103
  viscosity, 81–93
Connective tissue disease, 122–123
Contrast venography, 226
Cooperative Thrombolytic Trials, 207
Cor pulmonale, 291–320, 321–339
  see also Lung disease
Coumadin, 108
Council on Thrombosis of the American Heart Association, 230
CREST syndrome, 122–123
Crotalaria fulvia, 353
Crotalaria laburnoides, 353
Crotalaria spectabilis, 353
Cyanosis, 62–63, 129
  in the newborn, 61–62
Cyclo-oxygenase pathway, 264–266
Cyclosporin A, 156
Cyclotron, 215
Cystic fibrosis, 292
Cytochrome P-450, 275–276

Deep venous thrombosis and pulmonary embolism, 180–182, 226–231
Dermatomyositis, 122–123
Diabetes, 60, 151–152
Diaphragmatic hernia, congenital, 14
Diazoxide, 148, 151–152

438

Index

Diet *see* Nutrition
Digoxin, 308
Diltiazem, 150–151
Dipyridamole, 108, 144, 153–154, 371
Direct-acting vasodilators, 151–155
Disodium cromoglycate, 262, 267
Diuretics, 308–309
Dopamine, 376
Doppler, 19
Drug-induced pulmonary hypertension, 341–359
Ductus arteriosus, 62
Dyspnea, 6, 299

Echocardiography, 15–19, 131–139
Edema, 129–130, 151–152, 196
Eisenmenger's syndrome, 5, 6, 14, 130
Electrocardiogram, 11–13, 207–208
Embolectomy, 232
Emboli *see* Thromboembolism
Embolic and thrombotic pulmonary vascular lesions, 414–419
 morphology, 415–416
 reversibility, 416–416
Embryology of pulmonary vessels, 97–99
Endocarditis, 222
Endothelial cell function, 122, 262, 354–355, 380–382
Environmental influences, 259
Erythrocytosis, 329
Exercise testing, 34–37
Experimental artifacts in hypoxic pulmonary vasoconstriction, 259–260
Experimental models, 361–391

Familial factors, 123–124
Fatigue, 8
Fenfluramine, 349
Fibrinoid necrosis, 88
Fibrinolytic activity, 120, 124, 126, 356
Fibrinolytic therapy, intravenous, 156, 232–235
Fibrinopeptides, 195
5-hydroxytryptamine, 265, 349, 351–352, 375–376
Fluoroacetate, 268

Genetic influences in hypoxic pulmonary hypertension, 259, 272
German Society of Cardiology, 343, 349
Glycosides, 308
Greenfield filter, 239

Headache, 123
Heart disease
 aortic valve, 5
 congenital, 11, 14, 73–114, 402–415, 431–434
 mitral valve, 14
 rheumatic mitral, 5
 valvular, 5
Heart-lung transplantation, 156
Hematocrit, 82, 108, 303
Hemodynamics, 52, 75, 80–84, 94–96, 99–103 *see also* Catheterization
Hemoptysis, 8–9
Heparin, 186, 194, 231, 236–237
Hepatomegaly, 129–130
Herbal toxins, 353–354
High altitude, 143, 259, 361
High altitude pulmonary edema, 276
High flow pulmonary hypertension, 379–382
Hilar/thoracic index, 14
Hirsutism, 151–152
Histamine, 262, 351
Hoarseness, 9
Hormones, 57–59
Hunter-Sessions intracaval balloon, 239
Hyaline membrane disease, 14
Hydralazine, 40, 148, 150, 152, 309–310
Hyperplasia of vascular smooth muscle, 87–88
Hypocalcemia, 62
Hypoglycemia, 62
Hypotension, 65, 151–152
Hypoventilation, 321–339
 respiratory disorders of sleep, 327–336
 ventilatory drive, 321–326
 therapy, 336
Hypoxemia, 59–60, 63, 175, 195, 222, 253, 260–261, 297, 305–307, 330
Hypoxic pulmonary hypertension, 251–289, 361–374
 altered vascular tone, 252–254
 clinical correlations, 276–277
 hypoxic pulmonary vasoconstriction, 53–56, 105, 255–256, 293–295, 362–366
 mechanism of acute hypoxic pulmonary vasoconstriction, 260–276
 pathology, 425–428
 pathophysiologic significance, 251–252
 phylogeny, 254–255, 367–370
 pulmonary pressor response factors, 256–260
 site, 255–256

Idiopathic alveolar hypoventilation, 292
IgG, 376
Indomethacin, 108, 144, 155, 365, 376

International Multicentre Trial, 230
Iodoacetate, 268
Iron deficiency anemia, 81
Isoproterenol, 40, 148, 149, 308
Isovolumic hemodilution, 155

Jugular venous pulse, 9

Krebs cycle, 268
Kyphoscoliosis, 14, 292

Left recurrent laryngeal nerve, 9
Left stellate ganglion blockade, 156
Left ventricular dysfunction, 295–298
Left ventricular failure, 77–78
Leucotrienes see Lipoxygenase pathway
Lipoxygenase pathway, 127, 266–267, 365–366
Luminal radius, 85–96
Lung biopsy, 38–40, 94, 139, 345, 346, 393–437
  indications for, 399–400
  morphologic varieties, 401–433
  processing lung tissue, 396–398
  reporting, 398–399
  representation, 395–396
  risk, 394–395
Lung compliance, 128
Lung development, 362–364
Lung disease, 291–320
  chronic, 11
  clinical picture, 299–300
  definition, 291–292
  epidemiology, 292–293
  laboratory studies, 300–305
  pathogenesis, 293–299
  pathology, 428–430
  therapy, 305–315
Lung injury-induced pulmonary hypertension, 375–377
Lung scan, 201, 209–215

Meclofenamate, 365
Meconium aspiration, 61
Menstrual cycle, 124–125
Migraine headache, 123
Minoxidil, 153–154
Mitochondria, 271–274
Mitral stenosis, 11, 80
Mitral valve disease, 14
Mixed connective tissue disease, 122–123
Mobin-Uddin umbrella, 239
Models of pulmonary hypertension, 361–391
Monitoring, 65–66
Monocrotaline, 353, 375, 377
Mortality, 79–80
  in the newborn, 61–62

Neonates see Newborn
Neoplasm, 206
Neuromuscular disease, 292
Newborn, 45–71
  clinical syndrome and management, 61–66
  development of the pulmonary vasculature, 46–52
  fetal and neonatal circulations, 45–46, 362–364
  pathophysiology, 59–60
  physics of flow, 52
  postnatal pulmonary vasodilatation, 56–59
  pulmonary vascular resistance in the normal fetus, 52–56
Nifedipine, 148, 150–151, 309
Nitrates, 238
Nitroglycerine, 40
Nitroprusside, 40, 154
Nocturnal Oxygen Therapy Trial (NOTT), 307
Norepinephrine, 121, 262–263
Nutrition, 125–126
  diet composition, 354
  fetal and neonatal, 45–46
  and pulmonary hypertension, 341–359

Obesity hypoventilation syndrome, 292, 326–327, 336
Ohm's law, 73–74
Oral contraceptives, 126, 142, 174, 352
Oxidative phosphorylation, 268–271
Oximetazolin, 351
Oxygen
  pulmonary vasodilatation, 56–57, 252
  therapy, 62–63, 154–155, 231–232, 303–307, 336
  transcutaneous measurement, 65–66
  transport, 28–30, 53
Oxygen radicals, 274–275, 377

Pain, anginal-like, 8
p-chlorophenylalanine, 376
Perinatal asphyxia, 62–63
Persistent fetal circulation syndrome, 45–71, 124, 365–366 see also Newborn
Pharmacology, 64–65, 125–126, 292
  see also individual drug names
Phenformin, 352
Phenmetrazin, 348
Phenobarbitone, 376
Phenoxybenzamine, 150, 376
Phentolamine, 148, 149, 308–309
Pickwickian syndrome, 327, 336
Platelets, 66, 127–128, 144, 195–196, 258, 354, 371–372, 382
Pleurisy, 206

Index

Pleuropulmonary fibrosis, 292
Plexogenic arteriopathy, 402–414
  morphology, 403–411
  reversibility, 411–414
Pneumonia, 61, 206
Polycythemia, 81, 96, 307, 334
Polymyositis, 122–123
Portal hypertension, 126–127
Prazosin, 149
Pre-ejection period, 17
Pregnancy, 124–125, 142–143, 222, 259
Primary pulmonary hypertension
  catheterization, 137–139
  definition, 115–117
  differential diagnosis, 140
  epidemiology, 117–118
  etiologic possibilities, 119–128
  lung biopsy, 139, 399–400
  management, 142–157
  non-invasive assessment
    laboratory investigations, 130–139
    perfusion/ventilation lung scan, 133–136
    physical signs, 129–130
    symptoms, 128–129
  pathology, 140–142, 402–411
  prognosis, 118–119
Prostacyclin, 65, 90–91, 143, 148, 152–153, 267
Prostaglandins, 58, 65, 196, 264–266, 351–352
Protriptyline, 336
Pulmonary angiography, 138–139, 215–224
Pulmonary arterial pressure, 22
Pulmonary artery anomalies, 85, 94–99
Pulmonary artery banding, 156
Pulmonary blood flow, 45–46, 99–108
Pulmonary embolectomy, 232
Pulmonary embolism *see*
  Thromboembolic pulmonary hypertension, Thromboembolism
Pulmonary hypertension *see also* specific etiologies
  acute hypoxic, 251–289
  approach to the patient, 1–44
  classification, 5–6
  and cor pulmonale in hypoventilating patients, 321–339
  definition, 2, 73, 115, 291–292
  diagnosis and management, 6–40, 115–168
  drug and dietary induced, 341–359
  experimental models, 361–391
  incidence, 2–5
  invasive assessment, cardiac catheterization, 19–37
    evaluation, 28–33

  exercise testing, 34–37
  indications, 19–22
  quality control, 22–25
  technique, 25–28
  lung biopsies, 38–40, 139, 393–437
    see also Lung biopsy in the newborn, 45–71
  non-invasive assessment, 6–19
    chest roentgenogram, 13–15
    electrocardiogram, 11–13
    physical examination, 9–11
    symptoms, 6–9
    ultrasound, 15–19
  secondary to congenital heart disease, 73–114
  secondary to lung disease, 291–320
  symptoms, 5–9
  thromboembolic pulmonary hypertension, 169–249
  treatment, 38–40
  unexplained (primary), 115–168, 399–400
  and vascular disease, 395–439
Pulmonary valvular closure sound (P_2), 10
Pulmonary vascular disease, 393–437
Pulmonary vascular morphology, 46, 60, 84–93, 140–142, 187–191, 345–347, 398–434
Pulmonary vascular resistance, 80–99, 292–293
Pulmonary veno-occlusive disease, 423–425
Pulmonary venous hypertension, 75–80, 377–379, 420–423
Pulmonary wedge pressure, 23
Pyridine nucleotides (NADP), 273–274
Pyrolizidine alkaloids, 353, 374–377

Raynaud's disease, 120–123
Recruitment, 83–84
Redox status, 273–274
Rheumatic mitral heart disease, 5
Rheumatoid arthritis, 122–123
Right ventricular lift, 10
Ringer's lactate, 64
Roentgenogram, 13–15

Sarcoidosis, 292
Schistosomiasis, 140, 142, 169
Scleroderma, 122–123
Senecio Jacobaea, 354
Septal defects, 84–85, 87, 99–107
Serotonin, 351
Shear force, 88–93, 103, 382
Shunting, 62, 142
Sickle cell disease, 81, 140, 141, 206
6-OH dopamine, 376
Sleep apnea syndromes, 330

Sleep, and respiratory disorders, 327–336
Smoking, 143, 293
SQ 14225, 376
SQ 20881, 376
Steroids, 155
Streptokinase, 232
Sudden death, 175
Surgery, 156, 175, 228, 238–239, 240, 380, 411–414
Sulfhydryl groups, 273–274
Syncope, 8
Systemic lupus erythematosus, 122–123

Tachycardia, 299–300
Tachypnea, in the newborn, 61–62
Temperature, 123, 256–257
Terbutaline, 149
Testosterone, 371
Theophylline, 305
Thrombocytopenia, 237
Thromboembolic pulmonary hypertension, 169–249
  angiography, 174–175, 186, 215–224
  autopsy studies, 172–173, 178
  diagnosis, 205–229
  etiology and pathophysiology, 182–191
  incidence and prevalence, 171–182
  inferior vena caval interruption, 238–242
  lung scans, 209–215
  occult thromboembolism, 177–179
  pathogenesis, 191–204
  pathology, 191–196
  treatment, 229–242
Thromboembolism, 119–120, 298
Thromboendarterectomy, 239–240
Thrombolytic Trials, 186–187
Thrombophlebitis, 11
Thromboxane, 127–128, 155, 196, 354–355
Tolazoline, 40, 64, 65, 149
Total anomalous pulmonary venous connection, 78–80
Tricarboxylic acid (TCA), 268, 269
Tumor emboli, 140

Ultrasound, 15–19
Upper airway obstruction, 292
Urokinase, 194, 232
Urokinase Pulmonary Embolism Trial, 193, 199, 204, 212, 235

Valve, replacement, 40
Valvular heart disease, 5
Vascular lesions
  in diminished pulmonary flow, 431–433
  in hypoxic pulmonary hypertension, 425–428
  in lung disease, 428–430
  morphology, 420–423
  reversibility, 423
Vasoactive substances, 57–59, 193
Vasoconstriction, 85–87, 120–122, 195
Vasodilators, 22, 36, 39, 64–65, 77, 93–94, 145–155, 238, 309
Venography, 226
Venous pressure, 75–80
Venous stasis, 230
Ventilation, 63–64
Ventilation/perfusion scan *see* Lung scan
Verapamil, 150–152, 273–274
Vinblastine, 123
Viscosity, 59–60, 81–83
Vital capacity, 128
Vitamin K, 236, 237

Wedge angiography, 94–95
World Health Organization (WHO), 119, 142, 291

X-ray, 13–15, 131–139, 207–208

Zoxazolamine, 376